DEVELOPMENTAL STAGES IN
HUMAN EMBRYOS

DEVELOPMENTAL STAGES IN HUMAN EMBRYOS

*Including a Revision of Streeter's
"Horizons" and a Survey of
the Carnegie Collection*

———

RONAN O'RAHILLY

and

FABIOLA MÜLLER

*Carnegie Laboratories of Embryology,
California Primate Research Center,*
and
*Departments of Human Anatomy and Neurology,
University of California, Davis*

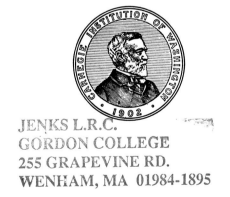

CARNEGIE INSTITUTION OF WASHINGTON
PUBLICATION 637
1987

Library of Congress Catalog Card Number 87-070669
International Standard Book Number 0-87279-666-3
Composition by Harper Graphics, Waldorf, Maryland
Printing by Meriden-Stinehour Press, Meriden, Connecticut
Copyright © 1987, Carnegie Institution of Washington

*Dem Andenken von Wilhelm His, dem
Älteren, der vor hundert Jahren die
Embryologie des Menschen einführte und dem
seines Protégé, Franklin P. Mall, dem
Begründer der Carnegie Collection.*

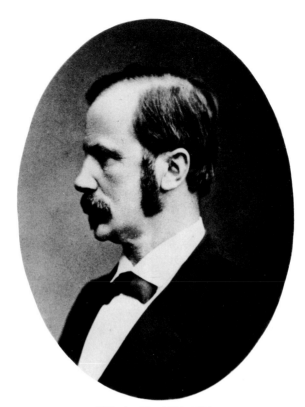

Wilhelm His, 1831–1904

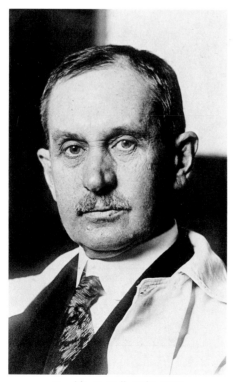

Franklin P. Mall, 1862–1917

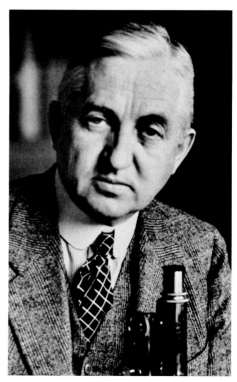

George L. Streeter, 1873–1948

PREFACE

During the past one hundred years of human embryology, three landmarks have been published: the *Anatomie der menschlichen Embryonen* of His (1880–1885), the *Manual of Human Embryology* by Keibel and Mall (1910–1912), and Streeter's *Developmental Horizons in Human Embryos* (1942–1957, completed by Heuser and Corner). Now that all three milestone volumes are out of print as well as in need of revision, it seems opportune to issue an updated study of the staged human embryo.

The objectives of this monograph are to provide a reasonably detailed morphological account of the human embryo (i.e., the first eight weeks of development), a formal classification into developmental stages, a catalogue of the preparations in the Carnegie Collection, and a reference guide to important specimens in other laboratories. The Carnegie staging system has now been accepted internationally and, when carefully applied, allows detailed comparisons between the findings at one institution and those at another.

The classifications and descriptions of stages 1–9 are based on light microscopy, and the criteria selected have stood the test of time. The present account is a revision of O'Rahilly's monograph of 1973. In stages 10–23, increasing attention is paid to external form, although internal structure is not, and should not be, neglected. Streeter's masterly account has been updated and is used here in treating stages 10–23. Many of Streeter's paragraphs have been left virtually unchanged (except for improvements in terminology) but others have been altered considerably, and much new material has been added.

Most of the drawings for stages 1–9 were prepared in the Department of Art as Applied to Medicine, the Johns Hopkins School of Medicine, under the direction of Ranice Crosby. Most of those for stages 10–23 are the work of James F. Didusch, although certain modifications in his terminology have been adopted.

A major change made here from Streeter's account is in the systematic inclusion of standard references. It should be stressed, however, that no attempt has been made to provide a comprehensive bibliography. Many more references can be found in a series of articles on the timing and sequence of developmental events, beginning in *Acta anatomica* in 1971 and continuing in the *Zeitschrift für Anatomie und Entwicklungsgeschichte* (now *Anatomy and Embryology*) from 1971 to 1983. For the nervous system, further references can be found in a continuing series of articles that began in 1981 in *Anatomy and Embryology*: stages 8–11 have already been published.

Particular attention has been paid to nomenclature throughout. Most of the terms used are in agreement with the *Nomina embryologica*. The latter, however, unlike the *Nomina anatomica*, is not exclusively human, and hence certain inappropriate terms have been replaced here.

It is appropriate to acknowledge here the great help provided by the National Institutes of Health, which have supported the writers' research (Grant No. HD-16702, Institute of Child Health and Human Development).

It is a particular pleasure to acknowledge the enthusiasm and collaboration of the late Dr. Ernest Gardner over many years, the friendship and assistance provided by Dr. Elizabeth M. Ramsey, and the continued encouragement of Dr. James D. Ebert, President of the Carnegie Institution of Washington, whose invitation to establish the first nine stages was made twenty years ago.

The authors wish to thank Mr. Ray Bowers and Miss Patricia Parratt of the Carnegie Institution's publications office for the exceptionally great care with which they brought this monograph to fruition.

R. O'R.
F. M.
January 1987

INTRODUCTION

*The norm should be established; embryos
should be arranged in stages.*

FRANKLIN P. MALL

The combined use of fixation, sectioning with a microtome, and reconstruction from the resultant sections first enabled Wilhelm His, Senior, to begin to elucidate thoroughly the anatomy of individual human embryos. Indeed, His may rightfully be called the "Vesalius of human embryology" (Müller and O'Rahilly, 1986a).

Although fixatives other than spirits were introduced early in the nineteenth century, formalin was not employed until the 1890s. His devised a microtome in about 1866. (A microtome had already been employed as early as 1770.) The wax plate reconstruction technique of Born (1883), introduced in 1876, has undergone numerous modifications over the years. These, as well as graphic reconstruction, have been discussed in a number of publications, e.g., by Gaunt and Gaunt (1978). Florian, who used graphic reconstruction of the human embryo to great advantage, elaborated the mathematical background in Czech in 1928. (See also Fetzer and Florian, 1930.)

It has been pointed out that "the idea of working out a complete account of the development of the human body was always before the mind of His," and his collaborator, Franz Keibel, proposed to provide "an account of the development of the human body, based throughout on human material" (Keibel and Mall, 1910) rather than from the comparative standpoint. The result was the *Manual of Human Embryology* edited by Keibel and Mall (1910, 1912), which was an important step in the goal of seeking precision in human embryology. The hope was expressed that, subsequently, a second attempt, "whether made by us or by others, will come so much nearer the goal" (*ibid.*).

The Carnegie Collection

Mall's collection of human embryos, begun in 1887, later became the basis of the Carnegie Collection (Mall and Meyer, 1921). Mall (1913) stated his indebtedness to His in the following terms: "We must thank His for the first attempt to study carefully the anatomy of human embryos, but his work was planned on so large a scale that he never completed it. . . . Thus we may trace back to him the incentive for Keibel's *Normentafeln*, Minot's great collection of vertebrate embryos and mine of human embryos."

In more recent years the Carnegie Collection has benefited enormously from the meticulous investigations of Bartelmez, the technical adroitness of Heuser, and the donation of, as well as research on, remarkably young specimens by Hertig and Rock. The microtomy of Charles H. Miller and William H. Duncan, the reconstructions by Osborne O. Heard, the artwork by James F. Didusch, and the photography of Chester F. Reather and Richard D. Grill, have each played a key role in the establishment of the superb embryological collection on which the present monograph is so largely based. In George W. Corner's apt comparison, the Collection serves "as a kind of Bureau of Standards."

Embryological Seriation

His had made the first thorough arrangement of human embryos in the form of a series of selected individual embryos, numbered in the presumed order of their development. The same principle was followed in the published plates known as the *Normentafeln*,

1

edited by Franz Keibel from 1897 onward; the volume on the human (by Keibel and Elze) appeared in 1908. The limitations of the method are (1) that individual embryos cannot be arranged in a perfect series, because any given specimen may be advanced in one respect while being retarded in another, and (2) that it may prove impossible to match a new embryo exactly with any one of the illustrated norms. The need for a more flexible procedure than a mere *Entwicklungsreihe* soon became apparent in experimental embryology.

Embryonic Staging

In the words of Ross G. Harrison (Wilens, 1969), "the need for standardized stages in the embryonic development of various organisms for the purpose of accurate description of normal development and for utilization in experimental work has long been recognized." Because "development is a continuous process with an indefinite number of stages" (*ibid.*), a certain number have to be chosen. Thus each stage "is merely an arbitrarily cut section through the time-axis of the life of an organism" (deBeer, 1958). It resembles, in Harrison's apt comparison, a frame taken from a cine-film. Stages are based on the apparent morphological state of development, and hence are not directly dependent on either chronological age or on size. Furthermore, comparison is made of a number of features of each specimen, so that individual differences are rendered less significant and a certain latitude of variation is taken into account.

Although embryonic staging had been introduced toward the end of the nineteenth century, it was first employed in human embryology by Franklin P. Mall (1914), founder of the Department of Embryology of the Carnegie Institution of Washington.

On the basis of photographs of their external form, Mall (1914) arranged 266 human embryos 2–25 mm in length in a series of fourteen stages, lettered from H to U. (A to G were to have been the earlier stages.)

Mall's successor, George L. Streeter, provided the definitive classification of human embryos into stages, which he termed "developmental horizons." Attention was concentrated on embryos up to about 32 mm greatest length because it was believed that, during the fetal period, the rate of increment in size and weight might be large enough to provide an adequate index of relative development.

The original plan was "to cover as far as possible the earliest specimens up to fetuses between 32 and 38 mm. long, the stage at which the eyelids have come together," and "twenty-five age groups" were envisioned (Streeter, 1942). Subsequently, Streeter (1951) decided that stage 23 "could be considered to mark the ending of the embryonic period" proper. The onset of marrow formation in the humerus was "arbitrarily adopted as the conclusion of the embryonic and the beginning of the fetal period of prenatal life. It occurs in specimens about 30 mm. in length" (Streeter, 1949). A scheme of the 23 stages, as modified and used in the present monograph, is provided in Table 0-1.

The term "horizon" was borrowed from geology and archaeology by Streeter (1942) in order "to emphasize the importance of thinking of the embryo as a living organism which in its time takes on many guises, always progressing from the smaller and simpler to the larger and more complex." However, the somewhat infelicitous term "horizon" has now been replaced by "stage" because the latter is the simple term employed for all other vertebrate embryos. Not only was the term "stage" used decades ago by Harrison for *Ambystoma* and subsequently by Hamburger and Hamilton for the chick embryo, as well as by others for a variety of reptiles, birds, and mammals, but, even in the case of the human, the term "stage" was employed by Mall (1914) when he first staged the human embryo more than half a century ago. The term is simpler, clearer, of widespread usage, and can be employed as a verb (to stage an embryo) as well as a participial adjective (a staging system). Furthermore, it should be pointed out that such expressions as "at the 3-mm stage" should be replaced by "at 3 mm." In other words, the length of an embryo is a single criterion that is not in itself sufficient to establish a stage. The term "stage" should be confined to its present-day usage in embryology (such as the 46 stages of Hamburger and Hamilton in the chick, and the 46 stages of Harrison in *Ambystoma maculatum*).

Additional alterations that have been made in the current work include the replacement of Roman by Arabic numerals and the elimination of the scientifically meaningless term "ovum."

Atlases based on the Carnegie system of staging have

been prepared by Blechschmidt (1973) and by Gasser (1975). Alternative systems of staging (discussed by O'Rahilly, 1973) are now obsolescent.

Stages 10–23 were published either by Streeter (1942, 1945, 1948, and 1951) or at least with the aid of his notes (Heuser and Corner, 1957). "The earliest age groups" were wisely "to be reserved to the last, so that advantage may be taken of any new material that becomes available" (Streeter, 1942). These groups, stages 1–9, which were to have been completed by the late Chester H. Heuser, became the task of O'Rahilly (1973).

Embryonic Length

Because most embryos are received already in fixative, it is more practicable for comparisons to use measurement after fixation as the standard (Streeter, 1945). The most useful single measurement is the greatest length (G.L.) of the embryo as measured in a straight line (i.e., caliper length) without any attempt to straighten the natural curvature of the specimen (Mall, 1907) and preferably (for purposes of standardization) after two weeks in 10 percent formalin (Streeter, 1920). Up to stage 10, measurements are frequently made on accurately scaled models, although the results (because of shrinkage in preparing the sections) are then smaller (by 25 percent, according to Streeter, 1942). A particularly interesting study has been made of the shrinkage of (pig) embryos in the procedures preparatory to sectioning (Patten and Philpott, 1921). Careful technique (see Heard, 1957) is naturally to be

TABLE 0-1. Developmental Stages in Human Embryos

Carnegie Stage	Pairs of Somites	Size (mm)	Age (days)*	Features
1		0.1–0.15	1	Fertilization.
2		0.1–0.2	1½–3	From 2 to about 16 cells.
3		0.1–0.2	4	Free blastocyst.
4		0.1–0.2	5–6	Attaching blastocyst.
5		0.1–0.2	7–12	Implanted although previllous.
5a		0.1	7–8	Solid trophoblast.
5b		0.1	9	Trophoblastic lacunae.
5c		0.15–0.2	11–12	Lacunar vascular circle.
6		0.2	13	Chorionic villi: primitive streak may appear.
6a				Chorionic villi.
6b				Primitive streak.
7		0.4	16	Notochordal process.
8		1.0–1.5	18	Primitive pit; notochordal and neurenteric canals; neural folds may appear.
9	1–3	1.5–2.5	20	Somites first appear.
10	4–12	2–3.5	22	Neural folds begin to fuse; 2 pharyngeal bars; optic sulcus.
11	13–20	2.5–4.5	24	Rostral neuropore closes; optic vesicle.
12	21–29	3–5	26	Caudal neuropore closes; 3–4 pharyngeal bars; upper limb buds appearing.
13	30–?	4–6	28	Four limb buds; lens disc; otic vesicle.
14		5–7	32	Lens pit and optic cup; endolymphatic appendage distinct.
15		7–9	33	Lens vesicle; nasal pit; antitragus beginning; hand plate; trunk relatively wider; future cerebral hemispheres distinct.
16		8–11	37	Nasal pit faces ventrally; retinal pigment visible in intact embryo; auricular hillocks beginning; foot plate.
17		11–14	41	Head relatively larger; trunk straighter; nasofrontal groove distinct; auricular hillocks distinct; finger rays.
18		13–17	44	Body more cuboidal; elbow region and toe rays appearing; eyelid folds may begin; tip of nose distinct; nipples appear; ossification may begin.
19		16–18	47½	Trunk elongating and straightening.
20		18–22	50½	Upper limbs longer and bent at elbows.
21		22–24	52	Fingers longer; hands approach each other, feet likewise.
22		23–28	54	Eyelids and external ear more developed.
23		27–31	56½	Head more rounded; limbs longer and more developed.

*Olivier and Pineau (1962) for stages 11–23; miscellaneous sources for stages 1–10.

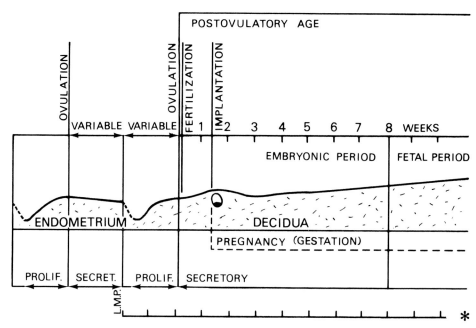

Fig. 0-1. Diagram of endometrial-decidual and embryonic-fetal relationships in relation to time. The second ovulation shown, which is followed by fertilization, is that from which postovulatory age is calculated. The last menstrual period (L.M.P.), which occurred a variable time previously, marks the beginning of the "gestational interval" (asterisk), as defined by Treloar, Behn, and Cowan (1967), who consider pregnancy (gestation) to begin with implantation, whereas others use fertilization as the starting point. Postconceptual hemorrhage in phase with menstruation would result in an apparently short gestational interval. On the other hand, an unrecognized abortion preceding pregnancy, if no menstruation intervened, would result in an apparently long gestational interval. Such possibilities, together with variability in both premenstrual and postmenstrual phases of the cycle, render menstrual data unsatisfactory in the assessment of embryonic age.

encouraged in order to keep artifactual changes to a minimum.

The crown-rump (C.-R.) length appears to have been introduced into embryology by Arnold in 1887 (Keibel and Mall, 1910), although the sitting height had been used as a measurement in the adult by Leonardo da Vinci. In the human embryo, from about stage 12 onward it becomes practicable to use the C.-R. length, but this measurement is less satisfactory than, and should be replaced by, the G.L., which can be used from stage 6 throughout the remainder of the embryonic and also the fetal period (O'Rahilly and Müller, 1984a). Other mensural criteria, such as foot length during the fetal period, may be employed, particularly if the specimen has been damaged. The G.L. (like the C.-R. length) should always be stated in millimeters. Particularly in the case of larger embryos and all fetuses, the G.L. of a given specimen should always be stated in preference to, or at least in addition to, its supposed age.

The embryonic lengths given in Table 0-1 indicate the suggested norms. Where possible they are based on specimens graded as excellent and after fixation. It should be stressed, however, that the figures do not indicate the full range within a given stage, especially when specimens of poor quality are included.

Body weight has been somewhat neglected within the embryonic period proper, although some data are available (Witschi, 1956a; Jirásek, Uher, and Uhrová, 1966; Nishimura et al., 1968). By stage 23, the embryo weighs about 2–2.7 grams.

Embryonic Age

The supposed age, as dubiously estimated from the menstrual history, is seldom useful within the embryonic period proper, and such expressions as "at the 18-day stage" should have no place in present-day embryology. Moreover, allowance should be made, but generally is not, for considerable variability in both premenstrual and postmenstrual (Stewart, 1952) phases of the menstrual cycle (Vollman, 1977), as well as for the possibility of incorrect identification of menstruation or erroneous interpretation of its absence (Treloar, Behn, and Cowan, 1967).

The ages of very early human embryos (those of the first 3–4 weeks) have been estimated chiefly by comparing their development with that of monkey conceptuses of known postovulatory ages (Rock and Hertig, 1944). Coital history, the condition of the corpus luteum, and the appearance of the endometrium are also taken into account (Rock and Hertig, 1948). More recently, ovulatory tests are providing additional information.

When an embryo has been staged, its presumed age in postovulatory days can be gauged from an appropriate table. The term "postovulatory age" (fig. 0-1) refers to the length of time since the last ovulation before pregnancy began. Because fertilization must occur very close to the time of ovulation, the postovulatory interval is a satisfactory indication of embryonic age. "Menstrual age," on the other hand, is a misnomer in that it does not indicate age. Furthermore, for precise timing, the words "gestation," "pregnancy," and "conception" should be avoided because fertilization is not universally accepted as the commencement: some authors use implantation.

In Table 0-1, the ages are based on Hertig, Rock, and Adams (1956) for stages 2–7, on Heuser (1932a) for stage 8, on Ludwig (1928) for stage 9, on Heuser and Corner (1957) for stage 10, and on Olivier and Pineau (1962) for stages 11–23.

The range is not indicated but (at least for stages 10–23) it was believed by Streeter to be ±1 day for any given stage. It should be noted, however, that from stage 14 onward, the ages become increasingly greater than those given by Streeter, which were based on comparisons with macaque embryos; it is now known that such comparisons are not warranted at these stages. Thus, by the time that the embryo reaches stage 23, there is general agreement that it is not 47 ± 1 days (Streeter, 1951) but rather at least 56 days (Witschi, 1956; Olivier and Pineau, 1962; Jirásek, Uher, and Uhrová, 1966; Jirásek, 1971). It has been confirmed ultrasonically *in vivo* that an embryo of 30 mm is normally aged 8 postovulatory weeks (Drumm and O'Rahilly, 1977).

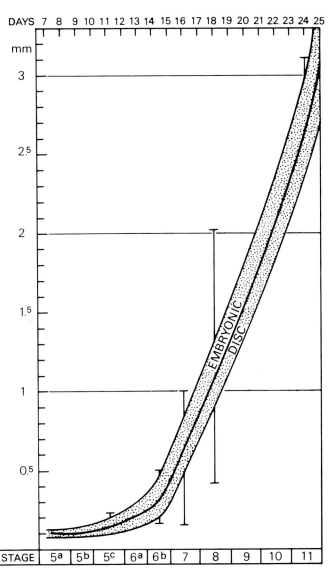

Fig. 0-2. The length of the embryonic disc from stage 5 to stage 11, approximately 1–3½ postovulatory weeks, based on the measurements of 81 embryos. Most of the specimens may be expected to fall within the shaded band, but extreme values are indicated by the five vertical lines. At 1 week the diameter of the disc is approximately 0.1 mm. At 2 weeks the disc is about 0.2 mm in length. At 3 weeks the embryonic length has increased to about 1.5–2 mm. The measurements at later stages are shown in figure 0-3.

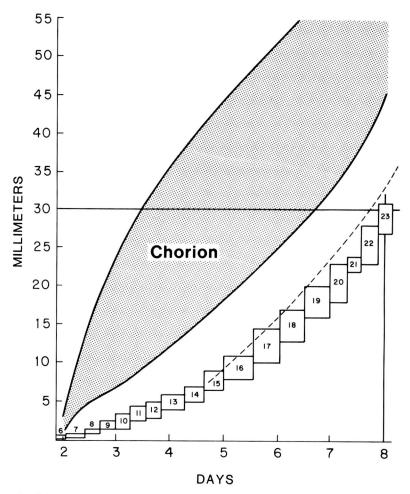

Fig. 0-3. The length of the embryo from stage 8 to stage 23, approximately 2½ to 8 postovulatory weeks, based on the measurements of more than 100 specimens that had been graded as excellent in quality. The measurements at earlier stages are shown in figure 0-2. The maximum diameter of the chorion has also been included (based on 200 specimens graded as either good or excellent): the shaded band includes approximately 80 percent of the specimens. At 4 weeks the embryo is about 5 mm in length and the chorion about 25 mm in diameter. At 8 weeks the embryo is about 30 mm in length, and the chorion is about 65 mm in diameter.

A table of "gestational age ... estimated from anamnestic data available for embryos in the author's collection" has been published by Jirásek (1971). With few exceptions (chiefly stage 15), the figures given by Jirásek resemble closely those provided by Olivier and Pineau. Although in a few instances (stages 17, 19, 20, and 21) Jirásek's ages are from one-half to one day older, in most cases the figures of Olivier and Pineau fall within the range listed by Jirásek.

Further details concerning menstrual data and embryonic age have been provided by Moore, Hutchins, and O'Rahilly (1981). Human growth during the embryonic period proper has been discussed by O'Rahilly and Müller (1986a).

Normality

The majority of the approximately 600 sectioned Carnegie embryos assigned to the 23 stages are listed as normal, although variations in, and even anomalies of, individual organs are known to occur. It should not be assumed, however, that every minor defect would

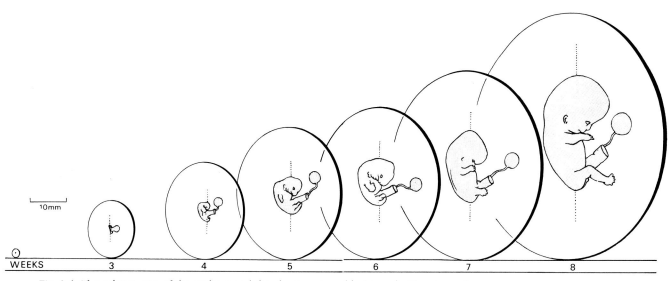

Fig. 0-4. The relative size of the embryo and the chorion at weekly intervals. The stages shown are 6, 10, 13, 16, 17, 20, and 23. The drawings are at approximately the scale of the actual specimens.

necessarily lead to a recognizable anomaly in later life. In the present investigation, an effort has been made to note specifically the presence of frankly abnormal specimens. Nevertheless, it is still true that "as our knowledge of the normal becomes more complete, we find that more and more young embryos which formerly were regarded as normal are not really so . . . it remains impossible even at the present time, to determine in all cases whether we are dealing with a normal or an abnormal specimen, even after it has been mounted in serial sections" (Meyer, in Mall and Meyer, 1921). It may be concluded that "The Borderland of Embryology and Pathology" (Willis, 1962) continues to be an important and fruitful area of investigation.

Terminology

In accordance with current practice in anatomical nomenclature, eponyms are avoided wherever possible.

The term anterior and posterior should never be used for the early embryonic period (stages 1–12) and are best avoided until considerably later. Terms considered unsuitable are listed in Table 0-2, together with suggestions for their replacement. Unfortunately the

TABLE 0-2.   List of Discarded and Replaced Terms

Alternative, Inappropriate, or Incorrect Terms	Terms Used Here
Blastocoel	Blastocystic cavity
Blastopore	Primitive pit
Blastula	Blastocyst
Branchial	Pharyngeal; visceral
Chorda dorsalis	Notochord
Embryonic shield	Embryonic disc (including cloacal membrane)
Formative cells	Epiblast
Gastrulation	Not used
Germ disc	Epiblast
Gestational age	Not used
Head process	Notochordal process
Horizon	Stage
Medullary groove and folds	Neural groove and folds
Menstrual age	Not used
Morula	Late stage 2 embryo
Ovum (egg)	Oocyte; ootid; embryo
Perivitelline space	Subzonal space
Placode	Plate or disc
Pronephros	Rostralmost part of mesonephros
Tail	Not used
Ultimobranchial	Telopharyngeal
Vitellus	Ooplasm; cytoplasm
Yolk sac	Umbilical vesicle

Nomina embryologica contains a number of inappropriate terms.

Graphs

Embryonic length is shown in figures 0-2 and 0-3, and the approximate diameter of the chorion is also provided in the latter. Relative sizes at weekly intervals are illustrated in figure 0-4.

Extension of Carnegie System

The attractive idea of using a standard system of staging throughout vertebrate embryology, as espoused by Emil Witschi, has been furthered by the recent appearance of an atlas for staging mammalian and chick embryos, based on the Carnegie system (Butler and Juurlink, 1987).

STAGE 1

Approximately 0.1–0.15 mm in diameter
Approximately 1 postovulatory day
Characteristic feature: unicellularity

Embryonic life commences with fertilization, and hence the beginning of that process may be taken as the *point de départ* of stage 1.

Despite the small size (ca. 0.1 mm) and weight (ca. 0.004 mg) of the organism at fertilization, the embryo is *"schon ein individual-spezifischer Mensch"* (Blechschmidt, 1972). The philosophical and ethical implications have been discussed briefly by O'Rahilly and Müller (1987).

Fertilization is the procession of events that begins when a spermatozoon makes contact with an oocyte or its investments and ends with the intermingling of maternal and paternal chromosomes at metaphase of the first mitotic division of the zygote (Brackett *et al.*, 1972). Fertilization *sensu stricto* involves the union of developmentally competent gametes realized in an appropriate environment to result in the formation of a viable embryo capable of normal further development (Tesařík, 1986).

Fertilization requires probably slightly longer than 24 hours in primates (Brackett *et al.*, 1972). In the case of human oocytes fertilized *in vitro*, pronuclei were formed within 11 hours of insemination (Edwards, 1972).

Given the availability of a mature oocyte (first meiotic division completed) and capacitated spermatozoa (permitting the acrosomal reaction), the criteria for fertilization generally adopted are (1) the presence of two or more polar bodies in the perivitelline space, (2) the presence of two pronuclei within the ooplasm, and (3) the presence of remnants of the flagellum of the fertilizing spermatozoon within the ooplasm (Soupart and Strong, 1974).

Fertilization, which takes place normally in the ampulla of the uterine tube, includes (a) contact of spermatozoa with the zona pellucida of an oocyte, penetration of one or more spermatozoa through the zona pellucida and the ooplasm, swelling of the spermatozoal head and extrusion of the second polar body,

(b) the formation of the male and female pronuclei, and (c) the beginning of the first mitotic division, or cleavage, of the zygote. The various details of fertilization, including such matters as capacitation, acrosomal reaction, and activation, are dealt with in special works.

When cortical granules are released, their contents appear to reinforce the structure of the zona pellucida (Sathananthan and Trounson, 1982). This is thought to be the morphological expression of the zonal reaction, and the cortical and zonal reactions may provide a block to polyspermy.

The three phases (a, b, and c) referred to above will be included here under stage 1, the characteristic feature of which is unicellularity. The sequence of events before and during the first three stages is summarized in Table 1-1.

The term "ovum," which has been used for such disparate structures as an oocyte and a 3-week embryo, has no scientific usefulness and is not used here. Indeed, strictly speaking, "the existence of the ovum . . . is impossible" (Franchi, 1970). The term "egg" is best reserved for a nutritive object frequently seen on the breakfast table.

At ovulation, the oocyte is a large cell surrounded by a thick covering, the zona pellucida, which is believed to be produced (at least largely) by the surrounding follicular cells. Processes of the follicular cells and microvilli of the oocyte both extend into the zona. The diameter of such a mammalian cell, including its zona, ranges from 70 to 190 μm. In the human, the ooplasm measures about 100 μm, and the thickness of the zona ranges from 16 to 18 μm (Allen *et al.*, 1930). Good photomicrographs and electron micrographs of human secondary oocytes are available (e.g., Baca and Zamboni, 1967, figs. 20 to 24; Kennedy and Donahue, 1969). The zona pellucida is covered externally by the corona radiata, which is a loose investment of granulosa cells from the ovarian follicle. On fixation

9

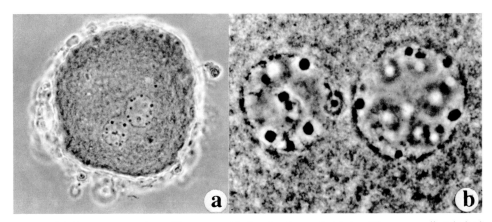

Fig. 1-1. (a) Phase contrast view of human ootid after fixation and staining. The zona pellucida had been dissolved during preparation of the specimen. (b) Phase contrast, oil immersion view of the pronuclei shown in (a). Both views, by courtesy of Dr. Z. Dickmann and Alan R. Liss, Inc. (*Anatomical Record, 152*, 293–302, 1965).

TABLE 1-1.   Tabulation of the First Three Stages

Stage	Event	Products
	Meiotic division 1	
		Oocyte 2 and polar body 1
	Beginning of meiotic division 2 and ovulation	
		Ovulated oocyte
1a	Penetration	
		Penetrated oocyte
	Completion of meiotic division 2 and formation of pronuclei	
1b		Ootid and polar body 2
	Pronuclei enter cleavage division	
1c		Zygote
	Cleavage continues	
2		2 to about 16 cells
	Formulation of blastocystic cavity	
3		Blastocyst, from about 32 cells onward

(Stages 1a, 1b bracketed as "Fertilization")

and embedding, the oocyte undergoes shrinkage; this affects the cytoplasm more than the zona, so that a subzonal (or perivitelline) space becomes accentuated. The polar bodies are found within that space. It is said that the first polar body may divide before the second is released, and it has been claimed that each of the three polar bodies is capable of being fertilized. Although it is not unusual for the second polar body to display a nucleus, the chromosomes of the first polar body are isolated and naked (Zamboni, 1971).

It is "likely that no more than one day intervenes between ovulation and fertilization. This time interval may be taken then as the possible error in age of [an] embryo when it is considered the same as ovulatory age" (Rock and Hertig, 1942).

(*a*) *Penetrated oocyte.* This term may conveniently be used once a spermatozoon has penetrated the zona pellucida and, strictly, "after gamete plasma membranes have become confluent" (Zamboni *et al.*, 1966). Penetration has been inferred from the presence of spermatozoa in the zona pellucida or in the subzonal space (Edwards, Bavister, and Steptoe, 1969). Moreover, *in vitro* examples showing portions of spermatozoa within the ooplasm are illustrated by Sathananthan, Trounson, and Wood (1986), in whose work are also

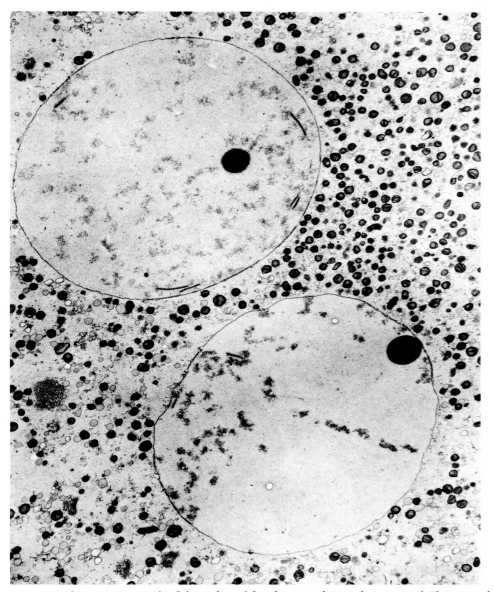

Fig. 1-2. Electron micrograph of the male and female pronuclei in a human ootid. The pronuclear material appears to be highly hydrated, although it is condensed in patches. A small black sphere, namely the nucleolus, and some annulate lamellae are visible within each pronucleus. Numerous organelles are present in the cytoplasm adjacent to the pronuclei, and portions of a Golgi complex are visible near the lower left-hand corner of the photograph. × 5,400. Reproduced through the courtesy of Dr. Luciano Zamboni, University of California, Los Angeles, and the Rockefeller University Press (*Journal of Cell Biology, 30*, 579–600, 1966).

detailed views showing the formation of the second polar body.

(*b*) *Ootid.* The cell characterized by the presence of the male and female pronuclei is termed an ootid (figs. 1-1 and 1-2). Several examples of human ootids have

been described. They are probably about 12–24 hours in age. The diameter, including the zona pellucida, is about 175 μm (Hamilton, 1946; Dickmann *et al.*, 1965), and the diameter of the subzonal space is approximately 140 μm. The cytoplasm of the ootid has a diameter of about 100 μm (Hamilton, 1946; Noyes *et al.*, 1965); each of the pronuclei measures about 30 μm (Zamboni *et al.*, 1966). The various ultrastructural features of the ootid have been described and illustrated (Zamboni *et al.*, 1966; Sathananthan, Trounson, and Wood, 1986).

Although "in most mammalian species, the male pronucleus has been reported to be larger than the female pronucleus," the converse has been found in one human specimen and, in two others, the pronuclei appeared to be of equal size (Zamboni, 1971).

(*c*) *Zygote.* The cell that characterizes the last phase of fertilization is elusive. The first cleavage spindle forms rapidly and has been used in identification. Such cells have probably been seen in certain mammals, e.g., the pig, cow, hamster, rat, and mouse.

Pronuclear fusion does not occur. Rather, the two pronuclear envelopes break down ("post-apposition envelope vesiculation," Szabo and O'Day, 1983), and the two groups of chromosomes move together and assume positions on the first cleavage spindle. Thus the zygote lacks a nucleus.

A human embryo "in syngamy just prior to cleavage" has been illustrated by Sathananthan and Trounson (1985, fig. 2). "The chromosomes, some associated in pairs, are located in an agranular zone in the central ooplasm."

In the human, the initial cleavage that heralds the onset of stage 2 occurs in the uterine tube "some time between twenty-four and thirty hours after [the beginning of] fertilization" (Hertig, 1968).

Specimens of Stage 1 Already Described

Embryos of stages 1–3 have been seen very frequently since the advent of *in vitro* fertilization in 1969.

Ootids have been described by the following authors:

Hamilton (1946 and 1949). Tubal. Diameter (including zona pellucida), 173 μm. Diameter of ooplasm, 100 μm. Sectioned serially at 7 μm. Two pronuclei, one larger than the other. Many spermatozoa in zona pellucida. Dickmann *et al.* (1965) have expressed some doubts about this specimen.

Khvatov (1959). Tubal. Two pronuclei, claimed to be distinguished as male and female.

Dickmann *et al.* (1965). Tubal. Diameter (including zona), 174 μm. Zona pellucida, 17.5 μm in thickness. Diameter of ooplasm, 103 μm (Noyes *et al.*, 1965). Two pronuclei, approximately equal in size (fig. 1-1b). Nucleoli visible. Tail of fertilizing spermatozoon identified over one pronucleus. Well illustrated (figs. 1-1a and b).

Zamboni *et al.* (1966). Tubal. Ootid estimated to have a maximum diameter of about 150 μm, and 110–120 μm without the zona pellucida (Zamboni, personal communication, 1970). Fixed and sectioned for electron microscopy. Zona seen and three polar bodies identified. Two pronuclei, of about equal size (30 μm), each with a spheroidal nucleolus. Remnants of penetrating spermatozoon identified near one pronucleus. Ultrastructural findings described in detail and well illustrated (fig. 1-2).

Edwards, Bavister, and Steptoe (1969). Seven ootids resulted from insemination *in vitro* of oocytes matured *in vitro*. Two had two pronuclei each, four had three each, and one had five. Photographs, but no cytological details, were provided.

Soupart and Morgenstern (1973). Two pronuclei and two polar bodies obtained *in vitro*.

Soupart and Strong (1974). Fourteen examples examined by electron microscopy. Two pronuclei (that near spermatozoal flagellum believed to be male) and two polar bodies.

Lopata *et al.* (1978, 1980). Several *in vitro* examples.

Sathananthan and Trounson (1982) studied the release of cortical granules at stages 1 and 2.

Pereda and Coppo (1984) found, by electron microscopy, light and dark follicular cells surrounding an ootid from the uterine tube.

Sathananthan, Trounson, and Wood (1986). Several *in vitro* examples are illustrated.

STAGE 2

Approximately 0.1–0.2 mm in diameter
Approximately 1½–3 postovulatory days
Characteristic feature: more than 1 cell but no blastocystic
cavity seen by light microscopy

Stage 2 comprises specimens from 2 cells up to the appearance of the blastocystic (or segmentation) cavity. The more advanced examples (from about 12 cells on) of stage 2 are frequently called morulae (L., *morus*, a mulberry). The term morula is not historically appropriate for mammals, however, because the amphibian morula gives rise to embryonic tissues only, whereas in mammals non-embryonic structures (such as the chorion and the amnion) are also derived from the initial mass of cells.

Size and Age

The diameter at stage 2 before fixation is of the order of 175 μm; after fixation, it is approximately 120 μm (Hertig *et al.*, 1954). Indeed, shrinkage of as much as 50 percent may occur in some instances (Menkin and Rock, 1948). Whether before or after fixation, the diameter at stage 2 may be expected to lie between 75 and 200 μm.

The volume of the protoplasmic mass diminishes during cleavage (O'Rahilly, 1973, table 5).

The age at stage 2 is believed to be approximately 1½–3 postovulatory days. The range is probably 1–5 days (Sundström, Nilsson, and Liedholm, 1981). *In vitro*, 2 cells may be found at 1½ days, 4 cells at 2 days, and 8 cells by about 2½ days.

General Features

The organism proceeds along the uterine tube by means not entirely understood (reviewed by Adams, 1960). It leaves the tube and enters the uterine cavity during the third or fourth day after ovulation, when probably 8–12 cells are present, and when the endometrium is early in the secretory phase (corresponding to the luteal phase of the ovarian cycle).

It has been shown experimentally (in the mouse, rat, and rabbit) that a blastomere isolated from the mammalian 2-cell organism is capable of forming a complete embryo. Separation of the early blastomeres is believed to account for about one-third of all cases of monozygotic twinning in the human (Corner, 1955). Such twins should be dichorial and diamniotic (fig. 5-2). The fact that nearly 60 percent of dichorial twins (whether monozygotic or dizygotic) have two unfused placentae "indicates that the zona pellucida . . . must have disappeared sufficiently long before implantation to allow the twins to become implanted in independent positions in the uterus" (Bulmer, 1970). Dizygotic twins, in contrast, are believed to arise from two oocytes, from a binucleate oocyte, or from a second polar body (Gedda, 1961).

The successive cleavage divisions do not occur synchronously, so that (in the pig) specimens of anywhere from 1 to 8 cells can be found. It has been suggested that the more precociously dividing cells may be those that give rise to the trophoblast. Moreover, differences in the size, staining, and electron density of the blastomeres are observed.

There is reason to believe, however, that the blastomeres are not determined very early in development. For example, it has been shown experimentally in the mouse that the ability to develop into trophoblastic cells is inherent in all blastomeres of the first two stages. Up to 16 cells, none of the blastomeres is yet determined to give rise to cells of the inner mass. It may be that the primary factor responsible for the determination of one of the two alternative routes of differentiation (trophoblast or inner cell mass) is simply the position (peripheral or internal) that a given cell occupies.

According to the "inside/outside hypothesis," micro-environmental differences influence the determination of blastomeres (between 8 and 16 cells in the mouse) so that those on the outside become more

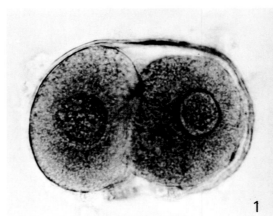

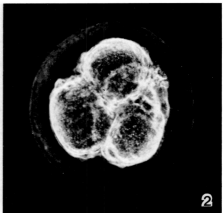

Fig. 2-1. Intact 2-cell embryo showing zona pellucida and two polar bodies, the larger of which is clearly visible at the lower end of the cleavage line. No. 8698.

Fig. 2-2. Intact 4-cell embryo. The granular zona pellucida can be distinguished. By courtesy of Dr. J. Lippes (Doyle *et al.*, 1966) and the C. V. Mosby Co. (*American Journal of Obstetrics and Gynecology, 95*, 115–117, 1966).

likely to form trophoblast (with more restricted potential) whereas those enclosed by other cells become more likely to form the inner cell mass. Another hypothesis accounting for early cellular diversity (in the mouse) is based on polarization of the larger, external cells, characterized by microvilli.

Furthermore, it has been possible in the mouse to unite two 16-cell organisms and obtain from them one giant, but otherwise perfectly normal, blastocyst. Fusion of mouse organisms with close to 32 cells each has also resulted in a single blastocyst.

It has been stressed that it is dangerous readily to infer normality on purely morphological grounds.

In the human, two significant specimens of stage 2 (Hertig *et al.*, 1954) will be cited.

A 2-cell specimen (No. 8698) was spherical and surrounded by a transparent zona pellucida (fig. 2-1). Two polar bodies were present. Each blastomere was nearly spherical. It has been maintained that the larger blastomere would probably divide first and hence may perhaps be trophoblastic (Hertig, 1968).

A 12-cell specimen (No. 8904) was perfectly spherical and surrounded by a clear zona pellucida. One blastomere, central in position and larger than the others, was presumed to be embryogenic, whereas the smaller cells were thought to be trophoblastic.

A number of human specimens of stage 2 found in atretic ovarian follicles were considered to be par-

thenogenetic by their authors (Häggström, 1922; Krafka, 1939; Herranz and Vázquez, 1964; Khvatov, 1968). Such a claim, however, has been disputed (Ashley, 1959), and it has been pointed out that polysegmentation, that is, cleavage-like conditions described as "pseudoparthenogenesis," are not infrequently encountered in moribund oocytes (Kampmeier, 1929). It is likely also that some instances of cleavage obtained *in vitro* may be pseudoparthenogenetic rather than caused by actual fertilization by spermatozoa.

The presence of a Y chromosome in a "spread from a replicating blastomere" (Jacobson, Sites, and Arias-Bernal, 1970) has been claimed "but not convincingly demonstrated" (Brackett *et al.*, 1972).

The embryonic genome probably becomes functionally active during stage 2. Activation of transcription of rRNA genes (contributed to the embryonic genome by the male and female gametes at fertilization) is indicated *in vitro* by the pattern of nucleologenesis, which changes in 6- to 8-cell embryos and becomes typical in 10- to 12-cell embryos (Tesařík *et al.*, 1986).

SPECIMENS OF STAGE 2 ALREADY DESCRIBED
(listed in order of numbers of cells present)

Specimens believed by their authors to have been parthenogenetic are indicated here by an asterisk.

2 cells, Carnegie No. 8260. Described by Menkin and Rock (1948). Produced *in vitro*. Diameter, 153 × 155 μm; cytoplasm, 100 × 113 (50 × 75 after fixation); thickness of zona pellucida, 23 (8 after fixation); blastomeres, 88 × 58 and 105 × 58 (63 × 39 and 66 × 36 after fixation); polar body, 18 × 10 after fixation.

2 cells, Carnegie No. 8698 (fig. 2-1). Described by Hertig *et al.* (1954). Tubal. Diameter, 178.5 μm (122 × 88 after fixation; 111.6 × 75 after sectioning); blastomeres, 71 (74 × 64 and 80 × 56 after fixation; 68.3 × 61.6 and 70 × 50 after sectioning); polar bodies, 20 × 18 after fixation. A few cells of the corona radiata were present. Thick zona pellucida (18 μm in thickness before fixation). No spermatozoa were seen in the zona, and the possibility of parthenogenetic cleavage "cannot be entirely ruled out" (Dickmann *et al.*, 1965). Two polar bodies. Whether the larger blastomere "is the one of trophoblastic potential is unknown but it is probable" (Hertig, 1968). Believed to be about 1½ days old.

2 cells. Illustrated by Shettles (1958 and 1960). Produced *in vitro.*

2 cells. Undergoing cytolysis, produced parthenogenetically by Edwards *et al.* (1966)* from an oocyte cultured *in vitro.*

2 cells and 4 cells. Described by Häggström (1922),* who found them in atretic ovarian follicles of a 22-year-old woman.

2 cells. Two *in vitro* embryos studied by electron microscopy (Dvořák *et al.*, 1982), both round. Surprisingly, one was surrounded by a large mass of cumulus cells.

2 cells. Illustrated by Pereda and Coppo (1985); believed to be 37 hours.

2–8 cells. *In vitro* examples are illustrated by Sathananthan, Trounson, and Wood (1986).

3 cells, Carnegie No. 8500.1. Described by Menkin and Rock (1948). Produced *in vitro.* Diameter, 170 × 183 μm; cytoplasm, 103 × 127 (50 × 86 after fixation); thickness of zona pellucida, 21; blastomeres, 97 × 73, 62 × 62, and 50 × 63 (66 × 49, 35 × 38, and 33 × 34 after fixation); a possible polar body, 14 × 9 after fixation.

3 cells. Produced *in vitro.* Petrov (1958) found spermatozoal penetration of the zona pellucida after 2 hours, polyspermy in all cases, the first cleavage furrow after 20 hours, and three blastomeres after 26 hours.

4 cells. Illustrated by Krafka (1939),* who found it (within a zona pellucida) in an atretic ovarian follicle of a 7-year-old child.

4 cells. Described by Herranz and Vázquez (1964),* who found it (within a zona pellucida) in an atretic ovarian follicle of a 20-year-old woman.

4 cells. Illustrated by Way and Dawson (1959). Found in a routine vaginal smear. Well-marked zona pellucida.

4 cells. Illustrated by Shettles (1960). Produced *in vitro.*

4 cells. Illustrated by Doyle *et al.* (1966). Found in middle third of uterine tube. Devoid of corona radiata. Granular zona pellucida (fig. 2-2).

4–10 cells. Eight *in vitro* examples, studied by electron microscopy (Sundström, Nilsson, and Liedholm, 1981). They ranged from 60 to 120 hours, and the average cleavage time varied from 24 to 86 hours.

5–12 cells. Pathological specimens of 5 (No. 8630), 8 (No. 8450), 9 (No. 8190), and 11 or 12 (No. 8452) cells, found by Hertig *et al.* (1954).

6 cells. Illustrated by Brackett *et al.* (1972). Produced *in vitro.* Other specimens consisted of 2–12 cells and "a questionable morula undergoing degeneration."

7 cells. Illustrated by Avendaño *et al.* (1975). Measured 201 × 197 μm. Zona intact (25 μm in thickness). Three polar bodies. Two of the seven blastomeres were metachromatic and electron-dense, and one polar body was metachromatic. Believed to be about 72 hours.

8 cells. Noted by Khvatov (1968)* in an atretic ovarian follicle. Diameter (after fixation), 110 × 95 μm.

8 cells. *In vitro* specimens of 8 cells and also some "early morulae and blastocysts" (Edwards and Fowler, 1970).

8 cells. Two *in vitro* specimens, studied by electron microscopy (Sathananthan, Wood, and Leeton, 1982). Zona intact. "A small cleavage cavity was already apparent within each embryo" (their fig. 1).

12 cells, Carnegie No. 8904. Described by Hertig *et al.* (1954). Uterine. Diameter, 172.8 μm (115.2 after fixation); blastomeres, 38.4 × 19.2. Clear zona pellucida (10 μm in thickness before fixation). Polar bodies not identified. No evidence of a blastocystic cavity. A large, central blastomere was thought to be embryogenic, the other cells trophoblastic. Specimen lost during preparation. Believed to be about 3 days old.

14–16 cells. Lopata, Kohlman, and Johnston (1983) found complex intercellular junctions in the blastomeres that "suggest that compaction was occurring." Tinctorial differences were noted among the cells of specimens of 5–12 cells. Multinucleated (probably abnormal) examples were also recorded.

16 cells. Specimens ranging from 1 to "16 or more" cells were produced *in vitro* (Edwards, Steptoe, and Purdy, 1970). Photographs of a 4- and an 8-cell specimen were included.

STAGE 3

Approximately 0.1–0.2 mm in diameter
Approximately 4 postovulatory days
Characteristic feature: free blastocyst

Stage 3 consists of the free (that is, unattached) blastocyst, a term used as soon as a cavity (the blastocystic, or segmentation, cavity) can be recognized by light microscopy. (The staging system is based on light microscopy and, in later stages, on gross structure also.)

The blastocyst is the hollow mass of cells from the initial appearance of the cavity (stage 3) to immediately before the completion of implantation at a subsequent stage. The blastocystic cavity, under the light microscope, begins by the coalescence of intercellular spaces when the organism has acquired about 32 cells. In *in vitro* studies, a cavity formed in some human embryos at 16–20 cells (Edwards, 1972).

It is necessary to stress that the cavity of the mammalian blastocyst is not the counterpart of the amphibian or the avian blastocoel. In the bird, the blastocoel is the limited space between the epiblast and the primary endoderm. The cavity of the mammalian blastocyst, however, corresponds to the subgerminal space together with the area occupied by the yolk (Torrey, personal communication, 1972).

The mammalian blastocyst differs from a blastula in that its cells have already differentiated into at least two types: trophoblastic and embryonic cells proper.

Heuser and Streeter (1941) emphasized an important point by using stage 3 as an example:

> The blastocyst form is not to be thought of solely in terms of the next succeeding stage in development. It is to be remembered that at all stages the embryo is a living organism, that is, it is a going concern with adequate mechanisms for its maintenance as of that time.

It is no less true, however, that changes occur "in the growing organism and its environment which provide critically for the future survival of the organism" (Reynolds, 1954). Indeed, such morphological and functional changes during development "critically anticipate future morphological and functional requirements for the survival and welfare of the organism" (*ibid.*).

Sex chromatin has been "tentatively identified" in two *in vitro* human blastocysts (Edwards, 1972).

Probably the first recognition of the inner cell mass of the mammalian (dog and rabbit) blastocyst was that by Prévost and Dumas in 1824. This and many other aspects of the blastocyst are considered in a book edited by Blandau (1971).

SIZE AND AGE

In the human embryo the maximum diameter increases from 100–200 μm at stages 2 and 3 to 300–450 μm at stage 5a.

Embryos of stage 3 are believed to be about 4 days in age. *In vitro* embryos of stage 1 have been recorded at 9–32 hours after insemination; stage 2 at 22–40 hours (2 cells), 32–45 hours (4 cells), and 48 hours (8 cells); stage 3 at 100 hours, and extruding from the zona pellucida at 140–160 hours, at which time they show differentiation into trophoblast, epiblast, and hypoblast (Mohr and Trounson, 1984).

HISTOLOGICAL FEATURES

Zona pellucida. In stage 3 the zona pellucida may be either present or absent. *In vitro*, the blastocyst emerges from the zona at about 6–7 days. The emergence is commonly referred to as "hatching."

Trophoblast. During stage 3 the trophoblastic cells, because of their peripheral position, are distinguishable from the embryonic cells proper. The trophoblastic cells that cover the inner cell mass are referred to as polar: i.e., at the embryonic pole or future site of implantation. The remaining trophoblast is termed mural.

Cavitation. It is believed that the blastomeres (in the mouse) attain the ability to secrete the blastocystic fluid after a definite number of cleavages, namely at the end of the fifth and at the beginning of the sixth

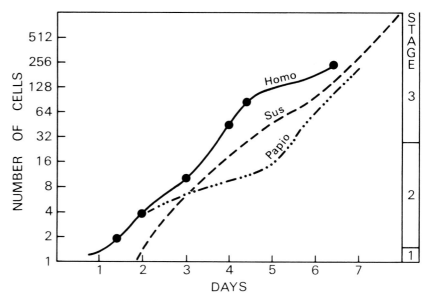

Fig. 3-1. Graph showing presumed age plotted against number of cells. The continuous line is based on six human embryos: 8698, Doyle *et al.*, 8904, 8794, 8663, and Krafka. The interrupted lines indicate pig (Heuser and Streeter, 1929) and baboon (Hendrickx, 1971) embryos. In each case the rate of cleavage during the first week is not much faster than one division per day.

mitotic cycle. In the mouse it has been shown that, when the organism consists of about 32 cells, small cavities unite to form the beginning of the blastocystic cavity. In other words, the solid phase of development (in the mouse) ends at about 28–32 cells, when fluid begins to accumulate beneath the trophoblastic cells. As the blastocyst develops, it undergoes expansions and contractions. When contracted, a "pseudomorula" of about 100 cells in the mouse can be seen.

Because no appreciable increase in size of the (cat) embryo occurs at first, it is thought that no mere flowing together of inter- or intra-cellular spaces or vacuoles is a sufficient explanation of the origin of the blastocystic cavity. Thus an additional factor, namely cytolysis of certain of the central cells, is also involved.

Electron microscopy has added further details. The formation of junctional complexes, which is regarded as the first sign of blastocystic formation, is found very early in the rat, when the embryo consists of only 8 cells, although the first indication of a cavity, as opposed to intercellular spaces, is not seen until after another series of cell divisions. In two human, 8-cell, *in vitro* embryos studied by electron microscopy, "a small cleavage cavity was already apparent within each

embryo" (Sathananthan, Wood, and Leeton, 1982).

Inner cell mass. The embryonic cells proper become surrounded by the trophoblastic cells and form an inner mass. Studies of various mammals have indicated that the inner cell mass represents more than the embryo itself, insofar as it constitutes a germinal mass of various potentialities which continues for a time to add cells to the more precociously developed trophoblast. The inner cell mass gives origin to the hypoblast, and its remainder (the "formative cells") constitutes the epiblast. The epiblastic cells soon become aligned into what was frequently described as the "germ disc." These various relationships are summarized in figure 6-2. It has been found that hypoblastic differentiation in the macaque occurred at about the same time that a basal lamina was found under mural trophoblast and epiblast (but not polar trophoblast or hypoblast) (Enders and Schlafke, 1981).

Duplication of the inner cell mass probably accounts for most instances of monozygotic twinning (Corner, 1955; Bulmer, 1970). Such twins should be monochorial but diamniotic (fig. 5-2). *In vitro*, "many blastocysts fail to hatch fully from their zona pellucida," and "two separate embryos could form if the inner

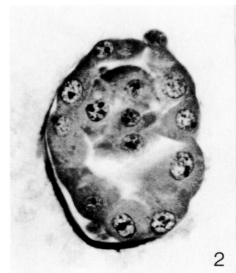 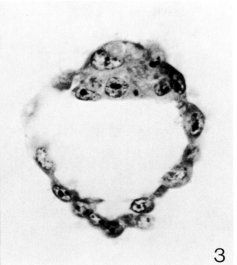

Fig. 3-2. Section through a 58-cell blastocyst (No. 8794). The zona pellucida is visible on the lower left-hand part of the mass, where a polar body can also be recognized. The inner cell mass can be seen above the blastocystic cavity. The more peripherally situated cells are trophoblastic.

Fig. 3-3. Section through a 107-cell blastocyst (No. 8663). The zona pellucida is no longer present. The blastocystic cavity is now quite large. The embryonic pole, characterized by the inner cell mass, is shown uppermost. The peripheral layer of cells constitutes the trophoblast.

cell mass was bisected during hatching" (Edwards, Mettler, and Walters, 1986).

Two significant specimens of stage 3 (Hertig *et al.*, 1954) are here cited.

In a 58-cell specimen (No. 8794), 53 of the cells were trophoblastic whereas 5 were embryonic. The latter composed the inner cell mass, which was located eccentrically within the blastocystic cavity but had not yet assumed a truly polar position.

In a 107-cell specimen (No. 8663), 99 of the cells were trophoblastic, and, of these, 69 were mural in position and 30 were polar (i.e., covering the embryonic pole). Eight of the 107 cells were embryonic, and were characterized by their larger size and by the presence of intracytoplasmic vacuoles. Moreover, the 8 cells comprised three types: "obvious primitive, vacuolated ectoderm [epiblast]; flattened primitive endoderm [hypoblast]; and a large indifferent cell, presumably a [primordial] germ cell" (Hertig, 1968). In addition, of the 30 polar trophoblastic cells, 4 which were situated "ventral and lateral to the formative cells . . . may actually be of primitive endodermal type" (Hertig *et al.*,

1954).

Dorsoventrality. A comparison of stage 3 embryos with those of stage 5 makes it clear that the surface of the inner cell mass that is adjacent to the polar trophoblast represents the dorsal surface of the embryo, and the surface of the mass that faces the blastocystic cavity represents the ventral surface. In other words, "dorsalization," or "dorsoventrality," becomes apparent during stage 3 (O'Rahilly, 1970). The possibility should be kept in mind, however, that the inner cell mass can perhaps travel around the inside of the trophoblastic layer.

Rate of division. In the pig embryo it has been shown that, in general, "during the first seven days the cells undergo about eight divisions, that is, they divide about once a day" (Heuser and Streeter, 1929). A similar generalization may be made for the human embryo during stages 1–3, and also for the baboon (Hendrickx, 1971). In the case of the baboon, "there is a close correlation between age and cell number," although "there is no consistent relationship between age and size for these stages of development" (*ibid.*).

Specimens of Stage 3 Already Described

(listed in order of number of cells present)

Ca. 32 cells. Described by Shettles (1956 and 1960). Produced *in vitro.* Zona pellucida denuded of corona and cumulus cells. "Early segmentation cavity."

Ca. 50 cells. Described by Shettles (1957) as caused by "parthenogenetic cleavage." Zona pellucida denuded of corona and cumulus cells. Diameter, including zona, 150 μm. "Early segmentation cavity."

58 cells, Carnegie No. 8794. Described by Hertig *et al.* (1954). Uterine. Diameter, 230 × 190 μm (108 × 86 after fixation; 101 × 73.3 after sectioning; diameters of blastomeres varied from 15 to 23 after sectioning; polar bodies, 18 μm after fixation. Zona pellucida intact while fresh but partly deficient after fixation (fig. 3-2). Two polar bodies. Early blastocystic cavity. Believed to be about 4 days old.

100 cells. Described by Khvatov (1967). Tubal. Diameter, 126 × 100 × 70 μm. Nuclei in trophoblastic blastomeres darker (with hematoxylin and eosin). Said to be female, "based on current studies concerning sex chromatin."

"More than 100 cells." In two such blastocysts produced *in vitro,* "bodies resembling sex chromatin were seen in a few nuclei" (Steptoe, Edwards, and Purdy, 1971; Edwards, 1972).

107 cells, Carnegie No. 8663. Described by Hertig *et al.* (1954). Uterine. No zona pellucida (fig. 8). Diameter, 153 × 115 μm (103 × 80 after fixation; 91.6 × 83.3 after sectioning); diameters of blastomeres varied from 8 to 21. Large blastocystic cavity (58 μm). Embryonic mass composed of 8 cells: epiblastic, hypoblastic, and a presumed primordial germ cell (Hertig, 1968). Believed to be about 4½ days old. Khvatov (1967), without further elaboration, claimed: "according to photographs, should be of the male sex." Smith (1970, fig. 15), without further justification, claimed that a cytoplasmic vacuole was "the first indication toward an amniotic space."

186 cells. Croxatto *et al.* (1972) suggested that "the unimplanted human blastocyst begins a process of expansion when it has between 107 and 186 cells," prior to shedding of the zona pellucida.

Ca. 200–300 cells. Described briefly by Krafka (1942). Tubal. Diameter, 120 × 180 μm. Zona pellucida intact. Some adherent granulosa cells. Described as "solid" but the large number of cells suggests that it should have had a blastocystic cavity (it may be a contracted blastocyst); hence it is included here in stage 3.

Unknown number of cells. Three blastocysts that failed to emerge from the zona were studied by electron microscopy (Lopata, Kohlman, and Kellow, 1982). One showed hypoblast.

STAGE 4

Probably approximately 0.1–0.2 mm in diameter

Approximately 5–6 postovulatory days

Characteristic feature: attaching blastocyst

Stage 4, the onset of implantation, is reserved for the attaching blastocyst, which is probably 5–6 days old.

Although the criteria for the first three stages are those of the first three horizons, it has not proved practicable in stages 4–10 to retain the criteria for horizons IV–X. This abandonment had already been begun by Hertig, Rock, and Adams (1956) and by Heuser and Corner (1957).

It should be noted that certain specimens that are now listed in stages 5a and 5b (Hertig, Rock, and Adams, 1956) were formerly included in horizon IV. In other words, because such specimens represent "significantly different stages of development" (*ibid.*), they have been transferred, and, as a result, stage 4 has been made more restricted. Healing of the uterine epithelium over the conceptus, for example, is too variable and has been eliminated as a criterion for stage 5; it usually occurs after horizon VI has begun (Böving, 1965).

Implantation is the specific process that leads to the formation of a specialized, intimate cellular contact between the trophoblast and the endometrium, or other tissue in the case of ectopic implantation (Denker, 1983).

Implantation is a highly complicated and ill-understood phenomenon "by which the conceptus is transported to its site of attachment, held there, oriented properly, and then attached by adhesion, trophoblastic penetration, spread, proliferation, envelopment of vessels, and other developments of the placenta, both conceptal and maternal parts" (Böving, 1963). In this broad sense, implantation includes at least stages 4 and 5.

Implantation, then, includes (1) dissolution of the zona pellucida, and contact and attachment (adhesion) between the blastocyst and the endometrium, (2) penetration, and (3) migration of the blastocyst through the endometrium. On the basis of comparative studies, it has been suggested (Böving, 1965) that stage 4 might be subdivided into these three phases. Human (but not macaque) implantation is interstitial in type: i.e., the blastocyst comes to lie entirely within the substance of the endometrium. In the human (as also in the macaque), implantation occurs into an edematous, non-deciduous endometrium. In other words, decidualization takes place at the end of implantation.

In his important study of the early development of the primates, Hill (1932) concluded as follows:

> The outstanding feature of the early human blastocyst is its extraordinary precocity as exemplified ... in the relations it very early acquires to the uterine lining and in the remarkably early differentiation of its trophoblast and its extra-embryonal mesoderm. It is no longer content to undergo its development in the uterine lumen as does that of all the lower Primates, but, whilst still quite minute, burrows its way through the uterine epithelium and implants itself in the very vascular subepithelial decidual tissue of the uterus. Therein it forms for itself a decidual cavity and undergoes its subsequent development, completely embedded in the maternal tissue. In this way the Primate germ reaches the acme of its endeavour to maintain itself in the uterus and to obtain an adequate supply of nutriment at the earliest possible moment.

The mammalian stage 2 organism and the early blastocyst are surrounded by an intact zona pellucida, which disappears at the beginning of implantation. Hence, implantation "is taken as beginning when the zona pellucida is lost and the trophoblast is in contact with the uterine epithelium throughout its circumference" (Young, Whicher, and Potts, 1968). Although claims have been made that the blastocyst emerges from its zona pellucida by "shedding" or by "hatching," it has also been maintained that, at least in the mouse, the zona undergoes rapid dissolution all around the blastocyst *in situ*, that is, at the actual site of implantation.

After the blastocyst becomes attached at random to the uterine epithelium in the mouse, it is believed that the inner cell mass can travel around the inside of the trophoblastic shell (presumably somewhat like a sat-ellite gear). Although the nature of the stimulus re-sponsible for the final orientation of the inner cell mass is unknown, it is postulated that the final position is determined either by a morphogenetic gradient across the vertical axis of the uterus or by changes in the trophoblast associated with its attachment to the un-derlying tissues, or by both.

The implantation site has been studied by electron microscopy in several mammals, such as the mouse. The cell membranes of the trophoblast and uterine epithelium become intimately related, and large cy-toplasmic inclusions are found in the trophoblastic cells. The ultrastructural changes taking place at im-plantation suggest that there may be a high degree of permeability between maternal and embryonic cells. In addition, there may be an exchange of cellular ma-terial between uterus and embryo.

After the zona pellucida has become dissolved, the surface membranes of the trophoblast and uterine ep-ithelium are separated by a very narrow interval (in the mouse). This first morphological sign of implan-tation can be detected only by electron microscopy.

In at least some macaque specimens a distinction between cytotrophoblast and syncytiotrophoblast can be made (Heuser and Streeter, 1941, e.g., No. C-520, their fig. 38). Moreover, amniogenic cells have been claimed to be "separating from the trophoblast above and . . . distinct from the germ disk" (*ibid.*, No. C-610, their fig. 53). Finally, epiblastic cells and hypoblast can be distinguished (*ibid.*, No. C-520, their fig. 40).

Of the several macaque specimens of stage 4 that have been described, in one instance (No. C-560), the uterine epithelium at the site of attachment showed a disturbed arrangement of its nuclei. Moreover, the cy-toplasm had become paler, which was taken to indicate beginning cytolysis. In the conceptus, the site of at-tachment was formed by syncytiotrophoblast, which is initially formed by the coalescence of polar trophoblast (Hertig, 1968). Some of the increased number of nu-clei appeared to have been released from the uterine epithelium and then engulfed by the rapidly expanding trophoblast. Within the cavity of the blastocyst, disin-tegrating embryonic cells were interpreted as a me-chanical accident caused by displacement of the cells.

At the site of attachment, fused multinucleated cells of the uterine epithelium constitute a "symplasma," which fuses with the syncytiotrophoblast (in macaque No. C-610, and also in the rabbit; in the latter it has been studied by electron microscopy by Larsen, 1970).

A specimen of stage 4 in the baboon has been il-lustrated (Hendrickx, 1971). The single layer of abem-bryonic trophoblast was continuous with the cyto-trophoblast dorsally. The syncytiotrophoblast was in contact with the uterine epithelium, which had lost its columnar appearance. Moreover, as much as one-half of the surface portion of the uterine cells had disap-peared at the site of attachment. The inner cell mass showed occasional "endoblastic" cells bordering the blastocystic cavity. The age of the specimen was esti-mated as 9 days.

Specimen of Stage 4 Already Described

In the human, the only report of stage 4 seems to be two not altogether satisfactory photographs in a Supplement to *Ovum humanum* (Shettles, 1960, figs. 65 and 66). One il-lustration is captioned "attachment of the blastocyst to the uterine epithelium during the sixth day after ovulation. The encapsulating zona pellucida has disappeared." The second figure is a high-power view to show that "pseudopodia-like protoplasmic projections from blastocyst traverse the adja-cent zona pellucida at area of contact with endometrium."

No specimen of stage 4 in the human has been recorded that would be comparable to those in the macaque illustrated by Heuser and Streeter (1941, plate 3, fig. 31, and plate 5, fig. 48).

STAGE 5

Approximately 0.1–0.2 mm
Approximately 7–12 postovulatory days
Characteristic features: implanted but previllous; solid trophoblast in 5a;
    trophoblastic lacunae, cytotrophoblastic clumps, and primary
    umbilical vesicle in 5b; lacunar vascular circle and some mesoblastic
    crests in cytotrophoblastic clumps in 5c

Stage 5 comprises embryos that are implanted to a varying degree but are previllous, i.e., that do not yet show definite chorionic villi. Such embryos are believed to be 7–12 days old. The chorion varies from about 0.3 to 1 mm, and the embryonic disc measures approximately 0.1–0.2 mm in diameter. The significant dimensions of Carnegie specimens of stage 5 are listed in Table 5-1. The external and internal diameters of the chorion are listed as "chorion" and "chorionic cavity," respectively. Additional features of stage 5 include the definite appearance of the amniotic cavity and the formation of extra-embryonic mesoblast. The appearances at stages 2 to 5 are shown in figure 5-1.

Implantation, which began in stage 4, is the characteristic feature of stage 5. It should be appreciated that both maternal and embryonic tissues are involved in the complex process of implantation: "in the normal process they are mutually supporting and neither can be regarded as chiefly responsible" (Boyd and Hamilton, 1970). An indication of a decidual reaction appears during stage 5 and, from this time onward, the term "decidua" (used by William Hunter) is commonly employed. The decidua, at least in the human, "is a tissue made up of endometrial connective tissue cells which have enlarged and become rounded or polyhedral due to the accumulation of glycogen or lipoids within their cytoplasm, and which occur either in pregnancy, pseudo-pregnancy or in artificially or pathologically stimulated deciduomata" (Mossman, 1937).

Successful implantation may depend on the ability of the embryo to produce an immunosuppressive factor (or factors) having a direct suppressive effect on the maternal immune response (Daya and Clark, 1986). Failure of implantation may result from rejection of the antigenic embryo by the maternal immune system.

Heuser's technique of opening the uterus laterally and searching for a young conceptus has been de-scribed on several occasions (e.g., by Heard, 1957, and by Hertig and Rock, 1973).

No correlation has been found between the side of the uterus on which the conceptus becomes implanted and the ovary from which the oocyte originated. Normal specimens, however, are more commonly found implanted on the posterior wall of the uterus, abnormal ones on the anterior wall (Hertig and Rock, 1949). Both walls are considered to be antimesometrial in comparison with a bicornuate uterus. Furthermore, "it is interesting to note that cases are known of a double discoid placenta in man very similar to that of the monkey. It seems entirely possible that in some cases the human blastocyst may attach both dorsally and ventrally and therefore fail to undergo complete interstitial implantation" (Mossman, 1937).

The trophoblast from stages 4 and 5 onward comprises two chief varieties, namely, cytotrophoblast and syncytiotrophoblast. That the latter is derived from the former had long been suspected and has been shown by organ culture and also indicated by electron microscopy (Enders, 1965).

An amniotic cavity is found by stage 5. If duplication of the embryo occurs after the differentiation of the amnion, the resulting monozygotic twins should be monochorial and monoamniotic (fig. 5-2). It has been estimated that the frequency of monoamniotic twins among monozygotic twins is about 4 percent (Bulmer, 1970). About once in every 400 monozygotic twin pregnancies, the duplication is incomplete and conjoined ("Siamese") twins (e.g., the second specimen of Shaw, 1932) result.

The following description of stage 5 is based largely on the work of Hertig and Rock, in whose publications (1941, 1945a, 1949) much additional information (including descriptions of the ovaries, uterine tubes, and uterus) can be found. Based on the condition of the

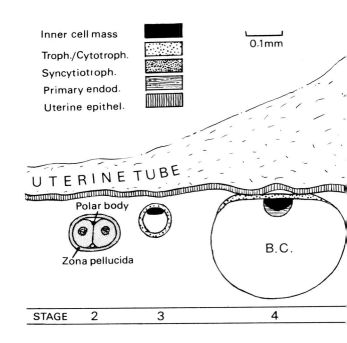

TABLE 5-1.   Significant Dimensions (in mm) of Carnegie Specimens of Stage 5

Stage	5a	5a	5a	5b	5b	5b	5b	5c	5c	5c	5c	5c
Serial No.	8225	8020	8155	8215	8171	8004	9350	7699	7950	7700	8558	8330
Age in days	7	7	8	9	9	9	9	11	12	12	12	12
Chorion	0.33 × 0.306 × 0.12	0.45 × 0.30 × 0.125	0.306 × 0.210 × 0.15	0.525 × 0.498 × 0.207	0.422 × 0.404 × 0.256	0.582 × 0.45 × 0.31	0.599 × 0.58 × 0.36	1.026 × 0.713 × 0.515	0.75 × 0.45	0.948 × 0.835 × 0.54	0.96 × 0.52	0.85 × 0.65
Chorionic cavity	0.228 × 0.20 × 0.03	0.288 × 0.186 × 0.044	0.168 × 0.082 × 0.066	0.228 × 0.21 × 0.10	0.164 × 0.138 × 0.08	0.312 × 0.185 × 0.12	0.3 × 0.1 × 0.1	0.48 × 0.336 × 0.276	0.40 × 0.26	0.55 × 0.498 × 0.425	0.58 × 0.36	0.46 × 0.40
Trophoblast	0.006– 0.086	0.003– 0.09	0.003– 0.08	0.013– 0.16	0.04– 0.13	0.035– 0.175		0.064– 0.153	0.04– 0.15	0.0125– 0.185	0.02– 0.28	0.10– 0.24
Embryonic disc	0.09 × 0.078 × 0.036	0.126 × 0.092 × 0.044	0.09 × 0.05 × 0.03	0.084 × 0.052 × 0.05	0.114 × 0.088 × 0.046	0.132 × 0.10 × 0.046	0.132 × 0.09 × 0.05	0.138 × 0.138 × 0.089	0.16 × 0.07	0.204 × 0.165 × 0.045	0.22 × 0.08	0.216 × 0.063
Amniotic cavity	0.06 × 0.054 × 0.006	0.025 × 0.024 × 0.003	0.048 × 0.032 × 0.02	0.05 × 0.048 × 0.022	0.04 × 0.036 × 0.024	0.078 × 0.066 × 0.012		0.108 × 0.099 × 0.024	0.02 × 0.014	0.174 × 0.14 × 0.0125	0.216 × 0.036	0.16 × 0.05
Primary umbilical vesicle				0.08 × 0.023	0.043 × 0.06	absent		0.246 × 0.168 × 0.124	0.33 × 0.19	0.474 × 0.41 × 0.29	0.49 × 0.30	0.35 × 0.31
Reference	Hertig and Rock (1945b)	Hertig and Rock (1945a)	Hertig and Rock (1949)	Hertig and Rock (1945c)	Hertig and Rock (1949)	Hertig and Rock (1945a)	Heuser (1956)	Hertig and Rock (1941)	Hertig, Rock, and Adams (1956)	Hertig and Rock (1941)	Hertig, Rock, and Adams (1956)	Hertig, Rock, and Adams (1956)

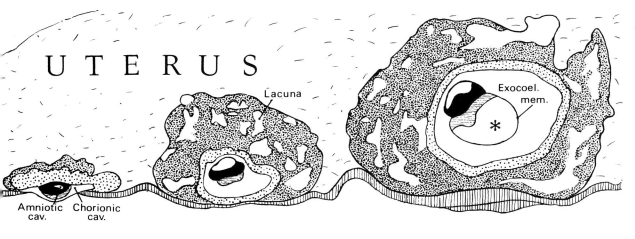

Fig. 5-1. Drawings of the embryo from stage 2 to stage 5c to show implantation. The drawings, which are all at the same scale of magnification, are based on human specimens, with the exception of stage 4, for which a macaque blastocyst was used. *B.C.*, blastocystic cavity. Asterisk, primary umbilical vesicle.

trophoblast and its vascular relationships, stage 5 is subdivided into three groups: 5a, 5b, and 5c (Hertig, Rock, and Adams, 1956).

Although a brief description of the trophoblast at each stage is provided in this account, the main emphasis is devoted to the embryo itself. This is justifiable inasmuch as comprehensive books on the human trophoblast (Hertig, 1968) and the human placenta (Boyd and Hamilton, 1970; Ramsey, 1975; Ramsey and Donner, 1980) have been published.

STAGE 5a

The characteristic feature of subdivision 5a is that the trophoblast is still solid, in the sense that definitive lacunae are not yet evident. Specimens of this stage are believed to be 7–8 days old. The chorion is less than 0.5 mm in its greatest diameter, and the embryonic disc is approximately 0.1 mm in diameter. Because of the collapse of the conceptus during implantation, the blastocystic cavity is flattened.

The rarity of specimens of stage 5a has been attributed to the circumstance that they are "impossible to discern in the fresh, and probably often unrecognizable even after fixation" (Hertig, 1968).

Endometrium. The endometrial stroma is edematous (fig. 5-4). Two specimens (Nos. 8020 and 8225)

show early, superficial implantation. The conceptus has eroded the surface epithelium of the uterus and has barely penetrated the underlying stroma (fig. 5-5). Apparently an attempt has been made by the maternal epithelium to repair the defect, and occasional mitotic figures are found. A portion of the conceptus, however, is still exposed to the uterine cavity. A third specimen (No. 8155) shows later, interstitial implantation. The conceptus is almost embedded within the endometrium, so that its abembryonic pole, which is barely exposed, is nearly flush with the epithelial lining of the uterine cavity (fig. 5-6).

Trophoblast. The trophoblast may encroach on the surrounding endometrial glands. At the abembryonic

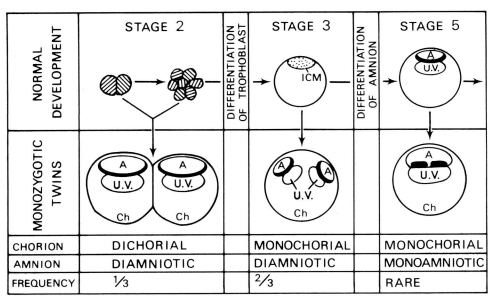

Fig. 5-2. Diagram to illustrate the presumed mode of development of monozygotic twins in the human. Based partly on Corner (1955). There exist "three critical stages at which the division of the embryo to form monozygotic twins may occur" (Bulmer, 1970). At stage 2, before the differentiation of the trophoblast, separation of the blastomeres would result in twins with separate choria and amnia. At stage 3 (and presumably at stage 4), before differentiation of the amnion, duplication of the inner cell mass would result in twins with a common chorion but separate amnia. At stage 5, duplication of the embryonic disc would result in twins with a common chorion and amnion. Deceptive fusion of the membranes may occur subsequently in certain instances but "the placenta and membranes, if subjected to skilled examination, including microscopic study of the chorionamniotic walls when necessary, will generally yield a correct impression of the type of twinning" (Corner, 1955; see also Allen and Turner, 1971). Partial instead of complete embryonic separation would result in conjoined twins of the various types classified by Wilder (1904).

pole, the wall of the conceptus is merely a thin layer of cells that resembles mesothelium. Because this region is not in contact with maternal tissue, it probably presents the structure of the wall of the blastocyst as it was at the time of implantation. Because of the collapse of the blastocyst during implantation, the mesothelioid layer is closely applied to the ventral surface of the embryonic disc (fig. 5-5).

As the mesothelioid layer is traced laterally, it becomes continuous first with indifferent trophoblastic cells, which, at the embryonic pole, become differentiated into cytotrophoblast and syncytiotrophoblast. Definitive trophoblast is found only in the area of endometrial contact, presumably under the influence of an endometrial factor. A ventrodorsal gradient of trophoblastic differentiation is noticeable. In other words, the most highly developed trophoblast tends to be found deeply (i.e., away from the uterine cavity).

The cytotrophoblast is located nearer the embryonic disc. The cells are large and polyhedral, and show distinct cell boundaries. Mitotic figures are moderately frequent.

The syncytiotrophoblast is described by Hertig (1968) as "invasive, ingestive, and digestive." It presents a dark, homogeneous cytoplasm, and large, densely stained nuclei. No mitotic figures are seen. Near the maternal tissue, the syncytiotrophoblastic mass displays numerous small nuclei, which appear to be formed amitotically, although some may perhaps be derived from the endometrial stroma. The syncytial masses project into, and frequently partly surround ("eat their way into"), the uterine stroma, giving the surface of the trophoblast a lobulated appearance. In only rare instances are vacuoles found in the syncytiotrophoblast, and they contain no maternal blood (No. 8020). Macroscopically, no congestion or hemorrhage is vis-

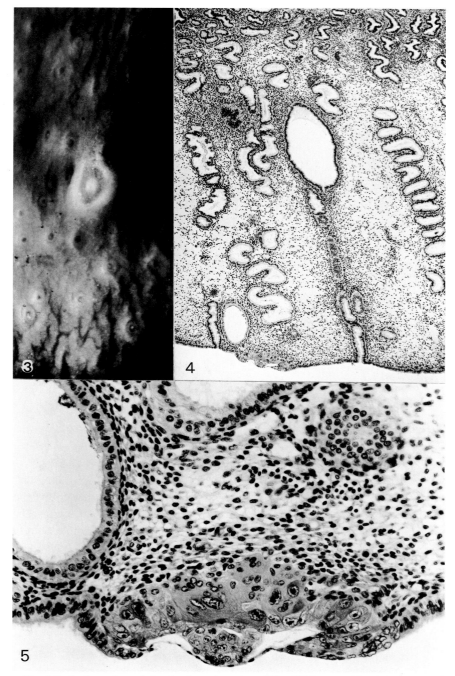

Fig. 5-3. Surface view of the implantation site of No. 8020, stage 5a, photographed under liquid. The dark ring indicates the chorionic cavity. The opaque area within the ring represents the embryonic mass, that outside the ring represents the trophoblast. The mouths of the endometrial glands appear as dark spots.

Fig. 5-4. General view of the tissues at and near the implantation site (No. 8020, stage 5a). The endometrium is edematous. Section 6-5-9.

Fig. 5-5. Section through the middle of No. 8020, stage 5a. The amniotic cavity and the bilaminar embryonic disc can be seen. The transition from the thin abembryonic trophoblast to the thick, solid layer at the embryonic pole is evident. Large multinucleated masses of syncytiotrophoblast project into the endometrial stroma. A dilated endometrial gland is cut through at the left-hand side of the photomicrograph. Section 6-5-9.

ible in the endometrium. Microscopically, the capillary plexus and sinusoids are moderately dilated but contain very few blood cells. It seems that the endometrium itself is adequate for the nourishment of the conceptus at this stage.

It has been found (in Nos. 8020 and 8225) that "the course of several capillaries can be followed through the syncytiotrophoblast. The endothelial walls of the capillaries are intact to the point where each vessel enters and leaves the trophoblast, but between these points red blood cells can be seen to occupy a series of irregularly shaped spaces, which are in continuity with one another" (Harris and Ramsey, 1966). These spaces, however, "are unlike the well-rounded vacuoles occasionally observed in syncytiotrophoblast," and they are "much smaller than the definitive lacunae" present within a couple of days. It is assumed that "the syncytium advances by a flowing movement that engulfs the blood vessels" in the capillary plexus of the adjacent stratum compactum (*ibid.*). Isolated endothelial cells in the lacunae may lend support to the supposition that capillaries have been engulfed (Dr. Ramsey, personal communication, 1972). In other words, the future lacunae, which are usually in continuity with maternal vessels (No. 8020), "are interpreted to be derived from engulfed maternal vessels" (Böving, 1981).

Trophoblast and endometrium (in No. 8020) are intimately related, and no cellular boundaries can be seen by light microscopy. It is probable that uterine epithelial cells have been phagocytized prior to autolysis, although it is possible that they are fused with the trophoblast (Enders, 1976). Indeed, it has been claimed that the appearances seen in the rabbit (fusion of a uterine "symplasma" with the syncytiotrophoblast) may apply also to No. 8020 in the human (Larsen, 1970). Implantation in the rhesus monkey has been studied by electron microscopy, including the spreading of trophoblast along the basal lamina of the uterine epithelium, the breaching of the basal lamina, and cytotrophoblastic proliferation (Enders, Hendrickx, and Schlafke, 1983).

Extra-embryonic mesoblast. The term mesoblast is preferred by Hertig and Rock (1941) to mesenchyme ("rather nonspecific"), primitive mesoderm ("one might unintentionally imply some connection with the embryonic mesoderm"), or magma reticulare (which "refers to the more mature characteristics of this tissue").

The magma has also been considered as merely a "degenerative remnant of primary yolk sac endoderm" (Luckett, 1978).

The formation of mesoblast begins in stage 5a. The theory that the extra-embryonic mesoblast develops *in situ* by "delamination" (i.e., without cellular migration) from the cytotrophoblast (Hertig and Rock, 1945a and 1949) remained current for many years, although other possible sources (embryonic disc, amniotic ectoderm, and endoderm) were also considered.

In his study of the Miller (5c) specimen, Streeter (1926) concluded that the primary mesoblast "must have either separated off from the inner cell mass during the formation of the segmentation cavity or have been derived from the trophoblast. Since it is, in reality, so largely concerned in the differentiation of the trophoblastic structures, the latter is the more probable explanation." From his investigations of the same specimen and more particularly of macaque embryos, Hertig (1935) believed in the "simultaneous origin of angioblasts and primary mesoderm by a process of delamination of differentiation from the chorionic trophoblast...."

According to the alternative view, namely that extra-embryonic mesoblast is not of trophoblastic origin, the trophoblast is considered to give rise to additional trophoblast only: i.e., cytotrophoblast, syncytiotrophoblast, and trophoblastic giant cells (Luckett, 1978).

Hill's (1932) studies of the primate embryo led him to believe in "the existence in early embryos of the Pithecoid and man of a mesodermal proliferating area involving the postero-median margin of the shield-ectoderm and the immediately adjoining portion of the amniotic ectoderm which contributes to, if it does not entirely form, the connecting stalk primordium. This proliferating area, it may be suggested, functionally replaces, if it does not actually represent, the hinder end of the primitive streak of the Tarsioid and the Lemuroid...." In pursuance of this idea, Florian (1933) concluded that, in the Werner (5c) embryo, an "area of fusion of the ectoderm of the caudal part of the embryonic shield with the primary mesoderm" was a site where "at least a part of the primary mesoderm originates."

This theory of Hill and Florian has been supported by Luckett (1978), who believes that "the caudal margin of the epiblast is a precociously differentiated pri-

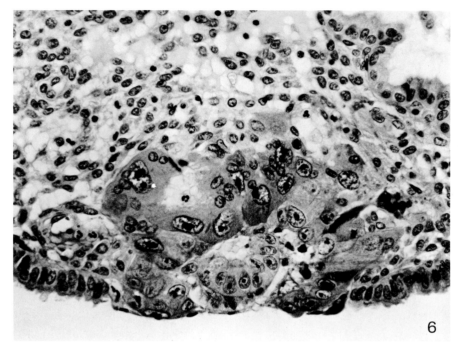

Fig. 5-6. Section approximately through the middle of No. 8155, stage 5a. The amniotic cavity ("tropho-epiblastic cavity?") and the bilaminar embryonic disc can be seen, although an amnion as such is not yet distinct. The thick, solid trophoblast at the embryonic pole is mainly syncytiotrophoblast. The endometrial stroma is edematous. Section 4-4-8.

mitive streak, which gives rise to the extraembryonic mesoderm of the chorion, chorionic villi, and body stalk." The term caudal mesoblast–proliferating area will be retained here and, as in previous studies, identification of the primitive streak will await stage 6b, an interpretation that has long met with general agreement.

Amnion. The cells of the inner cell mass that are adjacent to the mural trophoblast at stage 4 may already be those of the amniotic ectoderm. In stage 5a, the small space that appears within the inner cell mass, or in some instances seemingly between the mass and the trophoblast, represents the beginning of the amniotic cavity. Either the amnion itself or the amniotic cavity may be noticeable first.

In one instance (No. 8225), a single layer of flattened cells is found attached to the trophoblast although the amniotic cavity is scarcely present. In another case (No. 8155), by contrast, a prominent amniotic cavity (formed by the curved epiblast) is present although amniogenesis has not yet begun (fig. 5-6). In a third specimen (No. 8020), a small cavity is visible and amniogenesis is under way (fig. 5-5). The amniogenic cells, which

are believed by Hertig and Rock (1945a) to be delaminating from the trophoblast dorsal to the embryonic disc, appear to be in the process of enclosing the amniotic cavity by fusing with the margin of the germ disc. In summary, the roof and lateral walls of the amniotic cavity are, in Hertig's (1968) view, derived from the cytotrophoblast, and the cells are mesoblastic. The floor, however, is constituted by the epiblast.

In general terms, "two distinct methods of amnion formation are ordinarily considered: formation by folding and formation by cavitation, the latter being considered the more specialized" (Mossman, 1937). Both methods have been invoked by Luckett (1975), who, in an interpretation quite different from that of Hertig and Rock, has proposed that a primordial amniotic cavity appears within the embryonic mass (e.g., No. 8020), followed by opening of the roof to form a temporary tropho-epiblastic cavity (e.g., No. 8155). In stage 5b, it is maintained that the definitive amniotic cavity is formed by "upfolding of the margins of the epiblast" (e.g., No. 8215).

In a recent electron-microscopic study of the rhesus monkey (Enders, Schlafke, and Hendrickx, 1986) it was concluded that the amniotic cavity appears as a result of a rearrangement of epiblastic cells (a "change in cell association occurring within epiblast") whereby they are separated into amniotic ectoderm and epiblast proper.

The chief function of the amnion is not mechanical protection but rather the enclosing of "the embryonic body in a quantity of liquid sufficient to buoy it up and so allow it to develop symmetrically and freely in all directions" (Mossman, 1937).

Embryonic disc. The term "germ disc" was formerly employed for "the epithelial plate that is derived directly and exclusively from the blastomeric formative cells" (Heuser and Streeter, 1941). The plate may more conveniently be referred to as the epiblast. When the underlying primary endoderm is also included, the term "embryonic disc" (formerly "embryonic shield") is used.

The embryonic disc (figs. 5-5 and 5-6) is bilaminar, composed of the epiblast and the primary endoderm. It is concavoconvex from dorsal to ventral.

The epiblast consists of variably sized, polyhedral cells which either show no precise pattern of arrangement (No. 8020) or are in the form of a pseudostratified columnar epithelium (No. 8155). One or more mitotic figures may be encountered.

The primary endoderm consists of a cap of small, darkly staining, vesiculated cells without any specific arrangement. Mitotic figures are not noticeable.

SPECIMENS OF STAGE 5a ALREADY DESCRIBED

Carnegie No. 8225. Described briefly by Hertig and Rock (1945b). Hysterectomy (bicornuate uterus). Anterior wall of uterus. Chorion, 0.33 × 0.306 mm. Chorionic cavity, 0.228 × 0.2 mm. Embryonic disc, 0.09 × 0.078 mm. Perhaps more advanced than No. 8020 (Mazanec, 1959; Harris and Ramsey, 1966), but has also been interpreted as less advanced (Hertig, Rock, and Adams, 1956). Photomicrograph in Hertig, Rock, and Adams (1956, fig. 9). Presumed age, 7 days.

Carnegie No. 8020 (figs. 5-3 to 5-5). Described by Hertig and Rock (1945a). Hysterectomy. Posterior wall of uterus. Chorion, 0.45 × 0.3 mm. Chorionic cavity, 0.288 × 0.186 mm. Embryonic disc, 0.126 × 0.092 mm. New model of blood vessels at implantation site has been prepared (Harris and Ramsey, 1966). Presumed age, 7 days.

Fruhling, Ginglinger, and Gandar (1954) described briefly a specimen of about 8 days. Curettage. Early implantation. Few trophoblastic digitations. Beginning amniotic cavity. Most sections through embryonic disc lost.

Carnegie No. 8155 (fig. 14). Described by Hertig and Rock (1949). Hysterectomy. Anterior wall of uterus. Chorion, 0.306 × 0.210 mm. Chorionic cavity, 0.168 × 0.082 mm. Embryonic disc, 0.09 × 0.05 mm. "Tropho-epiblastic cavity" (Luckett, 1975).

STAGE 5b

Subdivision 5b is characterized by the appearance of definitive lacunae in the trophoblast (fig. 5-9). The lacunae communicate with endometrial vessels, and "this joining of maternal vessels to trophoblast is the essence of the uteroplacental circulation of the so-called hemochorial type" (Hertig, 1968). It will be recalled that "the normal mammalian placenta is defined as an apposition or fusion of the fetal membranes to the uterine mucosa for physiological exchange" (Mossman, 1937).

Amniogenesis is well under way, and the primary umbilical vesicle is developed to a variable degree. Cytotrophoblastic clumps begin to project into the syncytiotrophoblast. The chorion attains approximately 0.6 mm in its greatest diameter and hence is readily visible to the naked eye. The space outlined by the internal surface of the chorion is slightly flattened but is un-

dergoing distension. The embryo is about 9 days old, and the embryonic disc is approximately 0.1 mm in diameter.

Endometrium. The endometrial stroma shows an early decidual (commonly called "predecidual") reaction. The conceptus is imperfectly covered by the uterine epithelium. In one specimen (No. 8171), "moderate numbers of leucocytes in the predecidual stroma immediately surrounding" the specimen were noted (Hertig and Rock, 1949). These cells, because of their absence elsewhere, were interpreted as a physiological response to the conceptus. They were "mainly lymphocytes, with lesser numbers of macrophages and polymorphonuclear neutrophils."

According to Krafka (1941), "the decidual reaction is generally defined as the appearance of certain large, clear, epithelioid, vesiculated cells, 40 to 50 μm in di-

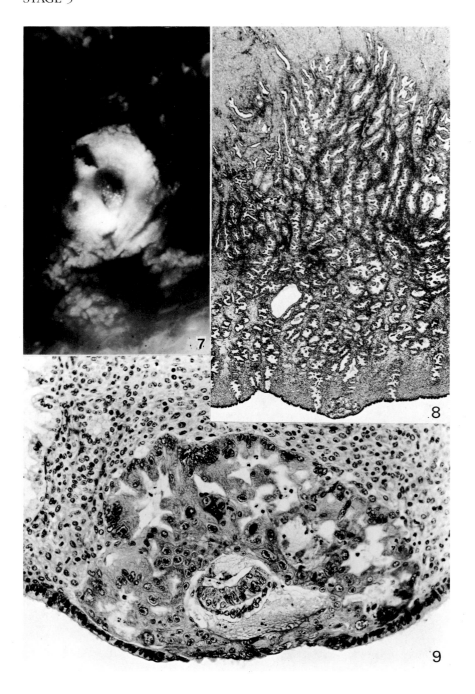

Fig. 5-7. Surface view of the implantation site of No. 8004, stage 5b, photographed under liquid. The dark area in the middle represents the abembryonic wall of the specimen.

Fig. 5-8. General view of the tissues at and near the implantation site (No. 8004, stage 5b). The endometrium is "predecidual." Section 11-4-4.

Fig. 5-9. Section through the middle of No. 8004, stage 5b. Some epithelial regeneration of the endometrium has taken place over the specimen. The large mass of syncytiotrophoblast shows intercommunicating lacunae. The chorionic cavity is surrounded by a thin layer of cytotrophoblast. The amniotic cavity and the bilaminar embryonic disc can be seen. Section 11-4-5.

ameter, ovoid or polyhedral in form, tightly compressed against one another (owing to imbibition of edema fluid or to storage of glycogen), having a conceded origin from the typical fusiform stroma cells primarily in the compacta." The cells are not peculiar to the uterus (they may be found at tubal or ovarian implantation sites, for example), and hence the term "stroma" (better, "stromal") reaction is preferred by Krafka.

Trophoblast. Although much of the trophoblast at the embryonic pole and at the equator is of the syncytial variety, an irregular inner rim of cytotrophoblast is present. In places, this rim has begun to form small, discrete masses (cytotrophoblastic clumps), which project into the syncytiotrophoblast and may be regarded as an indication of the future chorionic villi (fig. 6-3).

Various phases in the formation of lacunae within the syncytiotrophoblast are found (fig. 5-9). Most of these spaces have coalesced and, at several points, are in continuity with the dilated endometrial sinusoids. Few blood cells are seen in either the lacunae or the adjacent sinusoids, however, so that a uteroplacental circulation has scarcely been established. Rather, an ooze into the chorion occurs until chorionic villi appear at a later stage.

The origin of the lacunae has been investigated in the rabbit with the aid of electron microscopy. The study revealed "numerous vesicles in the cytoplasm of the syncytial trophoblast. These are the forerunners of larger cavities, approximately 30–40 µm in diameter," which "by their confluence are later transformed into the lacunae of the definitive placenta" (Larsen, 1970). When the trophoblast penetrates the maternal vessels, the lacunae gain access to maternal blood (*ibid.*). According to Harris and Ramsey (1966), however, "during the initial stages of implantation in the human it appears that the syncytiotrophoblast engulfs the capillary plexus in the adjacent *stratum compactum*. It is suggested that part of the plexus remains within the trophoblastic plate as a series of small spaces, which maintain continuity with the maternal circulation and subsequently enlarge to form the lacunae."

Extra-embryonic mesoblast. The mesoblast continues to develop.

Chorion. The term chorion is commonly used "for the outer fetal membrane made up of trophoblast and

somatic mesoderm" (Mossman, 1937), whether it be avascular (e.g., the "true chorion" of the pig) or vascular (e.g., the allanto-chorion of the human).

The mesoblastic lining of the trophoblast spreads during stages 5–7, and the combination of the two layers may now be termed chorion (Hamilton and Boyd, 1950). In stages 5b and 5c, however, the extent of the mesoblast is very slight, much or most of the extra-embryonic tissue is thought to be endoderm rather than mesoblast, and the chorionic cavity does not acquire a complete mesothelial lining until stage 6 or stage 7 (Luckett, 1978).

Amnion. The amniotic cavity, which is smaller than the umbilical vesicle, is almost closed by the amniogenic cells.

Embryonic disc. The bilaminar embryonic disc (fig. 5-9) resembles that seen at stage 5a.

The epiblast is a pseudostratified columnar epithelium in which the cytoplasm is beginning to become vacuolated ventrally.

The primary endoderm consists of either a single layer or a cap of cuboidal or polyhedral cells.

Umbilical vesicle. The primary umbilical vesicle is first seen in stage 5b and becomes limited by a layer that was formerly termed the exocoelomic membrane. This membrane is attached at the margin of the embryonic disc. The vesicle enclosed by the disc and the membrane "was first described and figured by Stieve (1931, 1936) in the Werner [5c] embryo" and, according to Davies (1944), he referred to this primary umbilical vesicle as the *Dottersackanlage*, although he made it clear that it is not the definitive umbilical vesicle as usually described.

The so-called exocoelomic membrane was described in the macaque as an "intrachorionic mesothelial membrane" that "must be regarded as a part of the primitive mesoblast" (Heuser, 1932a). In a later publication, however, the wall of the primary umbilical vesicle of the macaque was stated either to be derived from endodermal cells "which spread to line the chorion," or to "arise by delamination from the trophoblast" (Heuser and Streeter, 1941). Elsewhere in the same article, the exocoelomic membrane is said to be derived either by delamination from the endoderm (misprinted as "endothelium") or "by creeping in from the sides as a spreading membrane" of mesoblast.

In the human, the membrane and the embryonic

disc together enclose the primary umbilical vesicle. The suggested origin of the membrane *in situ* by delamination from the adjacent cytotrophoblast (Hertig and Rock, 1945a, 1949) and a similar mode of origin for scattered mesoblastic cells between the trophoblast and the membrane (Hertig and Rock, 1949) have been disputed. It has been reported that the primary umbilical vesicle "develops by the peripheral spread of extraembryonic endoderm," which forms an epithelial meshwork within the blastocystic cavity (Luckett, 1978). Thus the so-called exocoelomic membrane is considered to be merely the wall of the primary umbilical vesicle, and the surrounding meshwork is thought to be extra-embryonic endoderm rather than mesoblast.

SPECIMENS OF STAGE 5b ALREADY DESCRIBED

Carnegie No. 8171. Described by Hertig and Rock (1949). Hysterectomy. Posterior wall of uterus. Abnormal leucocytic infiltration of endometrium. Chorion, 0.422 × 0.404 mm.

Chorionic cavity, 0.164 × 0.138 mm. Embryonic disc, 0.114 × 0.088 mm. A cellular remnant within the umbilical vesicle, because it is probably derived from the endoderm, "may, in a sense, be regarded as an abnormal form of twin embryo" (*ibid.*). Presumed age, 9 days.

Carnegie No. 8215. Described briefly by Hertig and Rock (1945c). Hysterectomy. Posterior wall of uterus. Chorion, 0.525 × 0.498 mm. Chorionic cavity, 0.228 × 0.21 mm. Embryonic disc, 0.084 × 0.052 mm. Lacunae perhaps further developed than in No. 8171 (Mazanec, 1959), but specimen has been "considered to be slightly younger . . . because the decidual reaction is not yet apparent" (Hertig, Rock, and Adams, 1956). Photomicrographs in Hertig, Rock, and Adams (1956, figs. 15 and 17). Presumed age, 9 days.

Carnegie No. 8004 (figs. 5-7 to 5-9). Described by Hertig and Rock (1945a). Hysterectomy. Posterior wall of uterus. Chorion, 0.582 × 0.45 mm. Chorionic cavity, 0.312 × 0.185 mm. Embryonic disc, 0.132 × 0.1 mm.

Carnegie No. 9350. Described briefly by Heuser (1956). Hysterectomy. At junction of posterior and anterior walls. Chorion, 0.59 × 0.58 mm. Chorionic cavity, 0.3 × 0.1 mm. Embryonic disc, 0.132 × 0.09 mm. Presumed age, 9 days.

STAGE 5c

Stage 5c is characterized by the intercommunication of the trophoblastic lacunae. The contained blood is sufficient to appear as a discontinuous red ring, so that identification of the conceptus is possible on careful gross examination of the endometrial surface prior to fixation (fig. 5-12). Embryos of stage 5c are believed to be 11–12 days old, the chorion measures about 0.75 to 1 mm in its greatest diameter, and the embryonic disc is approximately 0.15–0.2 mm in diameter. Some cytotrophoblastic clumps are beginning to acquire mesoblastic crests. The space outlined by the internal surface of the chorion now appears distended again.

In their proposals to subdivide horizon V, Hertig, Rock, and Adams (1956) distinguished 5b, "formation of trophoblastic lacunae with amniotic and exocoelomic cavities," from 5c, "intercommunicating lacunae with beginning utero-lacunar circulation." In 5b, "although the vast majority of the lacunar spaces have coalesced they contain relatively little maternal blood, and that mostly plasma, since few adjacent capillary sinusoids of the endometrial stroma communicate directly with the lacunar network as yet." In 5c, "the lacunar spaces now intercommunicate and contain enough maternal blood" to enable specimens at this stage to be "easily identified on careful gross examination of the endometrial surface prior to fixation. Such lacunar blood appears as a discontinuous red circle about 1 mm in diameter" (fig. 5-12).

Because the quantitative changes between 5b and 5c may prove difficult to discern, and because a given specimen may not have been examined grossly prior to fixation, it was at first considered that the two substages should be combined here into one for reasons of practicality. Nevertheless, in order to avoid complicating further an already established system, and in order to continue the subdivision of an otherwise large and prolonged (4-day) group of embryos, it was decided to retain 5b and 5c. It is hoped that, perhaps by comparing the measurements and the appearances of given specimens in section with the photomicrographs of embryos already staged, it may be possible to assign new examples to their appropriate places. If not, they could be classified as merely stage 5.

The availability of human specimens, after reaching its lowest point at stage 4, increases greatly with the advent of stage 5c, and from now onward the account will be confined almost entirely to the human.

Endometrium. The endometrial stroma around the

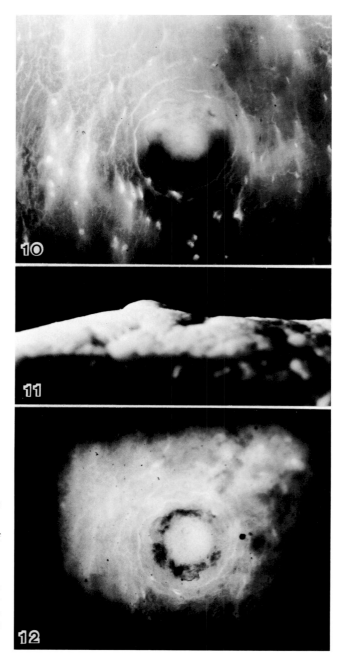

Fig. 5-10. Surface view of the implantation site of No. 7700, stage 5c.

Fig. 5-11. Side view of the implantation site of No. 7700, stage 5c.

Fig. 5-12. View of the implantation site of No. 7700, stage 5c, as seen in the cleared celloidin block. The irregular, dark ring is caused by maternal blood within the trophoblastic lacunae, and is a characteristic feature of subdivision 5c, as it has been defined by Hertig, Rock, and Adams (1956).

conceptus again shows an early decidual ("predecidual") reaction, and indeed decidua may be said to be present. The uterine epithelium continues its repair of the defect and, within the defect, a fibrinous, leucocytic, hemorrhagic coagulum may be present. Moreover, a "constant attempt on the part of maternal tissues to heal the endometrium persists until . . . the conceptus is of six weeks' developmental age" (Hertig, 1968).

The operculum, or closing plate, according to Krafka (1941), "is generally described as a simple organizing clot, including fibrin, fibrinoid, living and necrotic leucocytes, old and recent hemorrhage, and degenerating stroma." That it is something more than a simple organizing clot, however, is indicated by the circumstance that "both the aperture and the operculum increase in size" (*ibid.*). The nomenclature of this region (which includes *Verschlusspfropf, Schlusscoagulum*, and *Gewebspilz*) has been clarified by Hamilton and Gladstone (1942), who defined the operculum deciduae (of Teacher, 1925) as the flattened or dome-shaped head of the fungus- or mushroom-shaped structure, and the occlusion- or closing-plug as the part occupying and closing the aperture of entry.

Chorion. The cytotrophoblast, although it varies in thickness, is generally formed by a single layer of cuboidal cells. Masses of proliferating cytotrophoblast project into the syncytiotrophoblast. These cytotrophoblastic clumps (Davies, 1944), seen already at stage 5b, may be regarded as an indication of the future chorionic villi (fig. 6-3). In a few instances (in No. 7700) the beginning of a mesoblastic and angioblastic core has been detected. Such appearances may conveniently be termed mesoblastic crests (Krafka, 1941).

The syncytiotrophoblast forms about three-fourths of the total trophoblastic shell. It contains large, irregular, intercommunicating lacunae lined by a brush border and containing an increasing amount of maternal blood. The filling of the lacunae may result in a brilliant red circle (fig. 5-12), which enables the implantation site to be identified before fixation (Hertig, 1968). The presence of the lacunae gives the syncytiotrophoblast a spongy structure, and the lacunar system is primarily labyrinthine (Hamilton and Boyd, 1960). The implantation area presents intercommunicating capillaries, which, by several relatively large branches, communicate directly with the lacunae within the trophoblast. Also within the syncytiotrophoblast are found what appear to be phagocytosed maternal blood cells and possibly other tissues.

According to Park (1957), sex chromatin is absent up to 12 days, that is, during the first five stages. In one (abnormal) specimen (No. 8000) of 5c, an incidence of less than one percent was found in the trophoblast.

Extra-embryonic mesoblast. In addition to the continuing formation of mesoblast, angiogenesis is beginning at the abembryonic pole.

Amnion. The amniotic cavity seems to be nearly completely closed (fig. 5-14), although (in No. 7700) the appearances suggested to Hertig (1968, fig. 70) that amniogenic cells are still "being added to by the adjacent trophoblast." The amniotic cavity is still smaller than the umbilical vesicle.

Embryonic disc. The bilaminar embryonic disc (fig. 5-14) resembles that seen at stage 5b. It is either basically circular on dorsal view, so that a longitudinal axis is not yet evident (No. 7699), or it is pyriform or ovoid, so that an apparent axis may be more or less envisioned (No. 7700 and No. 8139). It is possible also that a condensation of extra-embryonic mesoblast may serve to indicate the caudal end of the disc (Hertig, Rock, and Adams, 1956, fig. 38).

The epiblast is a pseudostratified columnar epithelium in which vacuoles are seen, mostly ventrally. Some mitotic figures may be observed.

The primary endoderm is sharply demarcated peripherally from the adjoining cells of the "exocoelomic membrane." Mitotic figures, if found at all, are rare.

Umbilical vesicle. The so-called exocoelomic membrane (fig. 5-13), which was first figured by Stieve (1931) in the Werner embryo, is clearly formed, although it may be deficient in places.

Prechordal plate. It has been claimed that (chiefly in No. 8330) a thickening of the endoderm at the rostral end of the embryonic disc is the prechordal plate and is "the first clear evidence of a craniocaudal embryonic axis" (Luckett, 1978, fig. 19). The histological quality, however, does not permit definitive identification at this early stage.

SPECIMENS OF STAGE 5C ALREADY DESCRIBED

Davies-Harding. Described by Davies (1944). Hysterectomy. Anterior wall of uterus. Incomplete (almost one-half of embryonic disc missing). "No true villi." Primary umbilical vesicle present. Extensive extra-embryonic meshwork. Slightly later stage of development than No. 8004 (Davies, 1944, Addendum), which belongs to 5b. "Possibly pathological" (Boyd and Hamilton, 1970). Chorion, 1.18 × 0.55 mm. Chorionic cavity, 0.409 × 0.238 mm. Embryonic disc, 0.117 mm. May be regarded as transitional between 5b and 5c. Presumed age, 9–10 days.

Carnegie No. 7699. Described by Hertig and Rock (1941). Hysterectomy. Posterior wall of uterus. Chorion, 1.026 × 0.713 mm. Chorionic cavity, 0.48 × 0.336 mm. Embryonic disc, 0.138 × 0.138 mm. New model of blood vessels at implantation site has been prepared (Harris and Ramsey, 1966). Presumed age, 11 days.

Carnegie No. 4900, Miller. Described by Streeter (1926). Curettage. Angiogenesis described by Hertig (1935). Incomplete (some sections missing). Primary umbilical vesicle present. New graphic reconstruction made by Streeter (1939a,b). Chorion, 0.9 mm. Chorionic cavity, 0.4 mm. Pre-

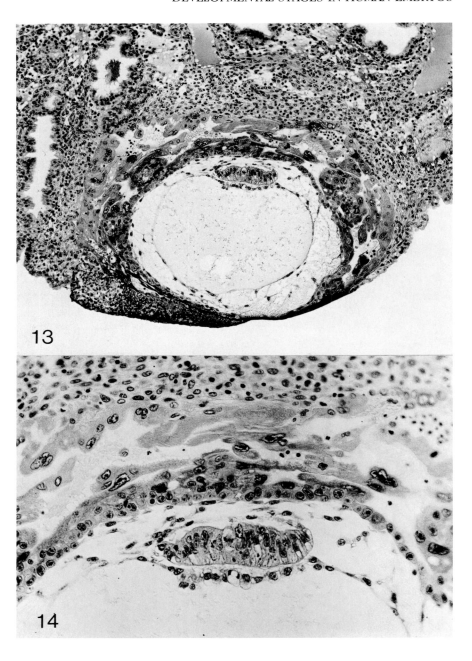

Fig. 5-13. Section through the middle of No. 7700, stage 5c. The space outlined by the internal surface of the chorion now appears distended again. However, a gradient of differentiating trophoblast from abembryonic to embryonic pole is still evident. Intercommunicating lacunae are visible in the syncytiotrophoblast. The primary umbilical vesicle, surrounded by a meshwork, can be seen. The endometrial stroma is edematous and decidua is developing. Section 6-1-5.

Fig. 5-14. The bilaminar embryonic disc of No. 7700, stage 5c. The amnion overlying the disc does not seem to be complete. The epiblast is a pseudostratified columnar epithelium. The surrounding cytotrophoblast is evident, and lacunae can be seen in the syncytiotrophoblast. Cytotrophoblastic clumps may be regarded as an indication of the future chorionic villi. Section 6-1-5.

sumed age, 10–11 days or perhaps even 12 days (Krafka, 1941).

Dible-West. Described by Dible and West (1941). Autopsy. Posterior wall of uterus. Incomplete. Chorionic cavity, 0.47 × 0.28 mm. Embryonic disc, 0.1 × 0.02 mm. Presumed age, 11–13 days.

Müller (1930) described an autopsy specimen. Only one section was near the embryonic disc.

Wilson (1954) found a specimen by endometrial biopsy. Chorion, 0.5 × 0.6 mm. Chorionic cavity, 0.47 × 0.24 mm. Between the amnion and the cytotrophoblast, "a small accumulation of fibroblastic cells . . . probably represents the earliest stage of the Bauchstiel." The endoderm is described as being "delaminated from the embryonic disc." Presumed age, 11 days.

Carnegie No. 7950. Described briefly by Hertig and Rock (1944). Chorion, 0.75 × 0.45 mm. Chorionic cavity, 0.4 × 0.26 mm. Embryonic disc, 0.16 × 0.07 mm. Slightly more developed than No. 7699, although embryo is a little less differentiated. Photomicrographs in Hertig, Rock, and Adams (1956; figs. 27 and 35). Presumed age, 12 days.

Carnegie No. 7700 (figs. 18–22). Described by Hertig and Rock (1941). Hysterectomy. Posterior wall of uterus. Chorion, 0.948 × 0.835 mm. Chorionic cavity, 0.55 × 0.498 mm. Embryonic disc, 0.204 × 0.165 mm. Presumed age, 12 days.

Carnegie No. 8558. Measurements and photomicrographs in Hertig, Rock, and Adams (1956; figs. 30 and 37). Chorion, 0.96 × 0.52 mm. Chorionic cavity, 0.58 × 0.36 mm. Embryonic disc, 0.22 × 0.08 mm. Presumed age, 12 days.

Carnegie No. 8330. Measurements and photomicrographs in Hertig, Rock, and Adams (1956; figs. 30 and 37). Chorion, 0.85 × 0.65 mm. Chorionic cavity, 0.46 × 0.4 mm. Embryonic disc, 0.216 × 0.063 mm. Condensation of extra-embryonic mesoblast perhaps indicates "the beginning of axis formation" (*ibid.*). Presumed age, 12 days.

Kleinhans. Described by Grosser (1922). Autopsy. Only one section. Embryonic disc not seen. Chorion, 0.8 × 0.65 mm. Chorionic cavity, 0.35 × 0.15 mm.

Barnes. Described by Hamilton, Barnes, and Dodds (1943), and further by Hamilton and Boyd (1960). Hysterectomy. Posterior wall of uterus. Pathological edema in endometrium (Davies, 1944). Chorion, 0.931 × 0.77 × 0.737 mm. Primary umbilical vesicle and perhaps early differentiation of secondary vesicle (Luckett, 1978). Presumed age, 10–11 days or perhaps 12 days (Davies, 1944).

Werner (Prof. Werner Gerlach). Described by Stieve (1936), with graphic reconstruction by Florian. Autopsy. Chorion, 0.78 × 1.36 × 0.72 mm. Embryonic disc, 0.18 × 0.12 mm. Some large, round cells in the epiblast are mentioned as possible primordial germ cells. Primary umbilical vesicle and perhaps early differentiation of secondary vesicle (Luckett, 1978). Primordia (mesoblastic crests) of chorionic villi (Her-

tig and Rock, 1941). "Connecting stalk" very indistinct. Rostrocaudal axis but no primitive streak; epiblast fused with extra-embryonic mesoblast caudally and perhaps is origin of latter (Florian, 1933 and 1945). Perhaps 12 days.

Knoth and Larsen (1972) studied an implantation site by electron microscopy. No villi, but "beginning" to form. Primary umbilical vesicle "not so easily seen." Probably 11 days.

Dankmeijer and Wielenga (1968) described a specimen of stage 5. Curettage. Incomplete.

Carnegie No. 8139. Described by Marchetti (1945), who admitted that it is "not entirely normal." Curettage. Chorion, 0.706 × 1.2 mm. Chorionic cavity, 0.635 × 0.582 mm. Embryonic disc, 0.126 × 0.048 × 0.116 mm. Embryo located centrally in chorionic cavity, which contains a meshwork. Embryonic disc, slightly ovoid (i.e., presents a longitudinal axis). Described originally as previllous, although "primitive villi" (stage 6) are mentioned by Boyd and Hamilton (1970): folds of undulating contour of cytotrophoblast are not yet "primitive unbranching villi, although they may be the primordia of them" (Marchetti, 1945; fig. 5). Primary umbilical vesicle present. May be regarded as transitional between stages 5 and 6. Presumed age, 13 days.

Bandler (1912) found a specimen embedded in tubal mucosa and which showed "as yet absolutely no suggestion of chorionic villi." No details available.

Pommerenke (1958) described a specimen of stage 5. Curettage. Incomplete. Embryo not included.

Macafee. Described by Morton (1949). Curettage. Probably belongs to stage 5. Embryonic disc not found.

Scipiades (1938) described a specimen that belongs either to stage 5 or to stage 6, probably the former, "but its preservation is so poor that accurate conclusions are impossible" (Hertig and Rock, 1941). Curettage. Chorion, 1.498 × 0.49 mm. Chorionic cavity, 0.99 mm. Embryonic disc (only two sections available), 0.18 × 0.048 mm. Presumed age, 11–12 days.

Thomas and van Campenhout (1963) found a specimen that probably belongs to stage 5, although some trophoblastic thickenings of a villous character were said to be present.

Teacher-Bryce I. A pathological specimen of stage 5 described by Bryce (1924).

Sch. (Schönig). A pathological specimen of stage 5 described by von Möllendorff (1921a).

Keller and Keller (1954) found a pathological specimen embedded in the stroma of the ostium uteri.

Several pathological specimens of stage 5c are in the Carnegie Collection. Nos. 8370, 7770, 8299 (malpositioned embryonic disc, Hertig, 1968, fig. 132), 8329, 8000 (superficial implantation), and 7771 (no embryo) were measured and illustrated by Hertig, Rock, and Adams (1956).

STAGE 6

Approximately 0.2 mm in size

Approximately 13 postovulatory days

Characteristic features: chorionic villi and secondary
umbilical vesicle in 6a; primitive streak in 6b

The appearance of recognizable chorionic villi is used as the criterion for stage 6. The villi begin to branch almost immediately.

The space bounded by the internal surface of the chorion begins to expand greatly toward the end of stage 5 and during stage 6 (fig. 6-1). The secondary umbilical vesicle develops.

Axial features are not evident, or at least have not been described, in all embryos of stage 6. Moreover, in some instances, their presence is in dispute. It is possible, however, if the fixation and plane of section were always suitable, the series complete and free from distortion, and an adequate search made, that axial features would be found. Thus, in the well-known Peters specimen, which is frequently considered not yet to show axial features, the possible presence of an allantois was raised originally (Peters, 1899); apparently Grosser believed for a time that a primitive streak was present.

Hence it is convenient to distinguish (a) those embryos in which little or no axial differentiation has occurred or been noted, from (b) those embryos in which axial features, particularly a primitive streak, have definitely been recorded (fig. 6-10). This distinction corresponds more or less to Mazanec's (1959) groups V and VI, respectively. In the latter, according to Mazanec, the chorionic villi have already begun to branch.

SIZE AND AGE

The maximum diameter of the chorion varies from 1 to 4.5 mm, that of its enclosed cavity from 0.6 to 4.5 mm. The embryonic disc varies from 0.15 to 0.5 mm in maximum diameter; the age is believed to be about 13 days.

It is of interest to note that those specimens (referred to here as 6a) in which definite axial features have not been described are characterized by a slightly smaller chorion (1–3 mm, as compared with 2–4.5 mm in the remainder, 6b), contained cavity (0.6–2.2 mm, as compared with 1.3–4.5 mm), and embryonic disc (0.15–0.22 mm, as compared with 0.15–0.5 mm).

HISTOLOGICAL FEATURES

A chart indicating the derivation of various tissues and structures is presented as figure 6-2.

Decidua. The decidua (fig. 6-8) varies considerably in thickness at the implantation site but is generally between 3 and 12 mm. A decidual reaction is present, a variable amount of edema and leucocytic infiltration is found, and actively secreting glands and prominent blood vessels are noticeable. Compact, spongy, and basal strata are distinguishable from superficial to deep (Krafka, 1941). At about this time the well-known subdivision of the decidua into three topographical components may be employed: (1) the decidua basalis is that situated at the deepest (embryonic) pole of the conceptus, (2) the decidua capsularis is reflected over the rest of the chorionic sac, and (3) the decidua parietalis lines the uterine cavity except at the site of implantation.

Chorion. The increasing structural complexity of the trophoblast from superficial to lateral and basal aspects has been attributed by Ramsey (1938) to the more advantageous nutritive conditions prevailing at the latter sites. The coalescence of the lacunae forms the intervillous space, which, placed as an offshoot on the uterine circulation, may be regarded as "a variety of arteriovenous aneurysm" (Hertig, 1968). The syncytiotrophoblast is more active enzymatically than the cytotrophoblast, and is believed, among other functions, to be responsible for the secretion of chorionic gonadotropin.

The cytotrophoblastic clumps and mesoblastic crests of stage 5 have now progressed to form processes that are commonly known as chorionic villi (fig. 6-3). Sev-

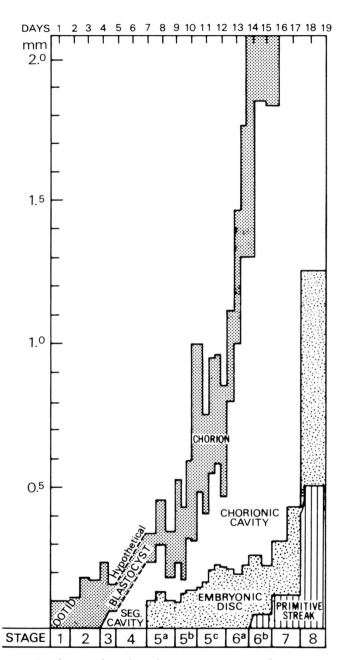

Fig. 6-1. Graph to show the progression in size from stage 1 to stage 8. Based on the measurements of 28 specimens. The interrupted lines indicate hypothetical values for stage 4. An enormous expansion of the chorionic cavity begins to take place toward the end of stage 5.

eral authors have pointed out that "the initial villi do not arise as free and separate outgrowths from the chorionic plate" into the lacunar spaces (Boyd and Hamilton, 1970). Trophoblastic trabeculae, which initially are syncytial in character, come to possess a central process of cytotrophoblast and are generally termed primary villi. None of the trabeculae, however, possesses a free distal end, because these "primary villous stems" do not arise as individual and separate sprouts from the chorion (Hamilton and Boyd, 1960) but rather by invagination of syncytiotrophoblast (fig. 6-3).

The mesoblastic crests form the cores of the villi, and the cytotrophoblastic clumps form caps from which cytotrophoblastic columns proceed externally. These columns, indications of which have been seen also at stage 5c, make contact with the stroma and form a border zone (penetration zone, Greenhill, 1927), the fetal-maternal junction, characterized by pleomorphic fetal cells (Krafka, 1941) and necrotic maternal cells. The columns also make contact with each other peripherally to form the cytotrophoblastic shell (fig. 6-3).

The cytotrophoblastic shell (of Siegenbeek van Heukelom) is the specialized, peripheral part of the cellular trophoblast in contact with maternal tissue. As the shell forms, syncytiotrophoblast is left both internally, where it lines the intervillous space, and externally, where it forms masses that blend with the decidua. The development and arrangement of the shell have been discussed by Boyd and Hamilton (1970). Defective development of the trophoblast, especially of the shell, results later in villous deficiencies (Grosser, 1926). Moreover, it is important to appreciate that, even in instances where the embryonic disc either fails to form or remains rudimentary, a large chorion with luxuriant villi may still be found.

Because the number of mitotic figures in the cytotrophoblastic covering of a villus is approximately equal to that in the mesoblastic core, Krafka (1941) suggested "that the mesoblast, once established, proliferates at the same rate as the Langhans layer, and hence furnishes its own growth zone." The layer featured by Theodor Langhans (in 1870 and subsequently) is the villous cytotrophoblast, "which constitutes the *cellular* (as opposed to *syncytial*) investment of the villi" (Boyd and Hamilton, 1970).

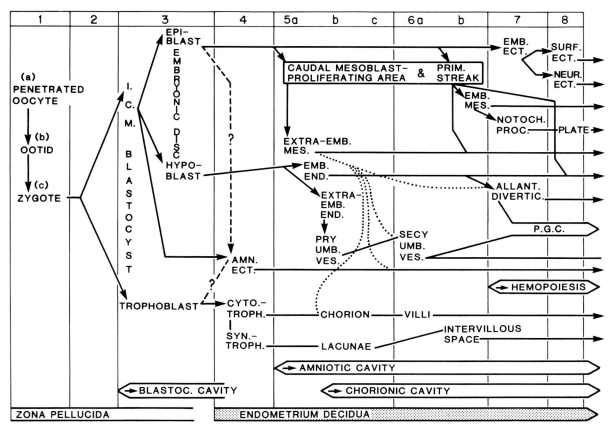

Fig. 6-2. Chart to show the probable sequence of development of various tissues and structures in the human embryo during the first eight stages. Some features are uncertain and others controversial, so that a definitive scheme will have to await further investigations. The various contributions of the extra-embryonic mesoblast to the chorion, amnion, secondary umbilical vesicle, and allantoic diverticulum are shown by dotted lines. In the mouse, it is now maintained that the hypoblast makes no contribution to the intra-embryonic endoderm. In the rhesus monkey, it is believed that the original epiblast gives rise to the amniotic ectoderm and the epiblast proper.

Park (1957) found a low incidence of sex chromatin in the trophoblast and chorionic mesoblast of an embryo (No. 7801) of stage 6, and in the chorionic mesoblast and umbilical vesicle of a second specimen (No. 7762).

Extra-embryonic mesoblast. The chorionic mesoblast is well formed and extends into the villi even in stage 6a, as seen clearly in the Linzenmeier and Peters specimens.

From his acquaintance with Hill's observations of primates and from his own studies of the Fetzer embryo, Florian (1933) believed in "the existence of an area in the most caudal part of the embryonic disc where the primary mesoderm is fused with the ecto-

derm." The zone in question may be the site "where primary mesoderm originates (at least in part). This area is situated close behind the primordium of the cloacal membrane" (*ibid.*), and involves the disc epiblast and the adjoining amniotic ectoderm. This theory of the origin of the primary mesoblast from a localized proliferating area has already been discussed under stage 5a.

At stage 6a, angiogenesis (see Hertig, 1935) is occurring in the chorionic mesoblast (Nos. 6900 and 6734), blood vessels are found in the villi (No. 6900), and blood islands are seen on the umbilical vesicle (No. 6734). By the end of stage 6b, vascularization of the chorion is almost constant and blood vessels are

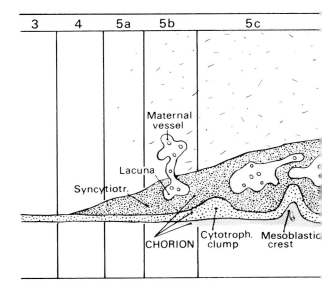

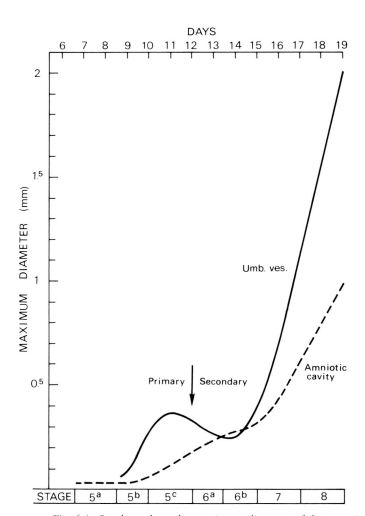

Fig. 6-4. Graph to show the maximum diameter of the amniotic cavity and of the umbilical vesicle from stage 5 to stage 8. Based on the measurements of 31 specimens. From stage 5c to stage 6, the primary is transformed into the secondary umbilical vesicle, although the mode of the transformation is not entirely clear. The secondary is at first smaller than the primary but soon enlarges considerably.

generally present in the villi (*ibid.*). Thus, the blood vascular system first arises in extra-embryonic areas. From his studies of chorionic angiogenesis, Hertig (1968) became convinced of "the independent *in situ* origin of angioblasts and mesoblasts from trophoblast."

Amnion. The amnion is well formed. At its upturned margins, the epiblast of the embryonic disc changes abruptly to the squamous cells of the amnion (fig. 6-9). Although the amnion appears largely as a single (ectodermal) layer, an external coat of mesoblast can also be detected and, in some places, it "runs along as a layer of mesothelium" (Heuser, Rock, and Hertig, 1945). The amniotic cavity may be either smaller or larger than the umbilical vesicle at stage 6 (fig. 6-4).

In the Fetzer embryo, among other specimens, Florian (1930a) was able to confirm von Möllendorff's finding in Op of enlargement of the amniotic cavity by epithelial degeneration. An active extension of the amniotic cavity toward the tissue of the connecting stalk took place in a dorsal and caudal direction from the embryonic disc.

The vault of the amniotic cavity may give rise to a diverticulum known as the amniotic duct. The appearances vary from a localized amniotic thickening (in No. 7801) to a pointed process directed toward the

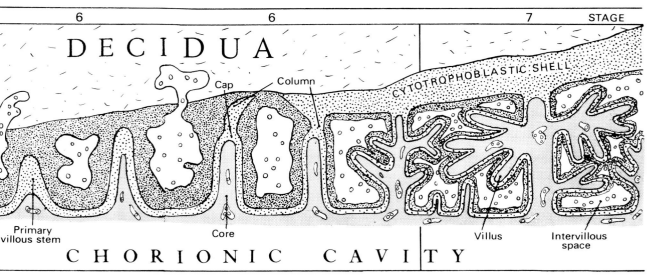

Fig. 6-3. Highly simplified scheme to show the preliminary events during stages 3–7 that lead to the development of the placenta. The cytotrophoblast (stage 3) gives origin to syncytiotrophoblast (stage 4), and lacunae appear in the latter (stage 5b). The appearance of a mesoblastic lining for the trophoblast results in a combination known as the chorion. Cytotrophoblastic clumps (stage 5c) acquire mesoblastic crests and become primary villous stems (stage 6). A cytotrophoblastic shell begins to form externally, and free villi project into the intervillous space (stage 7).

trophoblast (in No. 7634, Krafka, 1941, fig. 2, and in No. 7762, Wilson, 1945, fig. 8). The amniotic duct is generally regarded as an inconstant and transitory developmental variation.

Embryonic disc. Terms such as "embryonic disc," "embryonic shield," *Keimscheibe, Embryonalschild,* or "blastodisc" are used in measuring embryos from the rostral amniotic reflexion to, frequently, the caudal end of the primitive streak (Odgers, 1941). Although certain authors (e.g., Grosser, 1931a) therefore do not include the cloacal membrane, others (e.g., Florian and Hill, 1935) do include it. When the connecting stalk and allantoic diverticulum are also included, terms such as "embryonic rudiment," *Embryonalanlage, Keim-anlage,* or *Keimling* are employed. Many writers do not make clear their points of reference, nor do they always specify whether a measurement has been taken in a straight line (caliper length) or along the curvature of the disc (contour length). In the present work, the "embryonic disc" will be taken to include, where possible, the cloacal membrane, and, except where otherwise specified, the length will generally refer to that

measured in a straight line.

As seen from the dorsal aspect, the embryonic disc generally appears elongated, and the long axis of the disc usually (in ten out of twelve specimens of stage 6b) coincides with that of the primitive streak rather than lying at a right angle to it.

Although the dorsal surface of the disc may present some localized convexities and concavities, it is, as a whole, fairly flat. No. 7801, a particularly excellent specimen, is slightly convex (fig. 6-9), but the marked curvatures illustrated in some embryos (such as T.F.) may be assumed to be artifactual.

A detailed study of the "cytodesmata" in early human embryos was undertaken by Studnička (1929). In two specimens (Bi I and T.F.) of stage 6, cytodesmata were described between the germ layers ("interdermal cytodesmata") and between the mesothelial and the adjacent germ layer in both the amnion and the wall of the umbilical vesicle (Studnička and Florian, 1928).

With the appearance of the primitive streak during stage 6, a process is begun whereby certain cells of the epiblast enter the streak, and the remaining cells

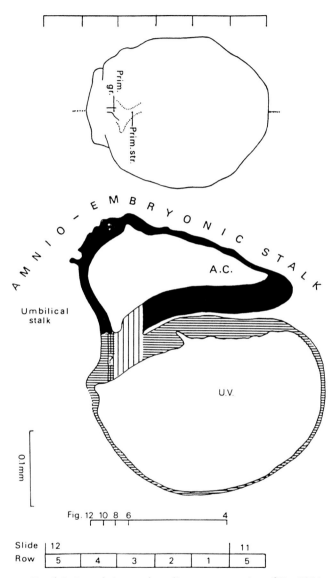

Fig. 6-5. Dorsal view and median reconstruction of No. 7801, stage 6, in alignment. The dorsal view, which is based on a graphic reconstruction by the present writers, shows the location of the primitive streak and primitive groove. The median reconstruction is based on a drawing by James F. Didusch (Heuser, Rock, and Hertig, 1945, Plate 3). The primitive streak is indicated by vertical lines, and the cross-hatched area (containing a question mark) suggests the site of the future cloacal membrane. The system of shading is further clarified in figure 7-1. The connecting stalk comprises amnio-embryonic and umbilical stalks. The figure references are to the sections reproduced by Heuser, Rock, and Hertig (1945, Plates 1 and 2).

on the dorsal aspect of the embryo will become the embryonic ectoderm. The epiblast is continuous with the amniotic ectoderm at the margin of the embryonic disc. The basement membrane (*membrana prima* of Hensen) of the epiblast is clearly visible in a number of embryos of stage 6, such as Harvard No. 55 (where it has been demonstrated histochemically by Hertig *et al.*, 1958), Peters, E.B., Bi I, etc.

The embryonic mesoblast will be discussed under the primitive streak.

The endoderm shows a marked concentration of glycogen, and some of its cells may be primordial germ cells (Hertig *et al.*, 1958). Rostral to the primitive streak, the endoderm consists of large vesicular cells (Heuser, Rock, and Hertig, 1945). It should be kept in mind that, in the chick embryo, it has been shown that the rostral part of the primitive streak (including the node) always contains a large population of presumptive endoblastic cells.

Primitive streak. The primitive streak is a proliferation of cells lying in the median plane in the caudal region of the embryonic disc (figs. 6-5 and 6-10). The streak on its first appearance and in narrow usage, is "the thick caudal end of the germ disk" (Heuser and Streeter, 1941). In a much broader and more functional sense, however, "the essential features of the primitive streak are the pluripotential nature of the cells that compose it and the continued segregation of more specialized cells which migrate or delaminate from the less specialized remainder" (*ibid.*).

The primitive streak enables cells from the outer layer of the embryo to pass inside and become mesoderm and endoderm (Bellairs, 1986). The process by which cells leave the epiblast, become part of the primitive streak, and then migrate away from the streak is termed ingression. It seems to depend on loss of the basal lamina beneath the streak.

On the basis of radio-autographic studies of grafts in chick embryos, the primitive streak is believed to be not a blastema but rather an entrance in which occur movement of epiblast toward the streak, invagination at the streak, and subsequent migration to both homolateral and heterolateral mesoderm. At primitive streak stages of the chick embryo, zones have been established for future ectoderm, mesoderm, endoderm, and notochord. It is likely that the mammalian pattern is basically similar. In the rabbit, the formation of the embryonic disc and primitive streak "is primarily achieved by migrations of cells that are being rapidly proliferated over the entire surface of the embryonic area. Cell death occurs but is an insignificant factor in this phase of embryonic growth" (Daniel and Olson, 1966).

In the human, the primitive streak appears first during stage 6. The possibility of a streak in some embryos (e.g., Peters) here classified as 6a has been raised. Conversely a streak in at least one 6b embryo (No. 8819) has been denied (Krafka, 1941).

Brewer's (1938) criteria for the presence of a primitive streak are (1) active proliferation of the cells (shown by a large number of cells in mitosis), (2) the loss of the basement membrane separating the epiblast and endoderm, (3) migration of the epiblastic cells, and (4) intermingling of the cells of the epiblast and endoderm of the disc.

The shape of the early streak is not entirely clear. Brewer (1938) described it as a crescentic formation at the caudal margin of the disc (similar to that seen in the pig), but, as already mentioned, the presence of a streak at all in his specimen (No. 8819) was denied by Krafka (1941).

In other young 6b embryos (Op, Fetzer, and Wo) the streak possesses the form of a node, and indeed initially "seems to correspond in its position with Hensen's knot" (Florian, 1930a). Thus, in the Fetzer specimen (Fetzer and Florian, 1930), the streak appeared almost circular in dorsal view, was situated not far from the middle of the embryonic disc, and did not reach the cloacal membrane. The question naturally arises whether the primordium is not in fact the primitive node rather than the primitive streak in these early specimens. This idea is supported by Dr. J. Jirásek (personal communication, 1970), who believes that the fusion of the epiblast with the endoderm found in this region indicates that the node rather than the streak is involved. According to this interpretation, the primitive node appears during stage 6 and the streak would not appear until the following stage. In the chick embryo, although the streak is said to appear before the node, there is reason to believe that the rostral end of the very young primitive streak already contains the material of the future primitive node.

When the primitive streak attains a rostrocaudal measurement of 0.1 mm or more, as in Beneke, Am. 10, Bi I, and T.F., its elongation fully justifies the name "streak." By the end of stage 6, both a node and a streak (separated by a "neck") have been recorded in one (somewhat abnormal) embryo (HEB-18, Mazanec, 1960).

In the first specimens of stage 6b (Liverpool I and II, No. 7801, No. 8819, No. 7762, Op, Fetzer), the length of the primitive streak is less than one-quarter that of the embryonic disc. In Wo and Beneke it is less than one-third, and in Am. 10, Bi I, and T.F. it is less than one-half. Finally, in the transitional and somewhat abnormal HEB-18 specimen, the streak attains one-half the length of the embryonic disc.

The primitive groove appears probably during stage 6b. At any rate its presence has been claimed in some specimens (Liverpool II, Op, and T.F.) of that stage (fig. 6-10).

Although it may be possible, at least in some instances, to ascertain the rostrocaudal axis of the embryo at stages 5c and 6a, unequivocal manifestation awaits the initial appearance of the primitive streak during stage 6b (O'Rahilly, 1970). With the establishment of bilateral symmetry, the embryonic disc, in addition to its dorsal and ventral surfaces, now has rostral and caudal ends and right and left sides. The median plane may be defined,[1] and the terms "medial" and "lateral" are applicable. Moreover, it is proper to speak of coronal (or frontal), sagittal, and transverse planes. The last-named, in anticipation of the erect posture, may be termed horizontal. Certain other terms, however, such as "anterior," "posterior," "superior," and "inferior," should be avoided at this period because of their special meaning in adult human anatomy.

Embryonic mesoblast. At first, the embryonic mesoblast is scarcely recognizable as such (Nos. 8819 and 7762) or is quite scanty in amount (No. 7801). Although the main bulk of the embryonic mesoblast is believed to come by way of the primitive streak, other sources are not excluded. Lateral to the streak, for example, it is possible that some epiblastic cells bypass the streak and migrate locally into the mesoblast (Heuser, Rock,

---

[1]The terms "median sagittal" and "para-sagittal" are redundant. The median plane is sagittal by definition and anything parallel with a sagittal plane is still sagittal. This usage has been accepted in all the recognized anatomical terminologies.

and Hertig, 1945). In addition, the possibility of contributions from the gut endoderm has been raised in the case of the macaque (Heuser and Streeter, 1941). Finally, the degree of incorporation of some of the primary mesoblast into definitive body mesoderm is unknown. Conversely, in the Beneke specimen, Florian (1933) "could trace the secondary mesoderm behind the caudal end of the primitive streak around the cloacal membrane into the connecting stalk." (The very closely arranged cells of the secondary mesoblast were distinguishable from the looser cells of the primary tissue.) Hence, the convenient distinction between primary and secondary mesoblast should not be interpreted too rigidly. A need exists for further detailed studies of the distribution and spread of mesoblast during these early stages.

In the chick embryo, at the stage of the definitive streak, it has been established that each topographical kind of mesoblast has a definite place along the rostrocaudal axis of the primitive streak, precise enough to be demonstrated experimentally.

Prechordal plate. The earliest human embryo in which a definite prechordal plate has been recorded seems to be Beneke at stage 6b. In that specimen, "in front of, and below the cranial extremity of the primitive streak . . . the endoderm is distinctly thickened and proliferative" in "a horseshoe shaped area"; that area "must be regarded as a mesoderm producing zone" (Hill and Florian, 1963). Study of later specimens, such as Manchester 1285 and Dobbin, led Hill and Florian to "regard the thickened area in question as prechordal plate." Dr. W. P. Luckett has called the writer's attention to several stage 5c specimens (Nos. 7950, 8558, and 8330) in which the endoderm appears to be thickened at one end of the embryo, as shown in the photomicrographs published by Hertig, Rock, and Adams (1956, figs. 35, 37, and 38).

It is of interest to note that, in *Tarsius*, the prechordal plate, which later adopts the form of an annular zone, is at first represented by a continuous sheet of thickened endoderm underlying most of the embryonic epiblast (Hill and Florian, 1963).

Umbilical vesicle (fig. 6-9). The umbilical vesicle functions "as a specialized nutritional membrane" (Streeter, 1937) and, in addition, serves as the site of origin of primordial germ cells as well as an important temporary locus of hematopoietic activity (Hoyes, 1969).

From stage 5c to stage 6, the primary is transformed into the secondary umbilical vesicle (fig. 6-4), although the mode of the transformation has long been disputed. (See Stieve, 1931; Heuser and Streeter, 1941; Strauss, 1945; Hamilton and Boyd, 1950; Starck, 1956.)

According to Hertig (1968), the primary vesicle "blows up" or "pops," and the torn edges that remain attached to the endoderm coalesce to form the secondary vesicle. The secondary sac "soon takes on a second or inner layer of epithelial nature" which is, in Hertig's view, derived from the wall of the sac itself. In other words, "endodermal" cells differentiate *in situ* from the wall of the umbilical vesicle (Streeter, 1937).

According to a number of other authors (such as Stieve, 1931), however, "it seems likely that endoderm from the edge of the embryonic disc proliferates and migrates round the interior" of the wall of the sac (Hamilton and Boyd, 1950), using that wall "as a guiding surface" (Mazanec, 1953).

A further possibility is the dehiscence of cells from the disc endoderm so that a new cavity is formed between the two endodermal layers or possibly between the disc endoderm and the dorsal part of the wall of the sac.

In any case, it appears likely that, at least in some embryos, the distal part of the primary umbilical vesicle becomes detached from the proximal part, thereby forming one or more isolated vesicles or cysts (see below). As a result of these processes, the secondary vesicle is at first smaller than the primary sac (fig. 6-4). Thus the secondary vesicle may develop "as a result of the collapse of the abembryonic and lateral walls" of the primary sac, "with subsequent pinching-off and vesiculation of the distal collapsed portion" (Luckett, 1978). The part of the primary vesicle immediately under cover of the embryonic disc persists as the secondary umbilical vesicle.

It is maintained that the secondary vesicle is unilaminar in stage 6 and that adherent epithelial remnants of the primary sac merely give an impression that the secondary vesicle has already acquired an external mesodermal layer (Luckett, 1978).

In a number of embryos of stage 6 (such as No. 7634) and some subsequent stages, a diverticulum of the umbilical vesicle has been recorded. These outgrowths arise generally at the abembryonic pole of the main sac. They vary from slight evaginations to long

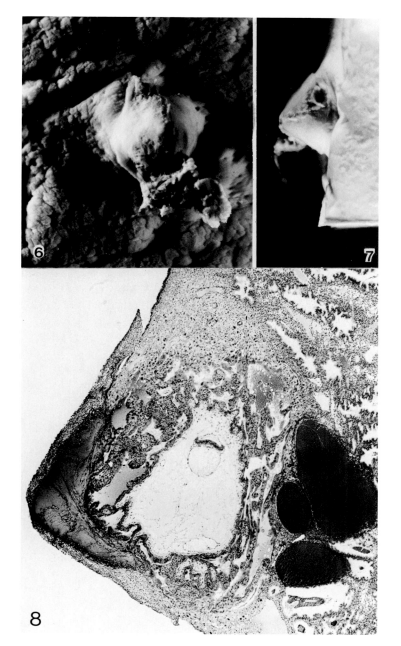

Fig. 6-6. Surface view of the implantation site of No. 7801. A small amount of maternal blood escaped and coagulated on one side of the elevated area.

Fig. 6-7. Side view of the implantation site of No. 7801.

Fig. 6-8. General view of the tissues at and near the implantation site (No. 7801) to show the scab (*Schlusscoagulum*) of hemorrhagic exudate, actual hemorrhage underlying the scab, primary villous stems, blood-filled uterine glands, and early decidua. The embryo is evident, and, near the opposite wall of the chorion, a vesicle presumed to be a detached part of the umbilical vesicle can be identified. Section 12-1-1.

processes (0.45 mm in Liverpool II, for example), and are frequently associated with cysts. It has been suggested that the diverticula and cysts are remnants of the primary umbilical vesicle (Heuser, Rock, and Hertig, 1945).

Cloacal membrane. The cloacal membrane appears during stage 6b. Although at least its site may be detected in the first specimens of that stage (such as No. 7801), the membrane is probably present in all spec-

imens that possess a primitive streak 0.05 mm or more in length. The membrane is at first a cell cord that connects the epiblast with the endoderm (Florian, 1933) and is of variable length (about 0.015–0.025 mm). Later (stage 7) it increases in size and begins to assume the form of an actual membrane.

Allantoic diverticulum. The existence of an allantois in the human remained controversial until the end of the nineteenth century (Meyer, 1953). In early embryos, the recognition of an allantoic primordium presents considerable difficulty. A recess of the umbilical vesicle, such as appears in embryo Op, should not be assumed to be necessarily the allantois. According to Florian (1930a), "the yolk-sac penetrates into the connecting stalk in the form of a narrow diverticulum which enlarges and eventually opens out again into the cavity of the yolk sac. This process may probably be repeated several times." Hence some reservations must be made concerning the "allanto-enteric diverticulum" of Liverpool I. In No. 7801, all that is found is merely "a tiny recess in the wall of the yolk sac at the spot where the allantoic duct presumably originates" (Heuser, Rock, and Hertig, 1945). In Wo, a solid *Allantoisanlage* has been claimed. In Beneke, the diverticulum of the umbilical vesicle is not the allantois (Florian and Beneke, 1931). In Bi I, the appearance of the diverticulum has been attributed to "a ventral down-bulging of the underlying wall of the yolk-sac" produced by the end node of the primitive streak (Florian, 1930a). The condition in T.F. may well be similar. In conclusion, it is difficult to find a convincing example of an allanto-enteric diverticulum at stage 6.

Connecting stalk. Florian (1930a) pointed out that the connecting stalk (as exemplified in embryo Op) comprises two portions (fig. 6-5): (1) the amnio-embryonic stalk, an attachment of the entire amnio-embryonic vesicle to the chorionic mesoderm, and (2) the umbilical stalk, by which the caudal end of the embryo is anchored to the chorion. The umbilical stalk, which is in all stages covered on its cranial surface by amniotic ectoderm, later becomes transformed into the umbilical cord.

The Peters embryo is situated in a thickening of the chorionic mesoderm but the connecting stalk is "not yet present" (Florian, 1930a). Although "a body stalk proper has not yet fully formed" in No. 7634 (Krafka, 1941), its primordium is present and comprises the amnio-embryonic and umbilical stalks of Florian. The condition is similar to that in Op, in which Florian has pointed out that the axis of the connecting stalk has already begun to form an acute angle (open caudally) with the embryonic plate. By the end of stage 6b, blood vessel primordia are present in the developing stalk and indicate the future umbilical vessels (Hertig, 1935). In the opinion of Hill and Florian (1963), the vessels of the connecting stalk in *Tarsius* "can arise directly as invaginations of the mesothelium" covering the stalk.

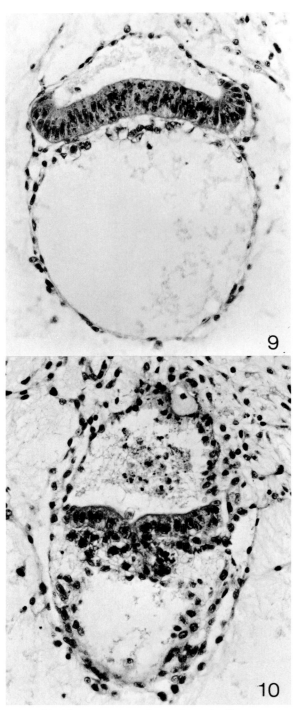

Fig. 6-9. The amniotic cavity, embryonic disc, and umbilical vesicle of No. 7801. The upturned margins of the epiblast change abruptly to the squamous cells of the amniotic ectoderm. The gut endoderm has a foamy appearance, whereas the cells lining the umbilical vesicle are squamous. The umbilical vesicle appears to be acquiring an external coat. Section 12-1-1.

Fig. 6-10. The embryonic disc of No. 7801, in the region of the primitive streak. The connecting stalk, the amniotic cavity, and the umbilical vesicle are also visible. Section 12-3-6.

SPECIMENS OF STAGE 6a ALREADY DESCRIBED

Carnegie No. 8905, Merrill. Unbranched villi. Although an abnormal leucocytic reaction is present, this specimen "represents the best example in the author's collection of formation of early primordial villi, active mesogenesis and angiogenesis, completion of the amnion and the transitional phase between the primary and definitive [secondary] yolk sac formation" (Hertig, 1968, who reproduced a photomicrograph as fig. 55). Presumed age, 12–13 days.

Carnegie No. 6800, Stöckel. Described by Linzenmeier (1914). Hysterectomy. Angiogenesis in chorion described by Hertig (1935). Photomicrographs reproduced by Hertig (1968), Figs. 56–58. Important as one of the youngest specimens having "true villi" (Hertig and Rock, 1941). Chorionic villi show "an occasional tendency to dichotomous branching" (Krafka, 1941). Indication of blood vessel formation in villi. Chorion, $2.75 \times 1.05 \times 0.9$ mm. Chorionic cavity, $0.75 \times 0.61 \times 0.52$ mm; capacity, 0.13 mm^3 (Odgers, 1937). Embryonic disc, 0.21×0.105 mm (Krafka, 1941). Allantoic diverticulum doubtful. Presumed age, 13 days.

Carnegie No. 8672. Photomicrograph illustrated by Hertig, Rock, and Adams (1956, fig. 40). Chorion, 1.14×1.08 mm. Chorionic cavity, 0.8×0.79 mm. Embryonic disc, 0.203×0.07 mm. Presumed age, 13 days.

Harvard No. 55. Studied histochemically by Hertig *et al.* (1958). Hysterectomy. Chorion, $1.77 \times 1.33 \times 0.598$ mm. Chorionic cavity, $0.73 \times 0.68 \times 0.221$ mm. Embryonic disc, $0.296 \times 0.196 \times 0.044$ mm. Chorionic villi essentially solid, with earliest suggestion of mesoblastic core formation. "Apparently without axial differentiation." Possesses "a very recently formed definitive [secondary] yolk sac." Possible primordial germ cells ("stuffed with glycogen") within endoderm near edge of disc. Presumed age, 13 days. For histochemical details, the original paper should be consulted.

Carnegie No. 8360. Photomicrographs illustrated by Hertig, Rock, and Adams (1956, figs. 42 and 46). Chorion, 1.466×1 mm. Chorionic cavity, 1×0.66 mm. Embryonic disc, 0.188×0.055 mm. Presumed age, 13 days.

Peters. Described in a monograph by Peters (1899). Autopsy. A famous embryo, for long the youngest known and the first to be described in detail. Photomicrographs have since been published (Rossenbeck, 1923, plate 42; Odgers, 1937, plate 2, fig. 2). The chorionic villi, some of which display a mesenchymal core, send cellular columns externally and these latter are beginning to form a cytotrophoblastic shell. Slight branching of villi (Krafka, 1941). Chorionic cavity contains magma réticulé of Velpeau (Mall, 1916). Blood islands on umbilical vesicle. Chorion, 1.5×2 mm. Chorionic cavity, $1.6 \times 0.9 \times 0.8$ mm; capacity, 0.7 mm^3 (Odgers, 1937). Embryonic disc, 0.18×0.24 mm (Krafka, 1941). The basement membrane (Hensen's *membrana prima*) of the epiblast was noted by Graf Spee. Allantoic diverticulum and primitive streak uncertain. Presumed age, 13 days (Krafka,

1941). A tabulation of normal human embryos compiled from the literature prior to 1900 and from Mall's own collection was published by Mall (1900, pp. 38–46). The least advanced specimen was the Peters embryo, and included in the list were 92 embryos of 0.19–32 mm, as well as 17 fetuses of 33–210 mm.

E.B. (E. Béla v. Entz). Described by Faber (1940). Curettage. Incomplete. Primitive villi. Chorionic cavity, 0.935×0.697 mm. Embryonic disc, 0.231 mm. No primitive streak, node, or groove. Secondary umbilical vesicle. No allantoic diverticulum. Said to resemble the Peters specimen closely.

Carnegie No. 7634, Torpin. Described in detail by Krafka (1941), who provided also an extensive discussion of the decidua. Hysterectomy. Posterior wall of uterus. Chorionic villi with mesoblastic cores, 0.1–0.2 mm in length. Villi "generally single, but two or more may arise from a common base," although no branching was recorded. Chorion (possessed 85 villi), $1.76 \times 1.7 \times 1.5$ mm. Chorionic cavity, $1.3 \times 1.1 \times 1$ mm. Embryonic disc, 0.216×0.21 mm. Amniotic duct. Neither primitive node nor primitive streak. Cloacal cord (rather than membrane) claimed, but doubted by Mazanec (1959). No allantoic diverticulum. Diverticulum of umbilical vesicle. Presumed age, 13 days. Dorsal and transverse projections published (Krafka, 1941, figs. 1 and 3, and plate 2).

VMA-1. Specimen of Knorre, summarized by Mazanec (1959). Chorion, 3.24×2.04 mm. Chorionic cavity, 1.53×1.02 mm. Embryonic disc, 0.23×0.2 mm. Development thought to be between Torpin and Yale specimens.

Carnegie No. 6734, Yale. Described in detail by Ramsey (1938). Necropsy. Left lateral uterine wall. Chorion, $2.75 \times 1.9 \times 0.76$ mm. Chorionic cavity, $1.3 \times 1.1 \times 1$ mm. Some of the chorionic villi "show dichotomous division, but no more complicated branching has occurred." Some angioblastic strands in villi. Embryonic disc (damaged and distorted), 0.15 mm. Allantoic diverticulum stated to be present but denied by Krafka (1941). Presumed age, 13–14 days. Drawings of model published (Ramsey, 1938, fig. 1).

Noback, Paff, and Poppiti (1968) described an autopsy specimen that possessed a chorion of $2.25 \times 1.25 \times 2$ mm. Chorionic villi avascular. Embryonic disc, 0.22×0.2 mm. No primitive node, notochordal process, cloacal membrane, or allantoic diverticulum. Axial differentiation, however, was suggested by the possible primordia of the prechordal plate and the primitive streak. Hence this specimen may be regarded as transitional between 6a and 6b.

SPECIMENS OF STAGE 6b ALREADY DESCRIBED
(listed in order of length of primitive streak)

Liverpool I. Described by Harrison and Jeffcoate (1953). Curettage. Chorionic villi "are only beginning to show evidence of branching" (*ibid.*, Plate 1, fig. 1). Chorion, 1.86×1.47 mm. Chorionic cavity, 1.5×0.84 mm. Embryonic disc, $0.161 \times 0.199 \times 0.033$ mm. Primitive streak, 0.021 mm. Allanto-enteric diverticulum claimed. Median projection published (*ibid.*, fig. 1; Mazanec, 1959, fig. 31).

Liverpool II. Described by Lewis and Harrison (1966), who, in view of "the dimensions, degree of differentiation and decidual appearances," assigned the specimen to horizon VII. Hysterectomy. The chorionic villi are localized to the embryonic pole, and their mesoblastic cores contain "isolated vascular primordia formed by coalescence of angioblasts." "The villi are branched; lacunae and intervillous spaces have formed." Chorion, 2.72 × 2.35 × 1.54 mm. Embryonic disc, 0.264 × 0.22 mm. Primitive streak, 0.024 mm. Amniotic duct and long duct of umbilical vesicle. Resembles Teacher-Bryce II embryo. Median projection published (*ibid.*, fig. 6).

Carnegie No. 7801 (figs. 6-5 to 6-10). Described in detail and illustrated by Heuser, Rock, and Hertig (1945). Hysterectomy. Posterior wall of uterus. "The primitive villi are short and stubby; a few reach a length of about 0.25 mm." Chorion, 2.6 × 1.9 × 1.4 mm. Chorionic cavity, 1.3 × 1.1 × 0.8 mm. Embryonic disc, 0.04 × 0.22 × 0.253 mm. Primitive streak, 0.04 mm. "Axial differentiation is just appearing." "In this embryo the site of the future [cloacal] membrane seems indicated, but not the structure itself." Probably no allantoic duct. Presumed age, 13–13½ days. Median projection published (*ibid.*, plate 3).

Carnegie No. 8819, Edwards-Jones-Brewer. Described in detail by Brewer (1937, 1938). Hysterectomy. "There is no branching of a mesodermal villus." Chorion, 3.6 × 3 × 1.9 mm. Chorionic cavity, 1.85 × 1.71 × 1.01 mm; capacity, 13.38 mm³. Embryonic disc, 0.209 × 0.177 mm; volume, 0.0814 mm³. Primitive streak, 0.04 mm, claimed, but its presence was denied by Krafka (1941). No allantoic diverticulum. Dorsal and median projections published (Brewer, 1938, plate 1, figs. 2 and 3; Mazanec, 1959, fig. 33). Some authors have attempted to identify a prechordal plate from the median projection.

Carnegie No. 7762, Rochester. Described by Wilson (1945). Curettage. Chorion, 2.3 × 2.2 × 2 mm. Larger villi have a mesoblastic core "and some show a tendency toward branching." Moreover, "no evidence of actual blood vessels is seen in the villi, but in many of them . . . groupings of angioblasts . . . are observed." Chorionic cavity, 1.75 × 1.3 × 1 mm. Embryonic disc, 0.313 × 0.22 mm. Primitive streak, 0.04 mm. No definite allantoic diverticulum. Amniotic duct. Median reconstruction published (*ibid.*, plate 3; Mazanec, 1959, fig. 36).

Op (Opitz). Described by von Möllendorff (1921b). Hysterectomy. Chorionic villi show first branching in many places. Chorionic cavity, 1.5 × 1.15 × 1 mm. Embryonic disc, 0.19 mm. Primitive streak, 0.045 mm. Allantoic diverticulum denied by Florian (1930a). Disintegrating epithelial proliferation of amnion behind caudal end of embryonic plate (*ibid.*). Median reconstruction published (Mazanec, 1959, fig. 34).

Fetzer. Described by Fetzer (1910) and by Fetzer and Florian (1929, 1930). Curettage. Chorionic villi "show a beginning tendency to branch" (Streeter, 1920). Chorion, 2.2 × 1.8 mm. Chorionic cavity, 1.6 × 0.9 mm. Embryonic

disc, 0.26 × 0.215 mm. Primitive streak (denied by Rossenbeck, 1923), 0.05 mm. Cloacal membrane (Florian, 1933) but no allantoic diverticulum. Area of mesoblastic proliferation from adjacent disc and amniotic ectoderm, "caudal" to cloacal membrane (Hill, 1932; Florian, 1933). Stated to lie between Wo and Bi I in development. Dorsal and median projections published (Fetzer and Florian, 1930, figs. 1a, 1b, 2 and 53; Florian, 1945, plate 4, fig. 40; Mazanec, 1959, fig. 37).

H.R. 1 (Hesketh Roberts). Described by Johnston (1940), who included Florian's divergent interpretation of the specimen. Hysterectomy. Chorion and endometrium described by Johnston (1941). According to Florian, the embryonic disc is 0.048 mm and the primitive streak is 0.06 mm in length. Primitive node, notochordal process, and prechordal plate all absent (but described as present by Johnston). Embryo abnormal in shape, the result of an abnormal growth process. Median projection published (Johnston, 1940, fig. 35).

Wo (Wolfring). Described by von Möllendorff (1925). Chorionic cavity, 2.52 × 2.16 × 2.06 mm. Embryonic disc, 0.25 × 0.22 mm. Primitive streak, 0.065 mm. Cloacal membrane rather than solid allantois (Florian, 1933). Median projection published (von Möllendorff, 1925, fig. 4; Florian, 1928a, fig. 40; Mazanec, 1959, fig. 38).

Beneke (Strahl-Beneke). Described originally by Strahl and Beneke in 1916 in a monograph and later by Florian and Beneke (1931). Chorionic cavity, 3.8 × 2.2 × 1.2 mm. Embryonic disc (narrow type), 0.375 mm (Florian, 1934a). Primitive streak (doubted by Rossenbeck, 1923, and denied by Fahrenholz, 1927, but acknowledged by Florian, 1928a), 0.1 mm. No notochordal process (Hill and Florian, 1931b). Prechordal plate, 0.066 mm. Dorsal and median projections published (Florian and Beneke, 1931, figs. 2 and 1; Florian, 1928a, fig. 42; Florian, 1945, plate 4, fig. 41; Mazanec, 1959, fig. 40).

Am. 10. Described by Krause (1952). Hysterectomy. Chorionic cavity, 3.6 × 2.5 × 2.5 mm. Embryonic disc (broad type), 0.32 × 0.3 × 0.06 mm. Primitive streak, 0.135 mm. No notochordal process (but see Mazanec, 1959) although a small lumen was suggested as a possible Anlage of "Lieberkühn's canal." Dorsal and median projections published (Krause, 1952, figs. 13 and 15; Mazanec, 1959, fig. 42). Could be stage 7.

Bi I (Bittman). Described by Florian (1927) and in 1928 in a Czech publication. (For general appearance, see Mazanec, 1959, figs. 95 and 112.) Chorionic cavity, 2.13 × 2.13 × 2.12 mm. Embryonic disc (broad type), 0.35 × 0.34 mm. Primitive streak, which appears as an "indifferent cellular knot" (Florian, 1928b, 0.135 mm). Possible primordial germ cell in ventral wall of umbilical vesicle (Politzer, 1933). Median projection published (Florian, 1928a, fig. 41; Florian, 1945, plate 5, fig. 42; Mazanec, 1959, fig. 41).

Lbg (Lönnberg). Described by Holmdahl (1939). Chorion, 16 × 15 mm. Embryonic disc, 0.285 × 0.236 × 0.032 mm. Primitive streak, 0.144 mm. No allantoic duct.

T.F. Described by Florian (1927, 1928a). Autopsy. Chorionic cavity, 4.578 × 3.078 × 1.76 mm. Embryonic disc, 0.468 × 0.397 × 0.485 mm. Primitive streak (Mazanec, 1959, fig. 100), 0.162 mm. No notochordal process. Median projection published (Florian, 1928a, figs. 27 and 43; Mazanec, 1959, fig. 43).

HEB-18. Described by Mazanec (1960). Abortion. Abnormal features. Chorionic cavity, 4.29 × 4 × 3.55 mm. Embryonic disc (broad type), 0.44 × 0.47 mm. Primitive streak, 0.187–0.22 mm, and node, 0.071 mm. No notochordal process. Dorsal and median projections published (*ibid.*, figs. 1 and 2). Regarded as transitional between stages 6 and 7.

ADDITIONAL SPECIMENS

Precise measurements of the primitive streak have not been provided in accounts of the following embryos. The specimens are listed in order of year of publication.

Minot. Described by Lewis in Keibel and Mall (1912). Primitive streak present. Median projection published (*ibid.*, vol. 2, fig. 229).

Schlagenhaufer and Verocay (1916) described an autopsy specimen that possessed an embryonic disc of 0.24 × 0.28 mm. Although a primitive streak was not found, the development of the specimen is such that it was probably present (Mazanec, 1959).

Teacher-Bryce II. Described by Bryce (1924) and M'Intyre (1926). Autopsy. Chorionic villi are "well developed but are still simple and little branched." Chorion, 4.5 × 4 × 3.5 mm. Chorionic cavity, 2.8 × 2.6 × 2.25 mm. Embryonic disc, 0.2 × 0.1 × 0.15 mm. Primitive streak present (Mazanec, 1959). Long stalk from umbilical vesicle. Blood vessel primordia in connecting stalk.

H 381. Described by Stump (1929). Chorionic villi branched. Chorion, 4.38 × 4.2 × 1.4 mm. Chorionic cavity, 3.48 × 3.44 × 0.81 mm. Embryonic disc, 0.58 × 0.3 mm. Primitive groove and streak or node believed to be present. Said to resemble Hugo and Debeyre specimens.

Andô. Described by Hiramatsu (1936). Hysterectomy. Chorion, 4.2 × 3.25 × 1.9 mm. Chorionic cavity, 4.2 × 2.4 × 1 mm. Embryonic disc, 0.24 × 0.26 × 0.04 mm. Some villi branched. Stated to resemble the Peters specimen. Described as possessing no primitive streak but Mazanec (1959) detected a very early Anlage of the primitive streak in one of the illustrations. Presumed age, 14–15 days. A median interpretation has been published (Mazanec, 1959, fig. 35).

Carnegie No. 6026, Lockyer. A pathological specimen described by Ramsey (1937). Necropsy. Branching villi. Chorionic cavity, 2.12 × 1.48 × 1.6 mm. Embryonic disc

degenerated. Primitive groove and embryonic mesoblast probably present. Formerly classified under horizon VIII.

Thomson. Described by Odgers (1937). Chorionic cavity, 2.1 × 1.51 × 0.7 mm; capacity, 1.55 mm³. Embryonic disc (which shows "a good deal of disorganization"), 0.26 × 0.31 (?) × 0.16 (?) mm. Compared by author to various embryos of stage 6.

Fife-Richter. Described briefly in an abstract by Richter (1952). Hysterectomy. Branching villi. Chorion, 3.44 mm. Chorionic cavity, 2.24 mm. Embryonic disc, 0.29 × 0.4 mm. "A poorly defined primitive streak with groove is present."

Kistner (1953) had only one slide through the embryonic disc. Curettage. Primitive streak thought to be present. Presumed age, 13 days.

Jahnke and Stegner (1964) described a specimen that possessed a chorionic cavity of 2.5 × 2.3 × 1.5 mm. Embryonic disc, 0.31 × 0.29 mm. Primitive streak not precisely ascertainable but thought to be present. Presumed age, 15–16 days. Median projection published (*ibid.*, fig. 2).

Hamilton, Boyd, and Misch (1967) described twins. Hysterectomy. Chorion 2.37 × 2 × 1.4 mm. Early villi. Embryonic disc with primitive node. Twin represented by (1) a vesicle interpreted as "a poorly developed embryonic disc and amnion," and (2) a detached umbilical vesicle. Monozygotic twinning here probably caused by unequal division of inner cell mass of blastocyst.

Carnegie No. 8290. Abnormal specimen illustrated by Hertig (1968, fig. 129). Polypoid implantation site, deficient polar trophoblast, and buckled embryonic disc. Presumed age, 13 days.

Carnegie No. 7800. Abnormal specimen illustrated by Hertig (1968, fig. 126). Trophoblastic hypoplasia with virtual absence of chorionic villi. Presumed age, 13 days. Thought to belong to either stage 6 or stage 7.

Liverpool III. Described by Rewell and Harrison (1976). Some chorionic villi branched. Embryonic disc, 0.238 mm. Primitive streak.

Several other unsatisfactory specimens (in poor condition or inadequately described or both) have been published but will not be referred to here. These include Bayer (Keibel, 1890) and von Herff (von Spee, 1896), and the specimens of Giacomini (1898), van Heukelom (1898), Jung (1908), Herzog (1909), Heine and Hofbauer (1911), Johnstone (1914), Greenhill (1927), and Thomas and van Campenhout (1953). These probably belong to stage 6, and further examples may be found in Mazanec (1959). Moreover, frankly pathological specimens have also been recorded, e.g., by Harrison, Jones, and Jones (1966).

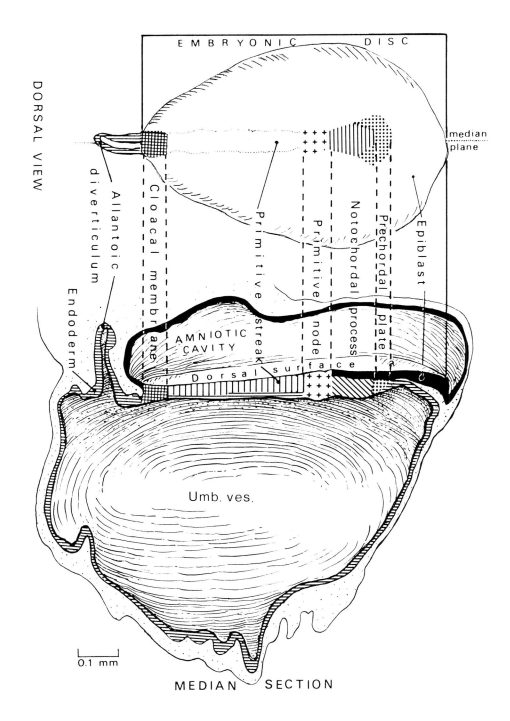

DORSAL VIEW

EMBRYONIC DISC

median plane

Allantoic diverticulum

Cloacal membrane

Primitive streak

Primitive node

Notochordal process

Prechordal plate

Epiblast

Endoderm

AMNIOTIC CAVITY

Dorsal surface

Umb. ves.

0.1 mm

MEDIAN SECTION

Fig. 7-1. Dorsal view and reconstruction of the left half of an embryo of stage 7 to show the general arrangement and the shading employed by Florian and Hill in their graphic reconstructions. Based on the Manchester embryo, No. 1285. The cloacal membrane is here included in the measurement of the length of the embryonic disc. The shading employed to indicate the epiblast (in the median view), prechordal plate, notochordal process (different in the two views), primitive node, primitive streak (in the median view), cloacal membrane, and the allantoic diverticulum and endoderm will be used again in subsequent drawings.

STAGE 7

Approximately 0.4 mm in length
Approximately 16 postovulatory days
Characteristic feature: notochordal process

The appearance of the notochordal process immediately rostral to the primitive node and streak is used as the criterion for stage 7 (fig. 7-1, facing page).

In Streeter's (1942) scheme, horizon VII was characterized by "branching villi, axis of germ disk defined." Such specimens are here classified in stage 6b because (1) some branching of villi has been recorded even in certain stage 6a (horizon VI) embryos (e.g., No. 6734: "occasionally they [the villi] show dichotomous division . . . ," Ramsey, 1938), so that this feature is of scant use as a criterion, and (2) the embryonic axis is defined in some embryos already admitted to horizon VI (e.g., No. 7801, which shows "the primordium of the primitive streak," Hertig, Rock, and Adams, 1956). Moreover, embryos already assigned to horizon VII (e.g., No. 7802) show additional differentiation in the presence of the notochordal process, which is not present in embryos of stage 6.

SIZE AND AGE

The maximum diameter of the chorion varies from 4 to 9 mm, that of the chorionic cavity from 1.5 to 8 mm. The embryonic disc is generally 0.3–0.7 mm in length but varies from 0.1 to 1 mm. The age is believed to be about 16 days.

EXTERNAL FORM

The dorsal surface of the disc is generally slightly convex (fig. 7-9). It varies in shape from oval (Biggart specimen) to pyriform (Manchester 1285) but may be almost circular (Hugo, Schö).

HISTOLOGICAL FEATURES

Decidua. The epithelial layer is intact. The glands are markedly tortuous (fig. 7-7) and lined by secretory epithelium. The stroma is edematous and shows a de-cidual reaction.

Chorion. The villi, which may reach a length of 0.5 or even 1 mm, are either present on the entire surface of the chorion (No. 7802, fig. 40) or are absent superficially (Biggart specimen). In one specimen (Hugo), 942 villi were counted (Stieve, 1926). The mesoblastic cores of the villi contain vascular primordia which are said to be derived from (1) cells arising by (the now disputed) delamination from the cytotrophoblast lining the chorionic cavity and then migrating into the villi, and (2) angioblasts differentiating from the cytotrophoblastic cells of the trophoblastic columns during the formation of early villi (Hertig, Rock, and Adams, 1956).

At this stage (in the Missen embryo) "the human placenta clearly presents a combination of labyrinthine and villous characters. It must be stressed that the main trabeculae, which we will call primary villous stems, were never free villi. From this stage forwards, however, it would be pedantic to avoid calling the lacunar system the intervillous space" (Hamilton and Boyd, 1960).

Secondary villi, i.e., those "branching or arising secondarily from a villus or the chorionic membrane itself" (Hertig, 1968), are seen by stages 7 and 8. Their formation involves all the elements of previously formed chorion (trophoblast, stroma, and blood vessels). They lack maternal attachment, and their limited movement has been compared to that of seaweed waving in a sheltered tidal pool (*ibid.*). These free villi (in the Gar embryo) may branch as often as three or four times (Hamilton and Boyd, 1960). At the periphery of the primary villous stems, the cytotrophoblast has broken through the syncytial layer and, by lateral expansion and fusion, constitutes a thick trophoblastic shell (fig. 6-3).

Amnion (figs. 7-9 to 7-11). The amnion consists of two layers of squamous cells: internally the amniotic ectoderm, and externally an interrupted stratum of cells resembling mesothelium. Between the two layers, some mesenchyme may be seen in places. An amniotic duct may be present (e.g., in No. 7802).

Primitive node and streak (figs. 7-10 and 7-11). At the rostral end of the primitive streak, "the ectodermal cells are loosely arranged and ... are disposed in a ventrolateral direction to form the primitive node" although a surface swelling is not necessarily present (Heuser, Rock, and Hertig, 1945). The primitive node (fig. 7-10), first described as a *Knoten* by Hensen in 1876, has been recorded as present in practically all stage 7 embryos, and varies in length from 0.02 to 0.1 mm. In some instances (e.g., Manchester 1285) the node appears to be separated from the streak by a slight constriction, or neck. From his studies of the pig embryo, Streeter (1927a) regarded the node as an additional, specialized center and not merely as the rostral end of the primitive streak. The idea that the node appears before the streak has been discussed under stage 6. Intercellular vacuoles in the primitive node

may presage the appearance of the notochordal canal (Jirásek, personal communication, 1970).

In the chick embryo, the primitive node has been shown to furnish simultaneously the axially located mesoblast and endoblast. At the stage of the notochordal process, the streak contains material destined for the formation of only the notochord, somites, lateral plates, and a small quantity of extra-embryonic mesoblast. Invagination remains active in the entire streak until at least the stage of the notochordal process, except in the node, where invagination has terminated already at the stage of the definitive streak.

Although the primitive streak (including the node) attains its maximum length (about 0.7 mm) in stage 8, its greatest relative length (about 50 percent of the total length of the embryonic disc) is probably reached during stage 7 (fig. 7-2). In the chick embryo, where the length of the streak is employed as a criterion of staging, the definitive streak extends over two-thirds to three-fourths of the area pellucida, whereas, in the

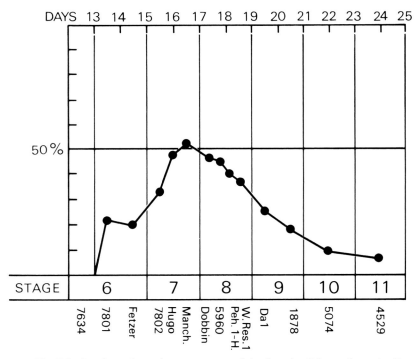

Fig. 7-2. Graph to show the percentage of the length of the embryonic disc occupied by the primitive streak and/or node during stages 6–11. Based on 14 specimens, which are listed below the graph. In the human, the primitive streak at its maximum development does not exceed about 50 percent of the total length of the embryonic disc.

human, it scarcely exceeds one-half of the length of the disc even at the height of its development.

The primitive streak is not necessarily straight, as has been shown in Hugo, Bi 24, and Manchester 1285 (Hill and Florian, 1963).

The presence of a primitive groove (which has already been seen in the previous stage) has been recorded in a number of embryos of stage 7: e.g., No. 7802, P.M., Robertson *et al.*, H. Schm. 10, and No. 1399 (Mateer). Its occurrence was used by Streeter (1920a) and by von Möllendorff (Meyer, 1924) in the grouping of human embryos. A primitive groove is never found in the absence of a primitive streak (Stieve, 1926a,b), although the converse does not hold.

Embryonic mesoblast. Mesoblastic cells accumulate ventral and caudal to the caudal end of the primitive streak, so that a temporary end node (*Endknoten* or *Sichelknoten*) may be formed: e.g., in Hugo (Stieve, 1926a,b) and in Bi 24 (Florian, 1933).

The embryonic mesoblast spreads laterally and rostrally from the primitive streak. Contributions to it are probably being made also by the gut endoderm and by the extra-embryonic mesoblast (Heuser, Rock, and Hertig, 1945). The limits between the primitive streak mesoblast and the endoderm of the umbilical vesicle are indistinct, and the two layers appear to be fused (Stieve, 1926a,b; Florian, 1933). In the Biggart specimen, according to Morton (1949), "in the angle between the anterior end of the shield and the yolk-sac there is a more loosely arranged mass of mesoderm which may well be the protocardiac area." As in the previous stage, localized mesoblastic proliferations directly from the disc epiblast have been recorded, e.g., in Bi I and in Hugo (Florian, 1945).

Notochordal process (fig. 7-9). The notochordal process gives an appearance of being a prolongation of the primitive streak in the direction of the future head region of the embryo. The unsatisfactory term "head process" (*Kopffortsatz*), objected to by Waldeyer (1929a) who proposed *der kraniale Mesoblastfortsatz des Primitivknotens*, is better handled by the French authors, who write of the *prolongement céphalique* of the primitive streak. However, because the cell column "is without question primarily concerned with the formation of the notochord . . . it seems therefore appropriate to refer to it as the notochordal process . . ." (Heuser, 1932b).

In the chick embryo, autoradiographic analysis has led to the conclusion that, at the definitive streak stage, all of the chordal cells are massed in the primitive node, and that the presumptive notochord may be responsible for somite formation. According to carbon-marking experiments, the notochordal process does not form out of nodal epiblast, although it does arise in part from the rostral end of the nodal mesoblast and also receives contributions from the endoderm. Removal of the primitive node results in complete absence of the notochord and in an apparent loss of control in the process of neurulation. In the mouse, X-ray destruction of the primitive node area before the appearance of the notochordal process results in absence of the notochord, although a certain degree of cerebral neurulation occurs.

The notochordal process, which is the characteristic feature of stage 7, varies in length from 0.03 to about 0.3 mm in the recorded specimens. In addition to a median cord, the notochordal process may also (in Bi 24 and Manchester 1285) possess lateral mesoblastic wings (Hill and Florian, 1931b). Moreover, the notochordal process "very early becomes intercalated in, or fused with, the endoderm."

Although the notochordal process appears to develop from the rostral end of the primitive node, Hill and Florian (1963) had no hesitation in identifying the notochordal process in *Tarsius* before the appearance of the recognizably differentiated primitive node. This again raises the question whether the node may not actually be present before the streak.

The notochordal process comprises "not only the primordium of a part of the mesoderm (which does not seem to be very extensive), but also that of the chorda" (Hill and Florian, 1931b). The notochordal process, however, is not synonymous with the notochord *sensu stricto*, which does not appear until stage 11.

Prechordal plate. This localized thickening of the endoderm, situated rostral to the notochordal process, has been recorded in certain embryos of stage 7, such as Bi 24 and Manchester 1285. It has already been mentioned under stage 6 and will be discussed under stage 8.

Umbilical vesicle. The cavity of the umbilical vesicle tends to be slightly larger than that of the amnion. The vesicle may project beyond the rostral limit of the embryonic disc (No. 1399), be approximately flush with it (Bi 24, Manchester 1285), or be receding in its relationship to it (No. 7802), although these variations may be caused, at least in part, by distortion.

A diverticulum of the umbilical vesicle may be present (e.g., in the Biggart specimen). In No. 7802, "detached vesicles observed in the chorionic cavity are regarded as transient parts of the earlier primary yolk sac" (Heuser, Rock, and Hertig, 1945).

Further spread of extra-embryonic mesoblast envelops the umbilical vesicle. The wall of the vesicle (figs. 7-9 to 7-12), like that of the amniotic cavity, may be said to comprise, at least in many areas, three layers: mesothelium, mesoblast, and endoderm, from external to internal. Clumps of cells, especially in the ventral wall of the umbilical vesicle, indicate that angioblastic tissue is differentiating. From their investigation of the Missen embryo, Gladstone and Hamilton (1941) conclude:

"The vascular spaces are partly developed by the fusion of small vacuoles, which are formed in solid angioblastic cords (intracellular spaces), and partly by direct transformation of mesodermal cells into flattened endothelium, which may either enclose the blood islands of the yolk sac, or form the walls of vascular spaces, which at first empty and incomplete, become secondarily filled with blood cells and enclosed by a continuous membrane."

Hematopoietic foci develop in the wall of the secondary umbilical vesicle, although it is not clear whether they are derived from the endoderm or from the embryonic mesoblast (Hertig, 1968). It seems that they are definitely seen only after such foci are already present in the chorion and the body stalk (ibid.). Moreover, "it appears certain that blood vessel precedes blood cell formation" (Gilmour, 1941). From their study of the Missen embryo, Gladstone and Hamilton (1941) conclude:

"The earliest generation of blood cells (haemocytoblasts and primitive erythroblasts) are formed in the wall of the yolk sac and in the umbilical segment of the connecting stalk in close connexion with the entoderm of the allanto-enteric diverticulum, and in the situation of the future umbilical vessels. A few rounded cells of endothelial origin were, however, found in the mesenchyme at the base, or amnio-embryonic segment, of the connecting stalk. These differ in type from the former cells which arise in close association with the entoderm of the yolk sac and its diverticulum."

Thus, although a number of workers have "suggested that the endoderm is the site of origin of the blood cells," nevertheless the blood cells may "depend for their normal development and haemoglobinisation upon their early release into the mesenchyme" (Hoyes, 1969).

At stage 7, three types of hemopoietic cells have been recognized in the blood islands of the umbilical vesicle (Robertson, O'Neill, and Chappell, 1948): modified mesenchymal cells, hemocytoblasts, and primitive erythroblasts.

A low incidence of sex chromatin has been recorded in the umbilical vesicle of No. 7802 (Park, 1957).

Cloacal membrane (figs. 7-4 and 7-12). The cloacal membrane is larger and better defined than in stage 6. It varies from 0.03 to 0.085 mm in length.

Allantoic diverticulum (figs. 7-4 and 7-12). Because of the considerable difficulty in finding a convincing example of an allantoic diverticulum at stage 6, it is safer to assume for the present that the allantoic primordium first appears during stage 7, where it can be identified with a reasonable degree of certainty in such embryos as No. 7802, Bi 24, and Manchester 1285. In his discussion of the diverticulum of the umbilical vesicle found in Peh. 1-Hochstetter (stage 8), Florian (1930a) referred to "the allanto-enteric diverticulum since its proximal part represents the later hind-gut, its distal portion the entodermal allantoic canal." In other words, "the very early primordium of the allantois does not arise directly from the hind-gut . . . but from an allanto-enteric diverticulum. The orifice of this diverticulum later comes to form a part of the hind-gut. It is only in the stage [10] when the insertion of the umbilical stalk has reached the ventral wall of the embryonic body that the allantois can be said to arise directly from the hind-gut . . ." (*ibid.*). This distinction was based largely on the relationship of the cloacal membrane to the orifice of the diverticulum. A comparison, however, of the wider choice of specimens now available would seem to indicate that, in stages 7–10, the diverticulum in question may be either allantoic or allanto-enteric at any given stage, as indicated in Table 7-1 and figure 7-3.

In the chick embryo, it has been maintained that the dorsal wall of the allantois is situated close to the epiblast, and the combination appears to be the cloacal

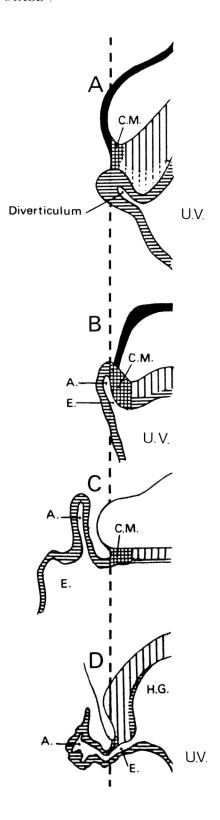

Fig. 7-3. The development of the allantoic diverticulum. In A (Bi 1 embryo, stage 6b), a diverticulum of the umbilical vesicle is present, but it is not the allantoic diverticulum. In B (Bi 24 embryo, stage 7), an allanto-enteric diverticulum (*A.* and *E.*) has formed and the cloacal membrane (*C. M.*) is incorporated in its wall. In C (Manchester 1285 embryo, stage 7), an allantoic diverticulum is present caudal to the cloacal membrane. In D (Da 1 embryo, stage 9), after the hindgut (*H. G.*) has begun to form, an allanto-enteric diverticulum can be seen. The system of shading is in agreement with that shown in figure 7-1. To aid in making comparisons, the caudal limit of the cloacal membrane has been placed on the same vertical line in each of the four examples. It is probable that, in stages 7–10, the diverticulum may be either allantoic or allanto-enteric at any given stage, as indicated in Table 7-1.

A+E = Allanto-enteric
         diverticulum
  A = Allantoic
        diverticulum
  E = Part of hindgut

Cloacal mem.
Endoderm
Primitive str.
Epiblast

(Median section)

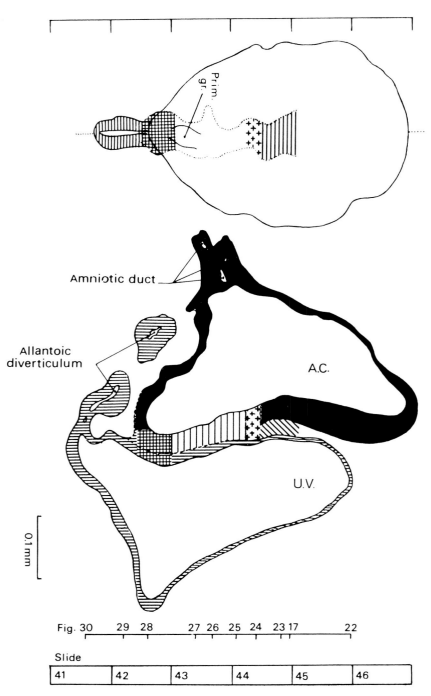

Fig. 7-4. Dorsal view and median reconstruction of No. 7802, stage 7, in alignment. The dorsal view, which is based on a graphic reconstruction by the present writers, shows the location of the notochordal process, primitive node, primitive streak and groove, cloacal membrane, and allantoic diverticulum. The system of shading is that shown in figure 7-1. The median reconstruction is based on a drawing by James F. Didusch (Heuser, Rock, and Hertig, 1945, plate 6). A section of the allantoic diverticulum appears detached because that structure is not entirely in the median plane. The figure references are to the sections reproduced by Heuser, Rock, and Hertig (1945, plates 4 and 5).

TABLE 7-1. Examples of Embryos of Stages 7–10 Showing either an Allanto-Enteric or an Allantoic Diverticulum

Stage	Allanto-Enteric Diverticulum	Allantoic Diverticulum
7	Bi 24	No. 7802
		Manchester 1285
8	No. 5960	No. 8820
	Peh. 1-Hochstetter	Western Reserve 1
9	Da 1 (No. 5982)	No. 1878
10	Bi II	No. 5074
		Bi XI
		Litzenberg (No. 6740)

membrane. These relationships do not appear to hold in No. 7802 or in Manchester 1285, although embryo Bi 24 (Florian, 1945, plate 5, fig. 43) does seem to resemble somewhat the conditions found in the chick, except that the hindgut has not been seen at such early stages in the human embryo. Embryo Bi I (stage 6) also bears some resemblance to the arrangement depicted in the chick but the diverticulum of its umbilical vesicle is not regarded as the allantois. It would seem that the above interpretation of the chick embryo is comparable to Florian's concept of an allanto-enteric rather than an allantoic diverticulum.

Primordial germ cells have been noted in the region of the allanto-enteric diverticulum in Bi 24 (Politzer, 1933).

"The essential part of the mammalian allantois from the physiological standpoint is its vascular mesoderm" (Mossman, 1937), and the question has been raised (George, 1942) whether "the precociously formed allantois in man may not have some inductor function in the origin and differentiation of the blood islands and blood channels of the body stalk." This would require the presence of the allantoic primordium at latest by stage 6b.

Specimens of Stage 7 Already Described
(listed in order of length of notochordal process)

HEB-37. Summarized by Mazanec (1959). Chorionic cavity, 2.25 × 1.29 × 0.4 mm. Embryonic disc, 0.4 mm. Primitive streak, 0.104 mm, and node, 0.04 mm. Notochordal process, 0.032 mm. Stalk of umbilical vesicle (*ibid.*, fig. 77). Median projection published (*ibid.*, fig. 45).

H. R. 1. Described by Johnston (1940), who believed that a notochordal process (0.04 mm) and a prechordal plate (0.075 mm) were present. Florian in an appendix to the

article disagreed, and his interpretation is followed here (see stage 6).

Biggart. Described by Morton (1949). Curettage. Embryonic disc (narrow type), 0.27 × 0.16 mm. Primitive streak and node, 0.059 mm. A notochordal process is not referred to in the text but is mapped on a dorsal projection of the embryo (*ibid.*, fig. 2) and is approximately 0.04 mm in length. The specimen is said to resemble the Yale embryo.

Guá (Guálberto). Described by Lordy (1931). Hysterectomy. Chorionic cavity, 8 × 7.5 mm. Embryonic disc, 0.776 × 0.0465 mm. Primitive streak, 0.09 mm. Notochordal process, 0.045 mm. Possible notochordal canal. Said to resemble Hugo embryo. Probably belongs either to stage 7 or to stage 8.

Carnegie No. 7802 (figs. 7-4 to 7-12). An important specimen described and illustrated by Heuser, Rock, and Hertig (1945). Hysterectomy. Chorion, 3.75 × 2.35 × 2.2 mm. Chorionic cavity, 2.3 × 1.4 × 1.1 mm. Embryonic disc (broad type), 0.42 × 0.35 × 0.05 mm. Primitive streak, 0.11 mm, and node, 0.03 mm. Notochordal process, 0.048 mm. Presumed age, 16 days. Median projection published (*ibid.*, plate 6; Mazanec, 1959, fig. 46) and dorsal projection has been prepared by the present writers.

P.M. Described by Meyer (1924). Curettage. Measurements have been criticized by Stieve (1926) but defended by Mazanec (1959). Chorion, 3.9 × 3.77 × 2.5 mm. Chorionic cavity, 2.7 × 2.6 × 2.1 mm. Embryonic disc (circular), 0.41 × 0.41 mm. Primitive streak, 0.12 mm, and node, 0.02 mm. Notochordal process, 0.06 mm, acknowledged by Mazanec (1959) although denied by Fahrenholz (1927). No notochordal canal. Median projection published (Mazanec, 1959, fig. 47).

Hugo. Described by Stieve (1926), who reproduced a photomicrograph of every second section. Hysterectomy. Surrounded by 942 chorionic villi ranging in length from 0.3 to 1 mm. Chorion, 6.4 × 5.9 × 5.6 mm. Chorionic cavity, 4.7 × 4.4 × 3.8 mm. Embryonic disc (broad type), 0.635 (Florian, 1931) × 0.63 mm. Primitive streak, 0.245 mm, and node, 0.05 mm. Notochordal process, 0.07 (0.11?) mm. (Florian, 1934c). No notochordal canal. Prechordal plate probably not yet developed (Hill and Florian, 1931a). Dorsal and median projections published (Florian, 1934c, fig. 1; Hill and Florian, 1931b, figs. 44 and 11; Mazanec, 1959, fig. 49).

Robertson, O'Neill, and Chappell (1948) described a hysterectomy specimen that possessed a chorion of 3.816 × 3.639 × 2.687 mm. Chorionic cavity, 2.718 × 2.239 × 1.679 mm. Embryonic disc (broad type), 0.462 × 0.485 mm. Primitive streak, 0.138 mm, and node (situated halfway), 0.03 mm. Notochordal process, 0.072 mm. Suggestion of notochordal canal in one or two sections. Assigned to horizon VIII by authors but probably belongs to stage 7. Median projection published (*ibid.*, fig. 12).

D'Arrigo (1961) described an embryonic disc of 0.47 mm, which showed a notochordal process of 0.075 mm. Canalization of the process is "doubtful," but the presence of a prechordal plate is "probable." The specimen "could be recorded in Streeter's horizon VII."

Goodwin. Described by Kindred (1933). Tubal. Chorion, 5.8 × 2.72 × 2.25 mm. Chorionic cavity, 2.44 × 2.25 × 0.75 mm. Embryonic disc, 0.588 mm in width. Primitive streak, 0.215 mm, and node, 0.078 mm. Notochordal process, 0.078 mm. No notochordal canal and no prechordal plate.

Pha I. Described by Mazanec (1949). Chorionic cavity, 7.872 × 5.475 × 2.032 mm. Embryonic disc, 0.66 × 0.52 mm. Primitive streak, 0.145 mm, and node, 0.06 mm. Notochordal process, 0.09 mm. No prechordal plate. Median projection published (*ibid.*, fig. 51).

H. Schm. 10 (H. Schmid). Described briefly by Grosser (1931c). Embryonic disc (almost circular), 0.51 × 0.58 mm. Primitive streak, 0.14 mm, and node, 0.1 mm. Notochordal process, 0.1 mm. Probably belongs to stage 7, although a cavity in one section was thought to represent "Lieberkühn's canal."

Bi 24 (Bittmann). Described by Hill and Florian (1931b). Chorionic cavity, 3.05 × 3.036 × 3.029 mm. Embryonic disc (narrow type), 0.62 × 0.39 mm. Primitive streak, 0.28 mm, and node (Mazanec, 1959, fig. 105), 0.05 mm. Notochordal process, 0.105 mm, consists of median chord and lateral mesoblastic wings. Prechordal plate, 0.03 mm. Possible primordial germ cells in endoderm of region of cloacal membrane and in endoderm of umbilical vesicle caudally (Florian, 1931). Politzer (1933) counted 41 germ cells in the region of the allanto-enteric diverticulum in this embryo, and 19 such cells in another presomite specimen (Bi 25). Dorsal and median projections published (Hill and Florian, 1931b, figs. 4 and 12; Florian, 1945, plate 5, fig. 43; Mazanec, 1959, fig. 50).

Manchester No. 1285 (fig. 7-1). Described by Florian and Hill (1935). Hysterectomy. Chorionic cavity, 4.28 × 3.28 mm. Embryonic disc (narrow type), 0.87 × 0.625 mm. Primitive streak, 0.39 mm, and node, 0.05 mm. Notochordal process, 0.125 mm. Prechordal plate, 0.03 mm. Connecting stalk attached to chorion at decidua capsularis (suggesting polar variety of velamentous insertion of umbilical cord). Dorsal and median projections published (Hill and Florian, 1931b, figs. 5 and 13; Florian and Hill, 1935, figs. 1–3; Mazanec, 1959, fig. 52). Specimen is housed in Department of Anatomy, University of Manchester.

Pha II. Summarized by Mazanec (1959). Chorionic cavity, 4.985 × 3.882 × 3.52 mm. Embryonic disc, 0.895 × 0.62 mm. Primitive streak, 0.37 mm, and node, 0.06 mm. Notochordal process, 0.13 mm. No prechordal plate. Median projection published (*ibid.*, fig. 53).

Thompson and Brash (1923) described a specimen that showed a notochordal process of 0.3 mm. It is described in the present work under stage 8.

ADDITIONAL SPECIMENS

Precise measurements of the notochordal process have not been provided in the accounts of the following embryos. The specimens are listed in order of year of publication.

Debeyre (1912) described in detail a specimen that possessed a chorionic cavity of 5.6 × 2.1 mm. Embryonic disc, 0.9 × 0.6 × 0.95 mm. Primitive streak stated to be 0.54 mm in length. Chorionic villi (0.4–1.6 mm) showed some branching. Unsuitable plane of section makes it impossible to assess the specimen precisely.

Carnegie No. 1399, Mateer. Described by Streeter (1920). Hysterectomy. Angiogenesis in villi described by Hertig (1935). Chorion, 9 × 8 × 3.5 mm. Chorionic cavity, 6.1 × 5.6 × 2.5 mm. Embryonic disc, 1 × 0.75 mm. Primitive streak and groove present. Although the notochordal process was originally thought probably to be absent, Hill and Florian (1931b) have no doubt that it is present. More advanced than Hugo (Florian and Völker, 1929). A very small twin embryo was originally described but that "interpretation has become open to doubt" (Corner, 1955). Drawing of every section reproduced by Turner (1920). A median drawing (Davis, 1927, fig. 5A) and a projection have been published (Mazanec, 1959, fig. 56).

Ho (Hodiesne). Described by Fahrenholz (1927). Abortion. Chorionic cavity, 6.5 × 6 × 3 mm. Embryonic disc (deformed), 0.6 mm (0.725 mm by flexible scale). Primitive streak, 0.22 mm (0.345 mm by flexible scale). Notochordal process just beginning ("undoubtedly present," Hill and Florian, 1931b). Possible prechordal plate claimed (disputed by Waldeyer, 1929a, but supported by Hill and Florian, 1963). "Lieberkühn's canal" (0.065 mm) is an artificial folding of the embryonic disc (Hill and Florian, 1931b). Dorsal and median projections published (Fahrenholz, 1927, figs. 32, 6 and 7; Mazanec, 1959, fig. 54).

Debeyre (1933) described a specimen (0.9 mm) that possessed a primitive streak and probably belonged to stage 6 or stage 7. Large cells near the opening of the allantois were identified as primordial germ cells.

Falkiner. Described by Martin and Falkiner (1938). Curettage. Embryo damaged and not in good condition. Measurements seem too small (see Mazanec, 1959). Chorionic cavity, 1.5 × 1.4 mm. Embryonic disc, 0.15 × 0.29 mm. Primitive streak, 0.07 mm. Notochordal process contains "no definite lumen." Cells rostral to notochordal process are "probably" the prechordal plate. Development "agrees most closely" with that of Bi I. Median projection published (Mar-

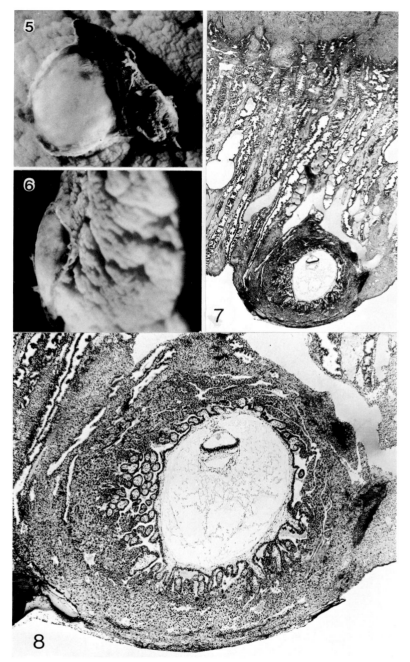

Fig. 7-5. Surface view of the implantation site of No. 7802, stage 7. Leakage of blood resulted in a clot which can be seen at the right-hand side of the photograph.

Fig. 7-6. Side view of the implantation site of No. 7802, stage 7.

Fig. 7-7. General view of the tissues at and near the implantation site (No. 7802, stage 7). A portion of the myometrium can be seen above. A cystic gland is present on the left-hand side of the mucosa. A large, branched vascular space partly surrounds the border zone of the specimen. Early decidua is present. Section 44-3-5.

Fig. 7-8. The chorionic vesicle of No. 7802, stage 7. The branched villi are evident. A cytotrophoblastic shell is forming. Section 44-3-5.

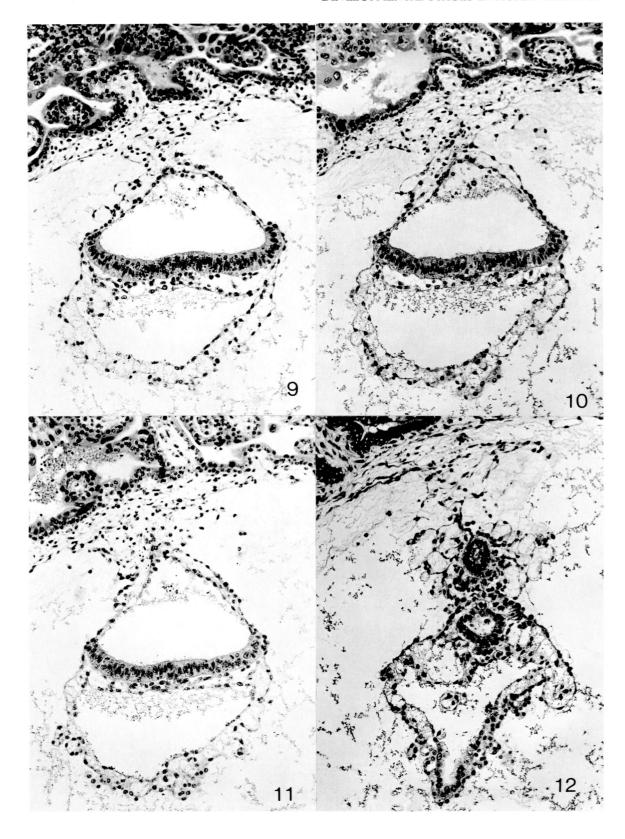

tin and Falkiner, 1938, fig. 8; Mazanec, 1959, fig. 39).

Gar (Green-Armytage). Described by West (1952). Hysterectomy. Chorionic cavity, 3 × 2.6 × 2 mm. Embryonic disc (broad type), 0.56 × 0.69 mm. Primitive streak, node, and groove present. Short notochordal process. No notochordal plate. Said to resemble Hugo embryo. Trophoblast described by Hamilton and Boyd (1960).

Mal (Maliphant). Described by West (1952). Hysterectomy. Chorionic cavity, 3 × 1.8 mm. Embryonic disc (broad type), 0.45 × 0.6 mm. Primitive streak, node, and groove present. Notochordal process present (Mazanec, 1959); small cavity in node (West, 1952) or in notochordal process (Mazanec, 1959) "hardly sufficient to warrant the name chorda canal." No prechordal plate. Belongs either to stage 7 or to stage 8

(said to resemble Jones-Brewer I, which is in stage 8).

Carnegie No. 8602. Photomicrograph reproduced by Hertig, Rock, and Adams (1956, plate 10, fig. 53). Chorion, 2.73 × 2.43 mm. Chorionic cavity, 1.83 × 1.33 mm. Embryonic disc, 0.3 × 0.06 mm. Presumed age, 16–17 days.

Missen. Trophoblast described by Hamilton and Boyd (1960). Curettage. Chorion, 1.66 × 1.43 mm. Embryonic disc, 0.28 × 0.214 mm. Primitive streak and node. Notochordal process. Said to resemble No. 7801 and Edwards-Jones-Brewer (stage 6). Presumed age, about 14 days.

Certain other embryos that probably belong to stage 7 but that have not been described in detail will not be referred to here. These include Fitzgerald, Fitzgerald-Brewer II, and Jones-Brewer II (Brewer and Fitzgerald, 1937).

Fig. 7-9. Embryo No. 7802, stage 7, to show the notochordal process, which appears as a clump of cells underlying the middle of the epiblastic plate. Some intra- as well as extra-embryonic mesoblast can be identified. Section 44-3-3.

Fig. 7-10. Embryo No. 7802, stage 7, to show the primitive node, which appears as a rearrangement of cells in and ventral to the middle of the epiblastic plate. A surface elevation is not present here. Section 44-2-2.

Fig. 7-11. Embryo No. 7802, stage 7, to show the primitive streak, which appears as a group of cells emerging from the ventral surface of the epiblastic plate. The wall of the umbilical vesicle is trilaminar. Section 44-1-2.

Fig. 7-12. The caudal end of embryo No. 7802, stage 7. A detached portion of the allantoic diverticulum can be seen above. Further ventrally, the caudal end of the amniotic cavity is evident, and the clump of cells in and on its ventral aspect represents the primordium of the cloacal membrane. The umbilical vesicle is readily visible in the lower half of the photomicrograph. Section 42-2-5.

STAGE 8

Approximately 1–1.5 mm in greatest length
Approximately 18 ± 1 postovulatory days
Characteristic features: presomitic; primitive pit; notochordal canal

Stage 8 is characterized by the appearance of one or more of the following features: the primitive pit, the notochordal canal, and the neurenteric canal. The embryo is presomitic, i.e., somites are not yet visible.

In Streeter's (1942) scheme, horizon VIII was characterized by "Hensen's node, primitive groove." Both these features, however, are present in embryos already assigned to horizon VII (e.g., No. 7802) and may even be found in at least some stage 6b specimens. It will be noticed, therefore, that the criteria employed here for stages 7 and 8 are *not* those of horizons VII and VIII, respectively; a similar statement will apply to stage 9 and horizon IX.

By this time, the third week of development, the uteroplacental circulation is well established, the decidua well formed, and the decidua capsularis healed over the conceptus (Hertig, 1968). Very much later, namely, at midterm, the decidua capsularis will fuse with the decidua parietalis, thereby obliterating the uterine cavity.

A fairly high incidence of sex chromatin has been recorded (Park, 1957) in the notochordal process and umbilical vesicle of two embryos of stage 8 (Nos. 7666 and 7701), and a lesser incidence in the amnion, trophoblast, and chorionic mesoblast, whereas none was found in two other specimens (Nos. 7949 and 8727).

Although doubts may be raised in regard to certain other specimens, the following definitely belong to stage 8 and may be taken as representative of that stage: Shaw, Kl.13, Dobbin, No. 5960, No. 7640, Peh. 1-Hochstetter, R. S., Western Reserve 1, Gläveke, and Strahl. Drawings of No. 5960 are provided in figures 8-3, 8-4, and 8-5.

A detailed investigation of this stage was undertaken by O'Rahilly and Müller (1981), who provided graphic reconstructions.

SIZE AND AGE

The maximum diameter of the chorion varies from 9 to 15 mm, that of the chorionic cavity from 3 to 10 mm (fig. 8-1). The embryonic disc is approximately 0.5–2 mm in length, and the age is believed to be about 18 days.

EXTERNAL FORM

The embryonic area is pyriform, being broader rostrally and tapering caudally. It may be possible to see the primitive node and the notochordal process from either dorsal (fig. 8-6) or ventral (fig. 8-7) view. The dorsal surface of the disc is slightly convex.

With the exception of those specimens that are either broad (No. 8820, Schö) or particularly elongated (Dobbin, Western Reserve 1), the dorsal surface of the embryonic disc appears ovoid (Wa 17) or pyriform (No. 5960). The interesting idea that two different types of young embryos occur was taken up and elaborated by Florian (1934a), who compared a "dwarf form" (*Zwergform:* Beneke, Bi 24, Wa 17, Western Reserve 1) with a "giant form" (*Riesenform:* Bi I, Hugo, Schö, Peh. 1-Hochstetter) at stages 6–8. O'Rahilly (1973) calculated an index (width × 100 ÷ length) for 55 specimens from stage 5c to stage 11. The result showed that eleven specimens had an index of more than 100 (broad specimens), one was at 100 (circular specimen), and 43 were below 100 (narrow specimens). Moreover, a gradual, relative elongation took place from stage 6 to stage 11. Specimens of stage 5c, which did not show definitive axial features, did not fit into the pattern. It may be concluded that Florian's study has served to emphasize that, from stages 6 to 8, wide

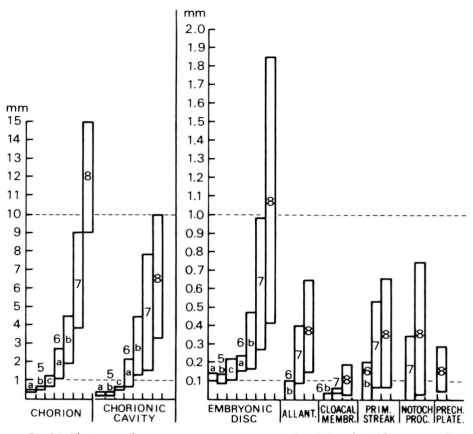

Fig. 8-1. The range of various measurements at stages 5 to 8. Based on 86 specimens (3 at stage 5a, 3 at 5b, 9 at 5c, 10 at 6a, 17 at 6b, 22 at 7, and 22 at stage 8). The two left-hand graphs are at a scale ten times greater than the others. It can be seen that the chorion attains a maximum diameter of 10 mm and the embryonic disc a length of 1 mm during stage 8.

variations in shape occur and embryos may be squat or, more commonly, elongated. As in the case of bodily habitus in the adult, however, a range is found, and it would be an oversimplification to attempt to force all examples into Laurel and Hardy types. Both the embryo and the adult are pleomorphic rather than dimorphic.

HISTOLOGICAL FEATURES

Decidua. The conceptus is embedded in the stratum compactum, which is sharply defined from the stratum spongiosum (No. 8820, Jones and Brewer, 1941, plate 4, fig. 10).

The first maternal vessels in communication with the lacunae appear to be venules or capillaries, so that the circulation in the lacunae is initially sluggish. It is said that "no direct arterial openings into the intervillous space are found in presomite embryos" (Hamilton and Boyd, 1960).

Amnion (figs. 8-8 and 8-12). The structure of the amnion resembles that seen in the previous stage. It is possible that "many of the cells of the amnion in the region of the peak undergo retrogressive changes and are sloughed into the amniotic cavity" (Jones and Brewer, 1941).

Embryonic disc (fig. 8-5). The ectodermal cells, mostly tall and columnar, rest upon a basement membrane except in the line of the axial formation. The transition to the flat cells of the amniotic ectoderm is sharp. Cells in mitosis are frequent. Small, deeply stained protein coagulatory granules are taken to be evidence of necrosis, which is said to be "noted in all normal young embryos" (Jones and Brewer, 1941). It may be men-

Stage 8

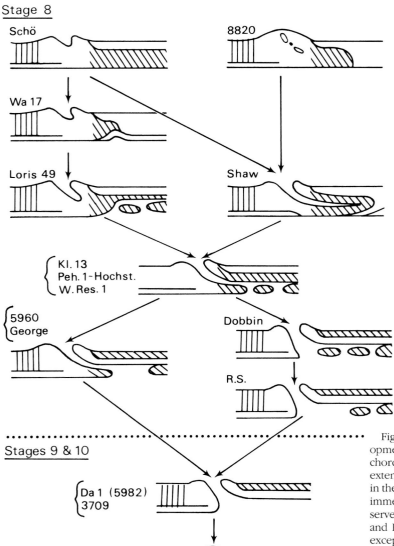

Fig. 8-2. Simplified scheme of the probable modes of development of canalization in the primitive node and in the notochordal process. The notochordal canal is formed at stage 8 and extends from the primitive pit into the notochordal process (as in the Shaw embryo). The floor of the canal breaks down almost immediately (as in Kl. 13, Peh. 1-Hochstetter, and Western Reserve No. 1), and the neurenteric canal appears (as in Dobbin and R.S.). All the specimens shown here are human, with the exception of *Loris* No. 49. The neurenteric canal, which first appears during stage 8, may still be found in certain embryos of stages 9 (Da 1) and 10 (No. 3709), but not in others (No. 1878 and No. 5074).

tioned in passing that cell deaths in normal human ontogeny have been studied chiefly in embryos from 3 mm in length onward (Ilieş, 1967).

Endoderm. The endoderm presents gentle elevations and depressions as seen from the ventral aspect, and its dorsal surface, "due to numerous extensions which lead toward the mesoderm, has the appearance of a range of mountains" (Heuser, 1932b).

By stage 5c the endoderm appears to be complete, i.e., it lines the umbilical vesicle and the ventral aspect of the embryonic disc. In stage 6b, when the primitive

streak and notochordal process form, the endodermal lining appears incomplete. No endoderm is present adjacent to the primitive streak (as shown by Brewer, 1938, in the Edwards-Jones-Brewer embryo) and notochordal process. The same is true for stage 7 (as shown by Hill and Florian, 1931b, Florian and Hill, 1935, and Florian, 1945, in the Hugo, Bi 24, and Manchester 1285 embryos). The situation becomes more complex in stage 8, when the endoderm begins to grow caudorostrally in the area of the primitive streak and node (as shown by Hill and Florian, 1931b, and

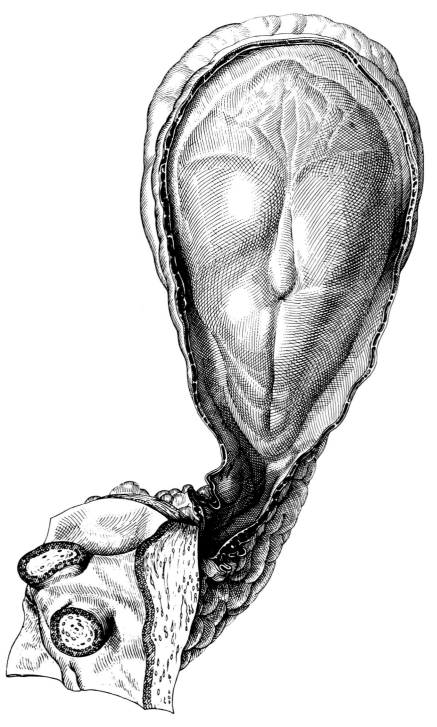

Fig. 8-3. Dorsal view of embryo No. 5960, drawn by James F. Didusch from a reconstruction. The amnion has been cut, and, on the dorsal surface of the embryonic disc, the neural groove, primitive node, and primitive groove can be identified in rostrocaudal sequence. A portion of the umbilical vesicle can be seen rostrally, and two chorionic villi appear in section in the lower left-hand corner.

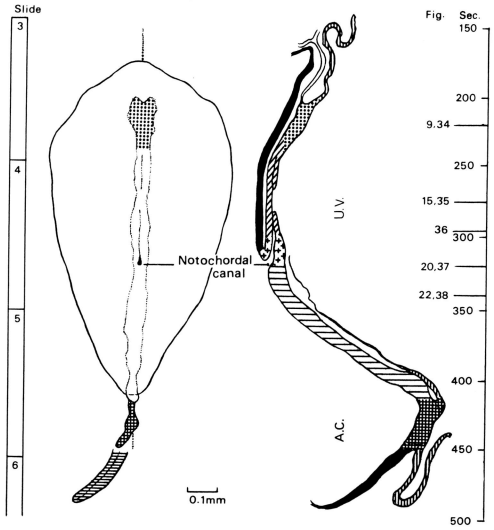

Fig. 8-4. Dorsal view and median reconstruction of No. 5960, stage 8, in alignment. The dorsal view, which is based on drawings by James F. Didusch (Heuser, 1932b, figs. 33 and 40), shows the prechordal plate, notochordal canal and primitive pit, cloacal membrane, and allanto-enteric diverticulum. The location of the prechordal plate is shown according to Heuser, and differs from the interpretation of Hill and Florian, who believed that the plate should be situated further rostrally. The system of shading is that shown in figure 7-1. The median reconstruction is based on a drawing by James F. Didusch (Heuser, 1932b, fig. 47). The notochordal canal can be seen to proceed from the primitive pit through the notochordal process, where the floor of the canal has disintegrated in its middle portion. Neither foregut nor hindgut is yet delineated. The allanto-enteric diverticulum can be seen caudally in close relation to the cloacal membrane. The figure references are to the sections reproduced by Heuser (1932b, plates 2 to 5).

Heuser, 1932, in the Dobbin, No. 5960, Peh. 1-Hochstetter, and Western Reserve 1 embryos). A clear succession is established whereby the least developed embryos have either no endoderm or a more restricted extent of it ventral to the primitive streak and node, as shown by O'Rahilly and Müller (1981, fig. 4): D (No. 9251), C (No. 9286), K (No. 9009B), E (No. 9123), B (No. 9009A), A (No. 8725), H (No. 5960), F (No. 8671), and G (No. 7545). In the last three cases the endoderm reaches as far as the primitive node. The most advanced embryos with regard to endodermal spread are also more advanced in other respects.

(Nos. 5960 and 7545 already show a neural groove.) It may be that this endoderm is derived from the caudal part of the primitive streak (fig. 6-2).

The area ventral to the notochordal process/plate remains free of endoderm also during stages 9 and 10. Only in stage 11, at the time when and in those places where the definitive notochord will form, does the endoderm become complete in the medial part of the embryonic intestinal roof. The mitotic figures giving rise to new endodermal cells are clearly found in the endoderm adjacent to the transforming notochordal plate (Müller and O'Rahilly, 1986c, fig. 2).

Neural plate and groove. The general area of the neural plate, comparable to that shown experimentally in the chick embryo, can be assessed (O'Rahilly and Gardner, 1971) at stages 7 and 8. Indeed, areas for the probable location of the future epidermis, neural crest, alar plate, and basal plate can be conceptualized in accordance with the scheme used for the chick blastoderm. In amphibian embryos it has been shown that the formation of the neural plate is "induced" by the "chordamesoderm," Spemann's organizer.

The neural groove (figs. 8-9 and 8-17) appears first in the more advanced specimens of stage 8: Nos. 5960, 7545, 7640, and 10157. These embryos possess a notochordal process longer than 0.4 mm. Another embryo (R.S.) is in very poor histological condition (Odgers, 1941), and further examples are either unconvincing (Triepel, 1916) or lack adequate mensural data (Cordier and Coujard, 1939). The neural groove has been recorded also in the M'Intyre and Gläveke embryos, which are very advanced in stage 8 and may even belong to stage 9.

The extent of the neural groove seems to be correlated not only with the length of the notochordal process but also with its shape. Four embryos that displayed a neural groove were also the only four out of eleven specimens in which the floor of the notochordal process was breaking down and a notochordal plate was present (O'Rahilly and Müller, 1981). Moreover, the neural groove was, in general, coextensive with the notochordal plate, reaching slightly more rostrally in two cases. Furthermore, the width of the neural groove corresponded approximately to that of the notochordal plate.

In summary, the first visible indication of the nervous system in the human embryo is the appearance of the neural groove during stage 8 (O'Rahilly and Müller, 1981). It appears before the heart or any of the other organs becomes visible.

Primitive node and streak. The primitive node has been recorded in most specimens. It varies from 0.03 to about 0.06 mm in length. The node may project above the surface, and it may (Nos. 5960 and 7640) be separated from the streak by a neck. In the intact embryo, the primitive node stands out as an opaque white spot (fig. 8-6). The node (fig. 8-2) may be merely indented by the primitive pit (Schö), possess some cavities (No. 8820), or be penetrated by a notochordal canal (Shaw). The cells of the node are large, possess more or less spherical nuclei, and tend to be arranged radially (Jones and Brewer, 1941). A plug (*Dotterpropf*) has been described immediately caudal to the dorsal opening of the notochordal canal (Rossenbeck, 1923).

The primitive streak (figs. 8-12 and 8-15) varies from 0.05 to 0.7 mm in length.

Embryonic mesoblast. Mesoblastic cells have by now spread beneath the entire surface of the ectoderm to reach the margin of the embryonic disc, where fusion with the extra-embryonic mesoblast occurs. The cellular density of the embryonic mesoblast is greatest near the primitive streak (Jones and Brewer, 1941, plate 5, fig. 11). Some mesoblastic cells are probably being contributed by the endoderm also (Heuser, 1932b). The extent of the mesoblast, however, is very variable (Grosser, 1934).

Somites. The initial appearance of somites is difficult to detect and is scarcely possible in transverse sections. Hence certain specimens that show very advanced features (e.g., a pericardial cavity) may well have possessed a pair of somites and may belong to stage 9 rather than to stage 8.

Coelom. Some isolated spaces are beginning to form in the mesoblast (in No. 5960) and, "from their position in the pericephalic region (figs. 6, 7, and 12) it is evident that they represent the pericardial cavities . . ." (Heuser, 1932b). Although such isolated spaces have been interpreted as the pericardial cavity, "no precardiac splanchnic cells could be identified in relation to such cysts," so that a pericardial cavity cannot be identified with certainty at stage 8 (de Vries, 1981). When the spaces coalesce, the typically U-shaped pericardial coelom is formed. This has been plotted by M'Intyre

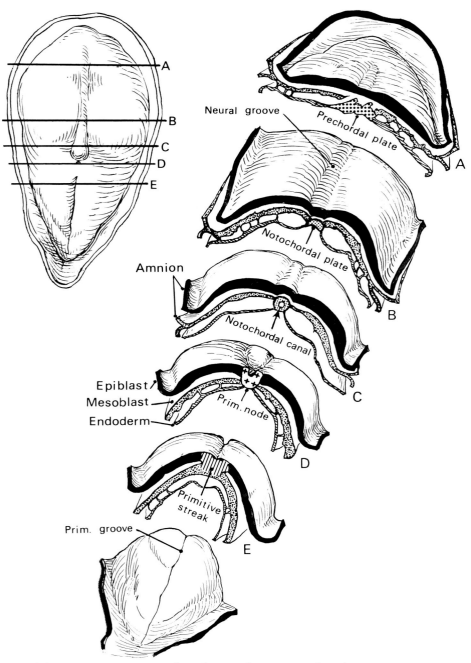

Fig. 8-5. Five transverse sections through No. 5960, stage 8, to show the arrangement of the germ layers and of the various axial features of the embryo. The levels of the sections *A* to *E* are shown also on a dorsal view of the intact embryo (inset drawing). The photomicrographs on which these sections are based are reproduced here in figures 8-8 to 8-12.

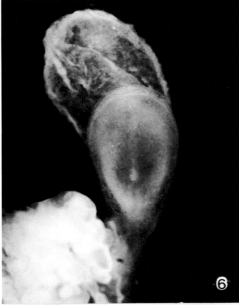

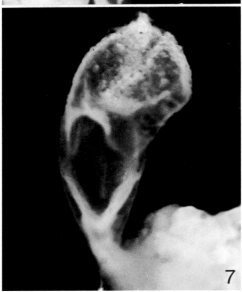

Fig. 8-6. Dorsal view of No. 5960, photographed in formalin. The primitive node appears as a conspicuous opaque knot from which the notochordal process extends rostrally. The umbilical vesicle is clearly visible in the upper third of the photograph, and the connecting stalk and adjacent chorion can be seen in the lower third.

Fig. 8-7. Ventral view of No. 5960, photographed in formalin. The notochordal plate can be detected. The umbilical vesicle is clearly visible in the upper third of the photograph, and the connecting stalk and adjacent chorion can be seen in the lower third.

(1926, text-fig. 7) but this advanced specimen may belong to stage 9. In another advanced embryo (Gläveke), which may also belong to stage 9, "a true typical endothelial anlage" of the heart, situated between the endoderm and the mesoblast, has been illustrated (Evans in Keibel and Mall, 1912, fig. 404). In summary, embryos that show a pericardial cavity or an indication of the heart belong probably to stage 9 rather than stage 8.

Notochordal process. The notochordal process, which varies from 0.01 to 0.8 mm in length, is fused with the endoderm and is in contact laterally with the mesoblast. Cytodesmata may be seen between the notochordal process and the overlying disc epiblast. The fully formed notochordal process, as seen in the Dobbin embryo, has been described as consisting of three portions (Hill and Florian, 1931b): (1) the rostral part, an undifferentiated cell mass, (2) the middle part, comprising a median, canalized process and two lateral mesoblastic bands, and (3) the caudal part, which lacks the lateral wings but possesses the notochordal canal.

Notochordal and neurenteric canals. The notochordal (or chordal) canal (of Lieberkühn) is initially indicated (fig. 8-2) merely by the primitive pit (in Schö) or by some cavities in the primitive node (in No. 8820). In its typical form, it extends from the primitive pit into the notochordal process (in Shaw), where the cells of the process are arranged around it in a radial manner (fig. 8-13). The intact canal is of very brief duration, however, and the floor of the canal, which becomes intercalated in the endoderm, begins to disintegrate at once in several places.

It should be stressed that the term "notochordal canal" is used for the canal in the notochordal process, that is, for the *Chordafortsatzkanal* or *Kopffortsatzkanal* (discussed by Springer, 1972), which is quite different from any cavity that may subsequently appear during the folding of the notochordal plate, an event that does not begin until during stage 10.

Already during stage 8 (fig. 8-2), in some areas (as many as seven in the Dobbin embryo) the floor of the notochordal canal may have disappeared (Kl.13, Peh. 1-Hochstetter, Western Reserve 1) so that the canal becomes replaced in part by a groove that opens ventrally into the umbilical vesicle. Rostrally, the canal reenters the tip of the notochordal process. The groove is situated in the notochoral plate, which is intercalated into the endoderm and, by increasing in thickness and breadth, appears to be more than "merely the remains of the dorsal wall of the chorda canal" (Odgers, 1941). Furthermore, "as Bryce and others have insisted, the breadth [of the plate] suggests that it must yield something more than simply the notochordal rudiment, i.e. that it probably helps to form the entoderm of the digestive" system (*ibid.*).

"It is probable that the disappearance of the ventral wall of the chorda-canal is subject to great individual variation, and cannot be used by itself as an infallible guide in estimating the stage of development" (Hill and Florian, 1931b).

The notochordal canal takes a course that goes from oblique to horizontal. With increasing breakdown of the canal floor a vertical (perpendicular to the disc) passage appears (in Dobbin and R. S.) and is known as the neurenteric canal (Odgers, 1941). Both canals commence in common dorsally in the primitive pit, and the neurenteric canal may be regarded as the remains of the notochordal canal at the level of the primitive node (Van Beneden, 1899).

Prechordal plate (figs. 8-8 and 8-16). The prochordal plate is a localized area of endoderm that becomes recognizable early in that part of the embryonic primordium destined to form the rostral region of the head of the vertebrate embryo, and with which the primordium of the notochord soon becomes continuous (Hill and Tribe, 1924).

The term "prochordal plate" (van Oordt, 1921) has been used above as a synonym for the inadvisable term "protochordal plate" (of Hubrecht), but it is also commonly employed (Gilbert, 1957) for a more restricted area known as the prechordal plate (*Praechordalplatte* of Oppel). Another and unjustified term sometimes found is the "completion plate of the head process" (*Ergänzungsplatte des Urdarmstranges* of Bonnet). The prochordal plate, in its wider sense, probably does not contribute to the notochord but gives origin to (1) cephalic mesenchyme, (2) at least a part of the lining of the foregut (all or a portion of the endodermal layer of the oropharyngeal membrane), (3) the preoral gut (Seessel's pocket), and (4) the prechordal plate in a restricted sense (Hill and Tribe, 1924). The production of mesenchyme by the prochordal plate in the human reaches its maximum only after the differentiation of the somites (Hill and Florian, 1931b).

In *Tarsius* (Hill and Florian, 1963), at a certain stage of development, the thickened endoderm becomes arranged as an "annular zone," the rostral part of which is constituted by the "prochordal complex" (prochordal plate of earlier stages). In the rabbit, on the other hand, a horseshoe-shaped zone of thickened endoderm has been found, and whether or not it corresponds with the rostral part of Hubrecht's annular zone remains an open question (Aasar, 1931). In the human also, a horseshoe-shaped band of thickened endoderm was detected by Hill and Florian (1931b) in some embryos of stages 6 (Beneke), 7 (Manchester 1285), and 8 (Thompson-Brash; Dobbin).

Either prechordal or prochordal, as used in a purely topographical sense, would seem to be a suitable term in the human embryo, and the former is employed in this study.

In most embryos of stage 8 the prechordal plate has been recorded as present, and it reaches its height of development (up to eight rows of cells) at that stage (O'Rahilly and Müller, 1981). It varies in rostrocaudal length from 0.03 to 0.3 mm. In No. 5960, for example, the plate (fig. 8-8) presents a very irregular dorsal surface "since cells are being given off to the surrounding tissue and some of them should no doubt be classified as mesodermal cells" (Heuser, 1932b). Chromatophil granules (as described by Bonnet) and small, isolated cavities, or perhaps even a channel (Odgers, 1941; George, 1942), may be found in the plate. Although the prechordal plate meets the notochordal process caudally, it does not ordinarily reach the rostral margin of the embryonic disc. Further detailed studies of the plate in the human embryo, however, are needed (Gilbert, 1957). The difficulties encountered in distinguishing and delimiting the prechordal plate can be seen from the fact that, in the case of one embryo (Manchester 1285), Hill and Florian changed their view concerning its limits and, in the case of a second specimen (No. 5960), these experts disagreed with another (Heuser) concerning its location.

The possible relationship of the prechordal plate to certain types of tumors, such as epignathus, was mentioned by Adelmann (1922). Defects in the prechordal plate may possibly result in holoprosencephaly or agenesis of the corpus callosum (Jellinger *et al.*, 1981).

In summary, the delimitation and first appearance

of the prechordal plate in the human embryo are not yet clear. It has been found in most embryos of stage 8, in some of stage 7 and even stage 6, and the possibility that it may be present at stage 5c has been raised.

Umbilical vesicle. The cavity of the umbilical vesicle is larger than that of the amnion, and the sac may project beyond the embryonic disc (No. 7640) or be approximately flush with it (Kl.13, No. 8820). The former relationship, however, is considered to be a distortion (George, 1942). Blood islands and blood vessels are seen in the wall of the umbilical vesicle, and an occasional cyst can also be found. Mesenchymal cells, hemocytoblasts, and primitive erythroblasts have been observed in the wall of the umbilical vesicle (No. 8820: Bloom and Bartelmez, 1940). A diverticulum of the vesicle may be present (Kl.13).

A rostrally situated fold of the umbilical vesicle (No. 5960) should not be mistaken for a precocious foregut. In more-advanced specimens (M'Intyre, Gläveke), which may, however, belong to stage 9, an indication of a foregut has been identified. A possible hindgut may be present in Peh. 1-Hochstetter (Florian, 1934b), but the assertion is not particularly convincing.

Primordial germ cells are probably not identifiable from the beginning of development, and probably arise from any of the totipotent or pluripotent cells of the early (e.g., 8-cell) embryo. The details of the arrival of the P.G.C. in the wall of the umbilical vesicle (perhaps by stage 8 and certainly by stage 11) are unknown.

In Bi 24, certain cells in the endoderm in the region of the cloacal membrane, as well as caudally in the endoderm of the umbilical vesicle, were thought to be probably primordial germ cells (Florian, 1931; Politzer, 1933). Such cells, although sought, were not found in some other specimens, however.

Cloacal membrane. The cloacal membrane varies from 0.02 to 0.185 mm in length. It has been suggested that "the cloacal membrane is early more extensive and that it later breaks down at the caudal end where the allantois is fused with the amniotic ectoderm" (Heuser, 1932b). The primitive groove may extend onto the cloacal membrane, as in the Dobbin embryo (Hill and Florian, 1931b).

Allantoic diverticulum (fig. 8-4). Either an allanto-enteric (No. 5960, Peh. 1-Hochstetter) or an allantoic (No. 8820, Western Reserve 1) diverticulum may be present. It varies in length from 0.14 to 0.65 mm. Vacuoles may be found in the cells of the rostral portion of the allantoic canal, and have been recorded there especially in later stages. The tip of the allantoic diverticulum may appear as a terminal vesicle and may even be separated from the remainder (Hill and Florian, 1931b).

Connecting stalk. The cells of the stalk are loosely arranged except in the proximity of the allantoic diverticulum. The stalk is covered by a layer of mesothelium, which forms thin-walled elevations that may be mistaken for blood vessels (Bremer, 1914), as may also certain vesicles within the stalk (Hill and Florian, 1931b). Because the vascular network comes in contact with the surface mesothelium in some areas, the latter may be a source, although not a very important one, of vascular endothelium (Heuser, 1932b). In other words, the mesothelium of the connecting stalk may possibly play some part in the formation of vessels (M'Intyre, 1926; but see also Hertig, 1935). Blood vessels are found in the wall of the umbilical vesicle, in the connecting stalk, and in the chorion and villi. Two anastomosing vessels (in Dobbin), one on each side of the allantoic diverticulum, are regarded as the primordia of the umbilical arteries, and a possible representative of the later primordium of the umbilical vein may be present (Hill and Florian, 1931b). The future umbilical arteries are the first channels that can be identified as vessels having a recognizable course (M'Intyre, 1926).

SPECIMENS OF STAGE 8 ALREADY DESCRIBED
(listed in order of length of notochordal process)

Pha XVII. Chorionic cavity, 3.317 × 2.79 × 0.714 mm. Embryonic disc, 0.412 mm. This embryo is said to resemble No. 7802 (stage 7). In addition to a notochordal process (Mazanec, 1959, fig. 104) of 0.01 mm, however, it is thought to show probably the Anlage of the notochordal canal and an unusually large prechordal plate. Possible primordial germ cells were seen in the wall of the umbilical vesicle. Presumed age, 16–17 days. Median projection published (*ibid.*, fig. 44).

Carnegie No. 8820, Jones-Brewer I. Described by Jones and Brewer (1941). Hysterectomy. Chorionic cavity, 6 × 5 × 2.5 mm. Embryonic disc (broad type), 0.58 × 0.78 mm (in straight line); 0.6 × 0.79 mm (over curve). Primitive streak, 0.22 mm. Primitive node (0.06 mm) situated somewhat rostral to midpoint of embryonic disc. Three small, discontinuous cavities in node "represent the beginning of a neurenteric canal" which has no dorsal opening and does not communicate with the umbilical vesicle. Notochordal

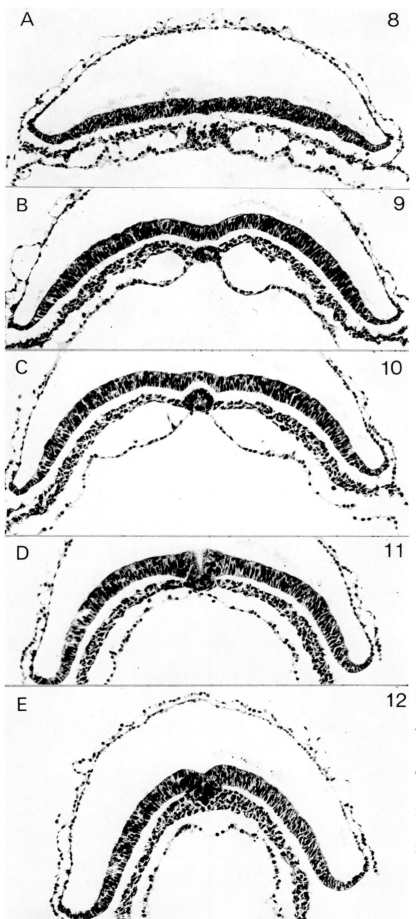

75

Fig. 8-8. The prechordal plate (Heuser's interpretation) of No. 5960.

Fig. 8-9. The notochordal plate of No. 5960. The developing neural groove can be seen.

Fig. 8-10. The notochordal process and canal of No. 5960.

Fig. 8-11. The primitive pit and node of No. 5960.

Fig. 8-12. The primitive streak and groove of No. 5960.

process, 0.0414 mm, but with no canalization. Hemocytoblasts and primitive erythroblasts identified in wall of umbilical vesicle (Bloom and Bartelmez, 1940). Presumed age, 18½ days. Dorsal and median projections published (Jones and Brewer, 1941, figs. 11 and 12; Mazanec, 1959, fig. 48).

Carnegie No. 9286. Embryonic disc, 1.13 × 0.77 mm. Primitive streak, 0.38 mm. Notochordal process, 0.15 mm. An excellent specimen reconstructed by O'Rahilly and Müller (1981, fig. 3), who give details of ten other Carnegie specimens.

Carnegie No. 9009. Described briefly in an abstract by Heuser (1954). Hysterectomy. Monozygotic twin embryos. Embryonic discs, 0.9 and 0.66 mm. In each: primitive node in middle of disc, notochordal process with first evidence of canalization. Notochordal processes, 0.16 and 0.07 mm. Assigned to horizon VIII by Heuser, who estimated the age as 17 days. Reconstructed by O'Rahilly and Müller (1981, fig. 2B,C).

Shaw. Described by Gladstone and Hamilton (1941). Hysterectomy. Chorion, 11 × 4.04 mm. Chorionic cavity, 8 × 3 mm. Embryonic disc (broad type), 1.05 × 1.34 mm. Notochordal process, 0.17 mm. Primitive pit and notochordal canal (which does not open into the umbilical vesicle). Prechordal plate identified but doubted by Mazanec (1959). No neural groove. Possible amniotic duct. Hemopoiesis (hemocytoblasts and primitive erythroblasts) under way in wall of umbilical vesicle and in connecting stalk. Chorionic villi and endometrium described by Hamilton and Gladstone (1942); trophoblast further described by Hamilton and Boyd (1960). Presumed age, 18 days. Median projection published (Gladstone and Hamilton, 1941; Mazanec, 1959, fig. 58).

Wa 17 (Wagner). Described by Grosser (1931a,b). Hysterectomy. Chorionic cavity, 8.5 × 8.5 × 7.5 mm. Embryonic disc (narrow type), 0.98 × 0.7 mm. Primitive streak, 0.5 mm. Notochordal process, 0.18 mm. Possible dorsal and ventral openings of the notochordal canal. Prechordal plate, 0.075 mm. Presumed age, about 19 days. Dorsal and median projections published (Grosser, 1931a, figs. 4 and 3; Hill and Florian, 1931b, fig. 7; Mazanec, 1959, fig. 59).

Carnegie No. 8671. Low-power photomicrographs reproduced by Hertig (1968, figs. 47 and 181). Notochordal process, 0.23 mm.

Kl. 13. Described by Grosser (1913). Traumatic abortion following salpingo-oophorectomy. Chorionic cavity, 8 × 6 mm. Embryonic disc, 0.67 × 0.5 mm. Primitive streak, 0.27 mm. Notochordal process, 0.2 mm. Notochordal canal, 0.25 mm (Florian, 1934c) with dorsal pit and ventral opening:

notochordal plate intercalated in endoderm. Possible prechordal plate. Presumed age, about 18 days. Median projection published (Grosser, 1913, plate 27, fig. 4; Mazanec, 1959, fig. 62). Compared with other specimens by Grosser (1934).

HEB-42. Described by Mazanec and Musilová (1959). Curettage. Embryonic disc, 1.17 × 0.72 mm; 1.43 mm by flexible scale. Primitive streak, 0.54 mm. Primitive node, 0.06 mm. Primitive pit. Notochordal process, 0.25 mm. Small cavity (primordium of notochordal canal) in notochordal process. Prechordal plate not mentioned. Presumed age, 17–18 days. Dorsal and median projections published (*ibid.*, figs. 1 and 2).

Dy (Dyhrenfurth). Described by Triepel (1916). Abortion. Embryonic disc, 1.6 × 1.04 mm. Primitive streak, 0.11 mm. Notochordal process and plate, 0.3 mm. Primitive pit, neurenteric canal, and neural groove believed to be present. Anlagen of hypophysis and optic vesicles claimed unconvincingly (plane of section unsuitable). Embryonic disc bent ventrally through a right angle (normality of specimen questioned). First somite probably not present.

Thompson and Brash (1923) described a hysterectomy specimen that showed a chorionic cavity of 10 × 7.5 × 4 mm. Embryonic disc (broad type), 0.68 × 0.9 mm. Primitive streak and groove present. Notochordal process, 0.3 mm, with no distinct lumen but notochordal canal about to appear. Mazanec (1959) considered that, on the basis of the reconstruction, the notochordal process could not be more than 0.23 mm. Definite prechordal plate (Hill and Florian, 1931b). Rough dorsal and median drawings included (Thompson and Brash, 1923, figs. 2 and 3) and median projection published (Mazanec, 1959, fig. 55). This embryo belongs either to stage 7 or to stage 8.

Schö (Schönholz). Described by Waldeyer (1929a,b). Hysterectomy. Embryonic disc, 0.99 × 1.03 × 0.11 mm. Primitive streak, 0.51 mm, and node. Primitive groove and pit: "indentation" is perhaps "first Anlage of [notochordal] canal." Notochordal process, 0.34 mm. Prechordal plate. Said to lie between Hugo (stage 7) and Peh. 1-Hochstetter (stage 8). Dorsal and median projections published (*ibid.*, figs. 6 and 5; Hill and Florian, 1931b, figs. 6 and 14; Mazanec, 1959, fig. 57).

Dobbin. Important specimen described in detail by Hill and Florian (1931a,b,c). Abortion. Chorion, 11.5 × 8.5 × 4.5 mm. Chorionic cavity, 9 × 5.5 × 2.5 mm. Embryonic disc (narrow type), 0.96 × 0.41 mm. Primitive streak, 0.42 mm to notopore. Notochordal process, 0.42 mm. Notochordal canal communicates with cavity of umbilical vesicle by seven openings, the caudalmost of which is the ventral open-

Fig. 8-13. The notochordal process and notochordal canal of No. 7545. Section 4-2-14. Cf. fig. 8-18.

Fig. 8-14. The primitive pit of No. 7545. Section 4-3-7. Cf. fig. 8-19.

Fig. 8-15. The primitive groove and primitive streak of No. 7545. Section 5-2-9.

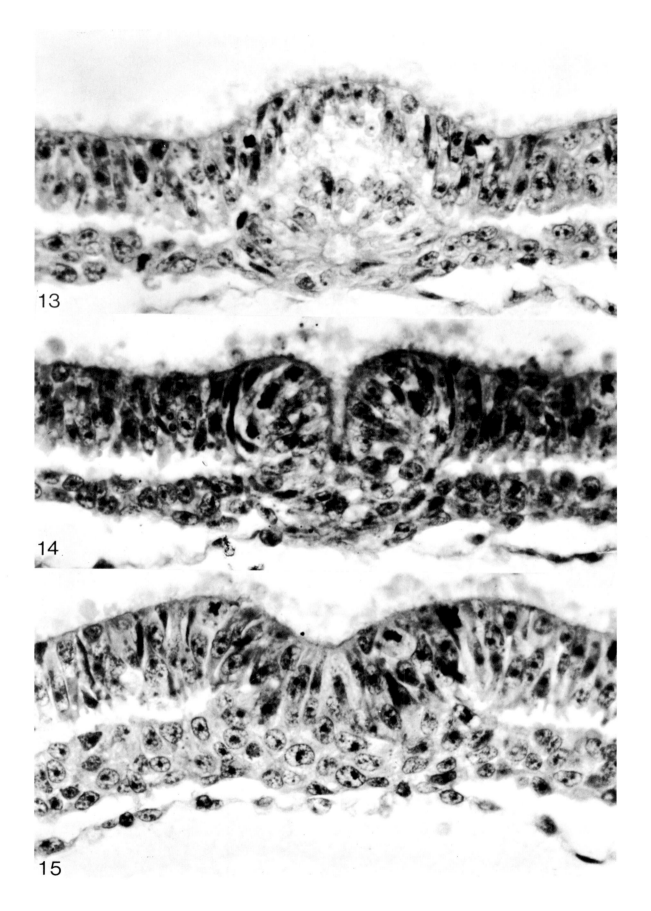

13

14

15

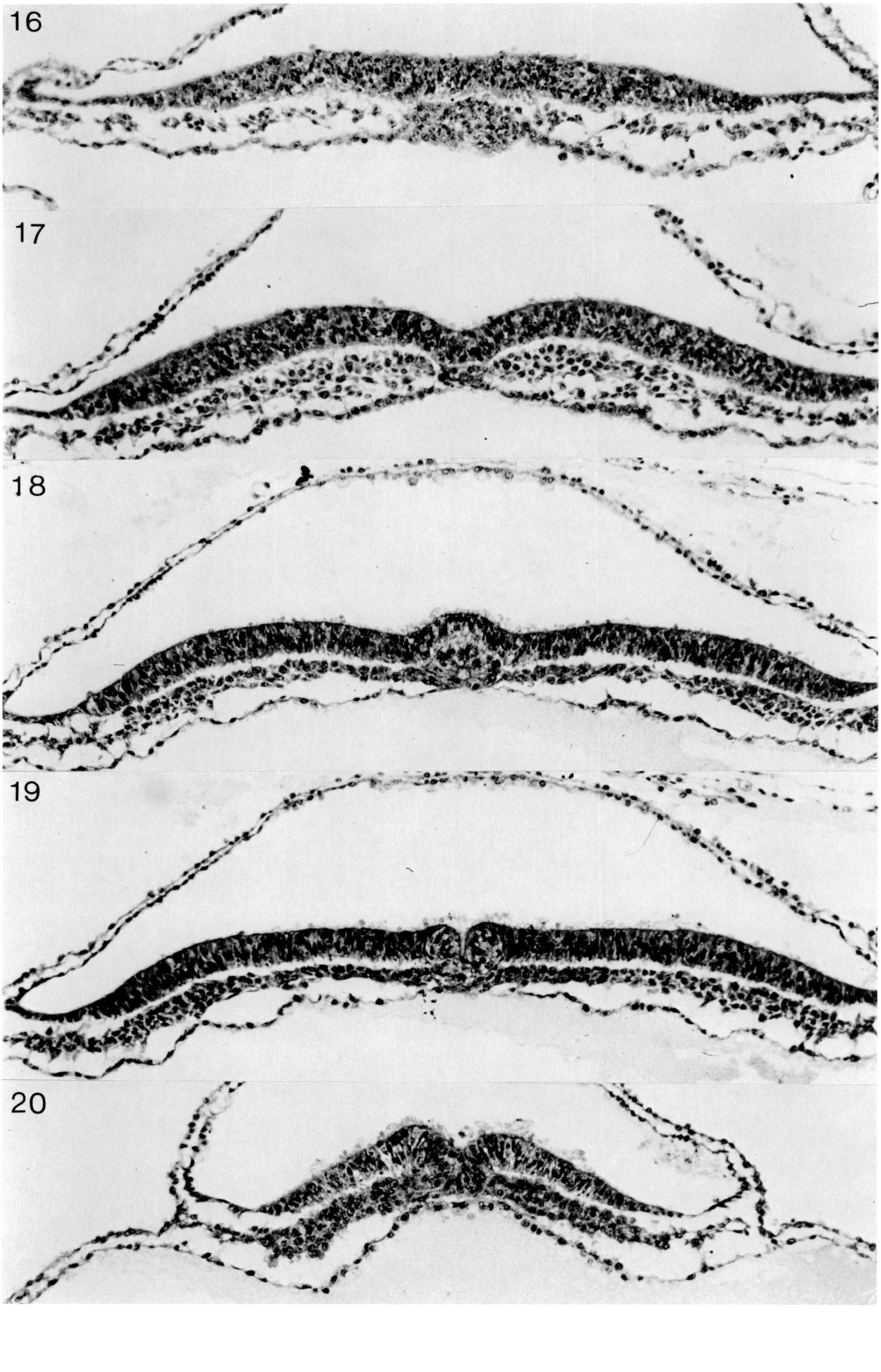
16
17
18
19
20

ing of a very short neurenteric canal. Prechordal plate, 0.03 mm; rostral end of notochordal process was at first mistaken for prechordal plate. Dorsal and median projections published (Hill and Florian, 1931b, figs. 1 and 2; Mazanec, 1959, fig. 60). The scale in fig. 3 of Hill and Florian (1931b) is incorrect (Florian, 1934c). Specimen is now housed in Hubrecht Laboratory, Utrecht (No. H91; HH 159).

Carnegie No. 5960 (figs. 8-3 to 8-12). Important specimen described by Heuser (1932b). Hysterectomy. Chorion, 15 × 14 × 9 mm. Embryonic disc (narrow type), 1.25 × 0.68 mm (in straight line); 1.53 × 0.75 mm (by flexible scale). Primitive streak, 0.5 (0.44?) mm. Primitive node, 0.2 (0.06?) mm, slightly caudal to midpoint of embryonic disc. Notochordal process, 0.42 mm (George, 1942). Notochordal canal (about 0.4 mm) opens ventrally. Prechordal plate, 0.15 mm. Florian (1934b), however, believed that the prechordal plate was situated further rostrally than shown by Heuser. Angiogenesis in umbilical vesicle, body stalk, and chorion. Angiogenesis in chorion described by Hertig (1935). Neural groove. Presumed age, 18 days. Dorsal and median projections published (Heuser, 1932b, figs. 33 and 47; Mazanec, 1959, fig. 63).

Carnegie No. 7545 (figs. 8-13, 8-14, 8-15, and 8-16 to 8-20). Embryonic disc, 1.52 × 1.03 mm. Primitive streak, 0.61 mm. Notochordal process, 0.43 mm. Reconstructed by O'Rahilly and Müller (1981, fig. 2E).

Carnegie No. 7640. Described by George (1942). Tubal. Embryonic disc (broad type), 1.01 × 0.83 mm (in straight line); 1.16 mm by flexible scale. Primitive streak, node, and pit present. Notochordal process, 0.44 mm. Notochordal canal continuous with primitive pit; floor of canal has disappeared in its middle quarter. Prechordal plate, 0.12 mm, said to contain continuation of notochordal canal. Neural groove. Dorsal and median projections published (*ibid.*, figs. 1 and 2).

Peb. 1-Hochstetter (Peham). Described by Rossenbeck (1923). Chorion, 10 × 7.7 mm. Chorionic cavity, 6.8 × 5.3 mm. Embryonic disc (broad type; this might be disputed, however), 1.77 (Florian, 1934) × 1 mm. Primitive streak, 0.69 mm. Notochordal process (Mazanec, 1959, figs. 107 and 108), 0.6 mm. Notochordal canal ready to break through into umbilical vesicle in one section. Prechordal plate (confirmed by Florian, 1931), 0.08 mm. Indication of hindgut (Florian, 1934b). Allanto-enteric diverticulum (Florian, 1930a). Dorsal

and median projections published (Hill and Florian, 1931b, figs. 9 and 16; Mazanec, 1959, fig. 61).

R. S. (Robb Smith). Described by Odgers (1941). Hysterectomy. Embryonic disc (broad type), 1.5 × 1.36 mm. Primitive streak, 0.4 mm. Notochordal plate (intercalated in endoderm), 0.7 mm. Neurenteric canal extends vertically from amniotic cavity to umbilical vesicle. Prechordal plate, 0.29 mm, containing perhaps remains of notochordal canal. Commencing neural groove. Dorsal and median projections published (*ibid.*, figs. 1 and 2).

Western Reserve No. 1. Described by Ingalls (1918). Abortion. Chorion, 9.1 × 8.2 × 6.5 mm. Chorionic cavity, 8 × 7 × 5 mm. Embryonic disc (narrow type), 2 (1.87?) × 0.75 mm. Primitive streak, 0.67 mm. Primitive pit present. Notochordal process, 0.75 (0.65?, Hill and Florian, 1931b) mm. Notochordal canal, 0.34 mm, with three ventral openings into umbilical vesicle. Prechordal plate identified (but not 0.4 mm in length, according to Mazanec, 1959). Dorsal and median projections published (Hill and Florian, 1931b, figs. 10 and 17; Mazanec, 1959, fig. 64).

ADDITIONAL SPECIMENS

Precise measurements of the notochordal process have not been provided in the accounts of the following embryos.

M'Intyre. Described by Bryce (1924) and M'Intyre (1926). Hysterectomy. Chorion, 14 × 13 × 8 mm. Embryonic disc, 1.37 × 0.5 mm. Primitive streak, 0.32 mm. Notochordal plate, neurenteric canal, and prechordal plate (with cavity) present. Neural groove, future foregut, U-shaped pericardial cavity, and "some general resemblance to somites" noted. Rough dorsal and median drawings included (Bryce, 1924, figs. 5 and 49). May belong to stage 9.

Frassi's specimen (Keibel, 1907; Frassi, 1908) was illustrated as *Normentafel* No. 1 by Keibel and Elze (1908). Embryonic disc, 1.17 × 0.6 mm. Primitive streak and neurenteric canal identified. Neural groove. No somites.

Gle., or *Gläveke* (von Spee, 1889 and 1896). Illustrated as *Normentafel* No. 2 by Keibel and Elze (1908). See also Kollmann (1907) and Keibel and Mall (1910, 1912). Chorion, 6 × 4.5 mm. Chorionic cavity, 5.3 × 3.8 mm. Embryonic disc, 1.54 mm. Primitive streak and node, notochordal plate, and

Fig. 8-16. The prechordal plate of No. 7545. Section 2-4-13.

Fig. 8-17. The neural groove of No. 7545. Section 3-3-9.

Fig. 8-18. The notochordal process and notochordal canal of No. 7545. Section 4-2-14. Cf. fig. 8-13.

Fig. 8-19. The primitive pit of No. 7545. Section 4-3-7. Cf. fig. 8-14.

Fig. 8-20. The primitive groove and primitive streak of No. 7545. Section 6-1-2.

neurenteric canal (Van Beneden, 1899) identified (Keibel and Mall, 1912, fig. 231). Neural groove. Indication of foregut and pericardial cavities. Anlage of endocardium. No somites detected, although a small cavity on the left side (Keibel and Elze, 1908, fig. 4f) could be considered as the first Anlage of a myocoele. May belong to stage 9.

Strahl (1916) described briefly a specimen that possessed a notochordal process and canal, and apparently a prechordal plate. A median drawing was included (*ibid.*, fig. a) but measurements were not provided.

Vuill., or *Vulliet.* Illustrated schematically by Eternod (1899a and 1909), Kollmann (1907), and Keibel and Mall (1912). Chorion, 10 × 8.2 × 6 mm. Chorionic cavity, 9 × 7.2 × 5 mm. Embryonic disc, 1.3 mm. Notochordal and neurenteric canals (Eternod, 1899b).

Cordier and Coujard (1939) described an embryo of 1.05 mm showing a neural groove and folds, notochordal canal, primordial germ cells, but no somites, no intra-embryonic coelom, and no cardiac rudiment.

Carnegie No. 8727. Photomicrograph reproduced by Hertig (1968, fig. 180). The partial duplication of the embryonic disc shown in this specimen would presumably have resulted in conjoined twins.

Certain other embryos that probably belong to stage 8 but that have not been described in adequate detail will not be referred to here. These include Krukenberg (1922) and Fitzgerald-Brewer I (Brewer and Fitzgerald, 1937). Boerner-Patzelt and Schwarzacher (1923) described an unsatisfactory specimen (embryonic disc, 0.47 × 0.43 mm) that showed a neurenteric canal. Broman (1936) described in detail an abnormal specimen ("Lqt") in which the primitive streak showed "overgrowth" in relation to the neurenteric canal, resulting in a dislocation within the embryonic disc.

STAGE 9

Approximately 1.5–2.5 mm

Approximately 20 ± 1 postovulatory days

Characteristic feature: 1–3 pairs of somites

Now that the neural groove and the first somites are present, the "embryo proper" may be said to have been formed (van Oordt, 1921). The criteria used in distinguishing stages 5–9 are shown graphically in figure 9-1.

Stage 9 is defined by the number of somites present, namely 1–3 pairs. Although the degree of development is in general agreement with the number of somites, exceptions do occur.

At a certain period in vertebrate development, the number of pairs of somites that are clearly visible constitutes a simple and fairly accurate criterion for staging. Thus, in *Ambystoma maculatum*, stages 17–23 of Harrison show 1–6 somite pairs, respectively. In *Gallus domesticus*, a stage has been assigned to every third pair of somites that is added: stage 7, 1 pair; stage 8, 4 pairs; stage 9, 7 pairs; etc. In the human, greater spans of somitic pairs have been assigned to each stage. Thus, after the first 3 pairs have appeared at stage 9, stage 10 shows 4–12 pairs, stage 11 presents 13–20 pairs, and stage 12 possesses 21–29 pairs, after which time counting becomes more difficult and other criteria are emphasized.

In Streeter's (1942) scheme, horizon IX was characterized by "neural folds, elongated notochord." The neural folds, however, can appear during stage 8 (O'-Rahilly and Gardner, 1971; O'Rahilly and Müller, 1981). Moreover, now that horizon X ("early somites present," Streeter, 1942) has been limited specifically to "4 to 12 somites" (Heuser and Corner, 1957), it follows that the first 3 pairs of somites must appear earlier, namely, during stage 9.

Stages 1–3 are sometimes referred to as pre-implantation stages, stage 5 as previllous, stages 6–8 as presomitic, and stage 9 to approximately stage 13 as somitic stages.

Embryos of stage 9 are very rare. Fortunately two have been described in considerable detail (figs. 9-2 and 9-5). A great need exists, however, for further

thorough accounts of specimens of excellent quality.

A detailed investigation of this stage was undertaken by Müller and O'Rahilly (1983), who provided graphic reconstructions.

SIZE AND AGE

Embryos of stage 9 vary from approximately 1.5–3 mm in length, and are believed to be about 20 days in age.

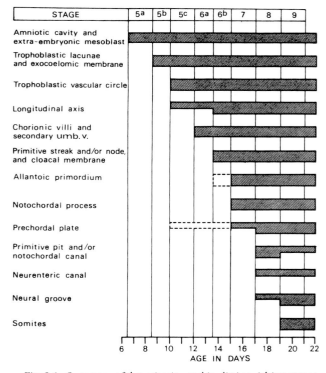

Fig. 9-1. Summary of the criteria used in distinguishing stages 5–9. The shaded bars indicate the stages at which a given feature is found. The following are not used: appearance of amniotic cavity, appearance of umbilical vesicle, branching of chorionic villi, cloacal membrane, allantoic diverticulum, prechordal plate, neural groove and neural folds.

81

EXTERNAL FORM

As seen from the dorsal aspect, the embryo is frequently described as shaped like the sole of a shoe (fig. 9-3).

Many, perhaps most, embryos of stages 9 and 10 display a dorsal concavity ("lordosis") which has been subject to considerable discussion (fig. 9-4). Although abrupt bends and kinks are artifacts, "anything from a gentle convexity to a moderate dorsal concavity must be considered normal" (Heuser and Corner, 1957). An excellent example can be seen in figure 9-8. At stage 9, the rostral and caudal ends of the embryo begin to be elevated "above" (dorsal to) the level of the umbilical vesicle. It should be kept in mind, however, that a dorsal concavity is augmented by the collapse of the umbilical vesicle; indeed, wrinkling of the vesicle and dorsal flexure increase *pari passu* during dehydration (Bartelmez and Evans, 1926).

Although an indication of a head fold may perhaps be detectable in a few embryos of stage 8, the caudal

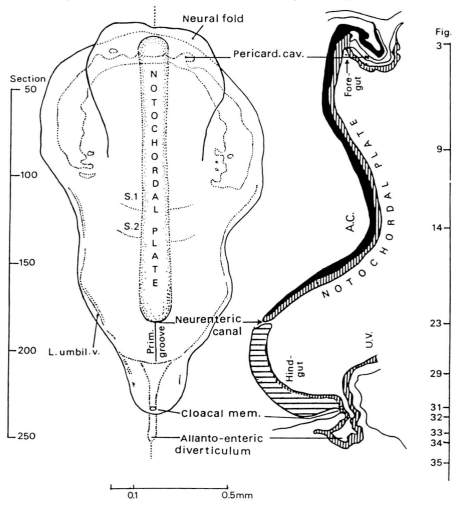

Fig. 9-2. Dorsal view and median reconstruction of embryo Da 1 (No. 5982), in alignment. The dorsal view, which is based on an illustration published by Ludwig (1928, fig. 2), shows the neural folds, pericardial cavity, notochordal plate, and somites. The median reconstruction is based on the same author (fig. 1). The foregut and hindgut are beginning to form, and the neurenteric canal and the allanto-enteric diverticulum are evident. The figure references are to the sections reproduced by Ludwig among an extensive series of photomicrographs.

fold does not appear until during stage 9 (in embryo Da 1). With the continuing elevation of the neural folds, lateral limiting sulci appear at first rostrally and then in the caudal part of the embryo (Da 1).

Studies of the chick embryo have led to the conclusion that "detachment of the head from the blastoderm is brought about to a lesser degree by independent head-fold formation, and to a greater degree by an influence of the fast-growing brain. Presence of detached fore-gut is a necessary prerequisite for head detachment" (Gruenwald, 1941a). Moreover, "we must abandon the conception of a simple folding of the blastoderm as the cause of detachment" not only for the rostral but also for the caudal end of the body and the corresponding gut. However, the process at the caudal end is "entirely different from that found in the head region. Here, too, the detachment is most probably due to growth of the body beyond its attachment to the blastoderm" (*ibid.*).

HISTOLOGICAL FEATURES

Amnion. An amniotic duct may be present (No. 1878).

Embryonic disc. Differentiation has now proceeded to the point where the various systems of the body can be discussed separately.

Primitive streak. The primitive streak extends from the cloacal membrane to the neurenteric canal. Rarely can its entire extent be appreciated in dorsal view (H3); usually it appears foreshortened (No. 1878) and may also be curved (Da 1). A primitive groove may be found but a distinct node may not always be readily distinguishable. When the obliquity and curvature of the streak are taken into account, the primitive streak occupies from one-third (Da 1; H3) to one-quarter (No. 5080; No. 1878) of the length of the embryo. This fraction becomes further reduced during stages 10 and 11 (Bartelmez and Evans, 1926).

Mesoderm. The mesoderm, as the mesoblast may now be termed, is arranged on each side as (1) a longitudinal, paraxial band (nicely shown in Ludwig's reconstruction, plate 2, figs. 3 and 4), and (2) a lateral plate. The paraxial mesoderm is beginning to become segmented in the junctional region with the spinal cord, i.e., RhD (Müller and O'Rahilly, 1983; O'Rahilly and Müller, 1984b).

Although no nephric structures are found until stage 10, the general region of the intermediate mesoderm can be made out in stage 9 between the paraxial mesoderm and the lateral plate. (It is particularly clear, for example, on the right side of sections 115–117 of embryo Da 1.)

Somites. Somites are first visible at stage 9, and the 1–3 pairs present are presumed to be occipital. The first pair appears immediately caudal to the level of the midpoint of the notochordal plate (No. 5080). The somites may differ in number on the two sides of the body (No. 1878). Cavities (the so-called myocoeles) may be detectable in the somites (fig. 9-11).

Coelom. The appearance of the coelomic cavity has the effect of splitting the lateral plate into somatopleuric and splanchnopleuric layers.

The pericardial cavity (figs. 9-2, 9-7, 9-9, and 9-10) is a constant finding. It appears as a horseshoe-shaped space, together with associated vesicles, within the mesoderm of the rostral half of the embryo (No. 5080, Davis, 1927, figs. 2 and 3; Da 1, Ludwig, 1928, fig. 2). The limbs of the horseshoe begin blindly on each side at the level of the first somite. Here the cavities closely approach the extra-embryonic coelom although the intra-embryonic coelom remains closed throughout. At first the right and left limbs do not intercommunicate (No. 5080) but soon do so (Da 1; No. 1878). The small, discrete vesicles associated with the limbs of the horseshoe are coelomic spaces that have not as yet joined the larger cavities. They suggest the mode of formation of the coelomic cavity, namely the fusion of discrete vesicles. Some indications of coelomic formation caudally may be detected (Ludwig, 1928), and distinct bilateral cavities are present in one specimen (fig. 9-13).

Notochordal plate. The notochordal plate (about 0.66 mm in length in Da 1) is intercalated into the endoderm (fig. 9-2). It extends rostrally almost as far as the oropharyngeal membrane, and, caudally, it blends with the primitive node. Extracellular granules in the prechordal plate, notochordal process, primitive streak, and neural plate have been noted in presomitic and early somitic embryos (Allan, 1963).

Neurenteric canal. The neurenteric canal (fig. 9-2) may be completely patent (Da 1; H3; see Wilson, 1914, fig. 7), only partly patent (No. 5080), or completely closed (No. 1878). The neurenteric canal appears first during stage 8 (e.g., in Dy, R.S., M'Intyre, Gläveke, Vuill.)

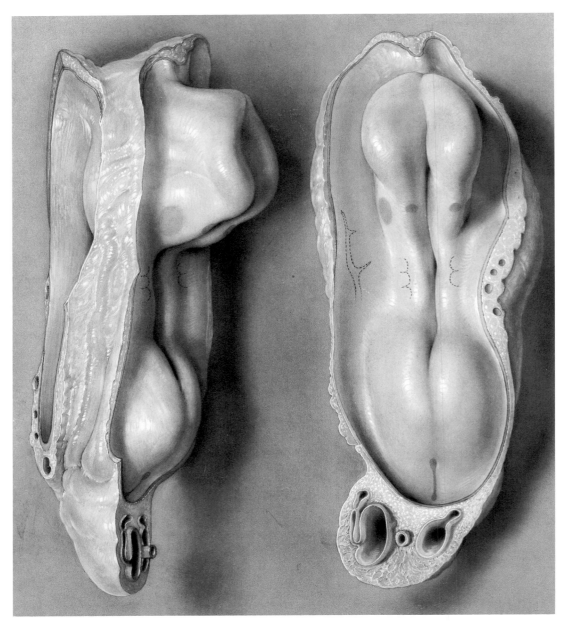

Fig. 9-3. Left lateral and dorsal views of No. 1878, as depicted by James F. Didusch in 1919. Cf. figures 9-4 and 9-5. Approximately one-half of the longitudinal extent of the neural groove represents the future brain.

and is found in some embryos of stages 9 and 10.

Persistence of the neurenteric canal (Dodds, 1941), associated with duplication of the notochord (Saunders, 1943), may be important in the production of combined anterior and posterior rhachischisis. Frequently a patent connection between gut and spinal cord is present (Gruber, 1926; Dénes *et al.*, 1967).

Prechordal plate. The prechordal plate consists of several layers of cells that resemble those of the neural plate. Rostrally, the prechordal plate usually separates from the neural plate and becomes continuous laterally with the cardiac mesoderm. The fusion of the rostral end of the notochordal plate with the mesoderm in Da 1 was thought by Hill and Florian (1931b) to be

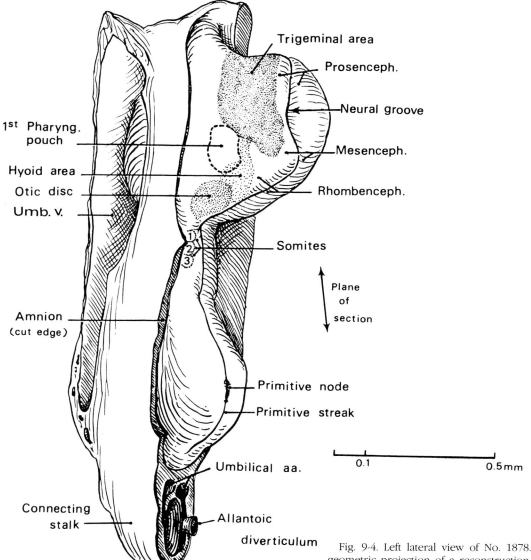

Fig. 9-4. Left lateral view of No. 1878. Based largely on a geometric projection of a reconstruction reproduced by Bartelmez and Evans (1926, plate 3, fig. 3). The ectodermal areas of the cephalic region are indicated by stippling. The mesencephalic flexure of the brain is evident.

the prechordal plate. It was believed to be identifiable in embryo Gv also.

The location of the prechordal plate in the human appears to correspond to "the axial mesoderm between the first pair of somitomeres" in the mouse (Meier and Tam, 1982). These authors found seven "segmental units" or "somitomeres" (derived from the primitive streak) in the paraxial region rostral to the first somite, so that "the cranial axis of the mouse

embryo is initially organized into segments like the rest of the body." Furthermore, their morphogenesis "is coordinate with neurulation."

The prechordal plate, which is in the longitudinal axis of the embryo at stage 8 (O'Rahilly and Müller, 1981, fig. 4), gradually becomes rotated in association with the head fold, so that it comes to lie at a right angle. The cardiogenic plate, which merges with the prechordal plate material, is also undergoing reversal.

Umbilical vesicle (fig. 9-9). Blood islands are numerous and a vitelline plexus is visible. A small diverticulum of the umbilical vesicle has been described (No. 1878).

Cloacal membrane. Even now, this union of ectoderm and endoderm "is in a way hardly a membrane" (Ingalls, 1920).

Allantoic diverticulum. Either an allanto-enteric (Da 1) or an allantoic (No. 1878) diverticulum may be present. It runs between the umbilical arteries (fig. 9-4).

In the chick, rotation at the caudal end of the embryo alters the allantois in such a way that it becomes partly unfolded (Gruenwald, 1941a). The allantois then becomes a shallow diverticulum of the hindgut (*ibid.*, fig. 6), although "it is highly probable . . . that the proximal part of the allantoic pocket contributes to the formation of the floor of the hindgut."

Connecting stalk. The vascular channels are well developed and occupy most of the stalk, which is quite thick. The right and left umbilical arteries are readily distinguishable, one on each side of the allantoic diverticulum. The future umbilical veins are represented by a vascular plexus which communicates with the arteries. Blood islands have been identified in the connecting stalk as well as over the umbilical vesicle.

CARDIOVASCULAR SYSTEM

Blood vascular system. Blood vessels are arising in several separate regions (Ingalls, 1920): the chorion, the connecting stalk, the umbilical vesicle, and the embryo proper, together with its amnion. The connections between these vessels are secondary, and they are established at various times and in a number of different places.

Within the body of the embryo, the two omphalomesenteric veins are distinguishable. Each enters the corresponding horn of the sinus venosus. Also present within the body are the first pair of aortic arches, the beginning of the internal carotid arteries, and, at least in an interrupted course, the two dorsal aortae (Ingalls, 1920). A closed circulation, however, is not yet present. The aortae constitute medial vascular tracts, whereas lateral tracts consist of the vitelline veins and the cardiac rudiments (Ludwig, 1928, plate 3, fig. 6). It seems that the connection of the vitelline plexus with the aorta caudally antedates the connection with the heart rostrally (Ingalls, 1920). In No. 1878 the sole union of

intra- and extra-embryonic vessels is provided by the aorta, which communicates (at least unilaterally) with the vitelline plexus. Either no blood cells (Da 1) or a few cells in the aorta (No. 1878) are found within the body of the embryo.

Heart

From his study of No. 5080, Davis (1927) concluded that, whereas the possibility of an extra-embryonic origin for the cardiac primordium could not definitely be excluded, "it can be stated with certainty that no connection exists between the well-differentiated angioblastic tissue of the yolk-sac and that of the heart." In brief, "the evidence strongly leans toward an intra-embryonic origin, that is, from the cardiogenic plate." The cardiogenic plate (of Mollier) is the ventral (splanchnic) wall of the pericardial cavity, and from it the myocardium is believed to be derived.

The endocardium (fig. 9-7) is represented at first by a network of mesenchymal cells between the cardiogenic plate and the endoderm. This endocardial plexus, which is at first (Da 1) mostly solid and paired, soon becomes divisible into three parts: atrial, ventricular, and conal (bulbar). The cellular cords that form the plexus become canalized, and their cavities become confluent (Orts Llorca, Jiménez Collado, and Ruano Gil, 1960).

A heart may be said to be present in Nos. 1878 and 7650 (Müller and O'Rahilly, 1983, fig. 7). The development of the cardiac region of one or both of these embryos has been discussed by Davis (1927), de Vries and Saunders (1962), and de Vries (1981). The endocardium at stage 9 may be in the plexiform phase of Davis (1927), as in embryo Gv (Orts Llorca *et al.*, 1960; Jiménez Collado and Ruano Gil, 1963). In Nos. 1878 and 7650, however, the heart would appear already to have entered the paired tubular phase (despite a statement to the contrary by Davis). Intra-embryonic blood vessels are most advanced in these same two embryos.

The conoventricular region (see O'Rahilly, 1971, for terminology) occupies the median plane in No. 1878, in which two ventricular roots unite with each other. Rostrally, the cardiac plexus gives way to the first pair of aortic arches, which in turn lead to the dorsal aortae. The atrial components remain bilateral until a subse-

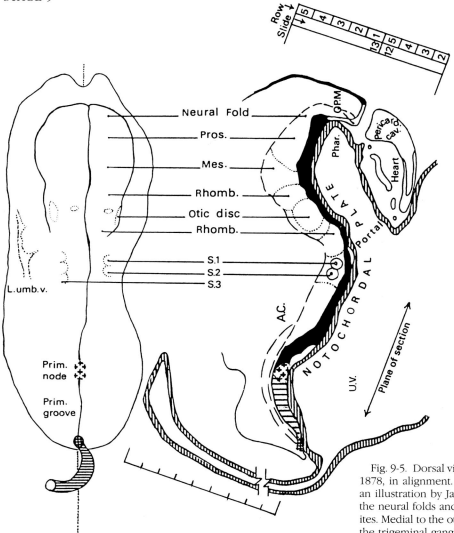

Row
Slide
5 4 3 2 1 13 12 5 4 3 2

O.P.M.

Neural Fold

Pros.

Mes.

Rhomb.

Otic disc

Rhomb.

Pericard.
Cav.

Phar.

Heart

S.1

S.2

S.3

L.umb.v.

A.C.

NOTOCHORDAL PLATE

Portal

U.V.

Plane of section

Prim.
node

Prim.
groove

Fig. 9-5. Dorsal view and median reconstruction of No. 1878, in alignment. The dorsal view, which is based on an illustration by James F. Didusch (see fig. 9-3), shows the neural folds and groove, the otic discs, and the somites. Medial to the otic discs, areas that possibly represent the trigeminal ganglia are indicated without a label. The median reconstruction is based on an illustration by James F. Didusch (Ingalls, 1920, plate 2) and on a drawing reproduced by Bartelmez and Evans (1926, plate 5, fig. 9). Various features are shown: pericardial cavity, oropharyngeal membrane (*O.P.M.*), developing pharynx (*Phar.*), rostral intestinal portal, and allantoic diverticulum.

quent stage.

With regard to the external appearance of the heart, three sulci have appeared in No. 1878: (1) atrioventricular, (2) interventricular (bulboventricular), and (3) conotruncal (interbulbar; infundibulotruncal). It should be kept in mind, however, that the cardiac region of this embryo appears to be distorted.

Other features that have been identified by stage 9 include the "cardiac jelly" (Davis, 1927), the mesocardium, and the septum transversum (Ingalls, 1920).

DIGESTIVE SYSTEM

The foregut develops during stage 9 (or possibly but doubtfully at the end of stage 8) as a recess of the umbilical vesicle. The midgut and hindgut, however, are either still combined (No. 1878 and No. 5080) or else (fig. 9-2) the hindgut is making its appearance as a separate recess (Da 1). In the former case, the cloacal membrane is still in the roof of the gut and, immediately caudal to it, the allantoic diverticulum arises

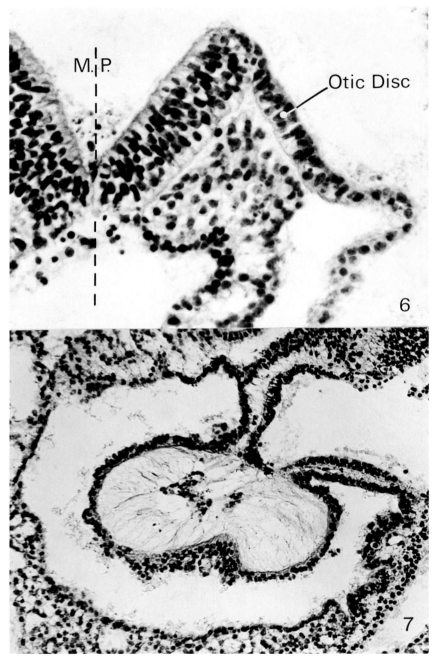

Fig. 9-6. The neural groove and one of the neural folds of No. 1878 in the region of the rhombencephalon. The otic disc is found on the lateral aspect of the neural fold. The basement membrane is visible. The interrupted line (M. P.) indicates the median plane. Section 12-5-7.

Fig. 9-7. Oblique section through the heart of No. 1878. The foregut appears near the upper right-hand corner of the photomicrograph. The U-shaped space is the pericardial cavity. The myocardial mantle, the "cardiac jelly," and the endocardial plexus are evident centrally. Section 12-3-5.

(fig. 9-5). In brief, although a rostral intestinal portal is present at this stage, a caudal portal may or may not be. In an excellent specimen that should be published *in extenso* (Prague No. 2008; 3 pairs of somites; embryonic disc, 1.73 mm), which one of the present writers examined through the kindness of Dr. J. E. Jirásek, the caudal fold, the hindgut, the caudal intestinal portal, and caudal coelomic cavities are all well marked (figs. 9-8 to 9-14).

From a study of abnormal chick embryos it has been concluded that, although "elevation of the head and proper development of the head fold largely depend on the condition of other structures of the head region," the foregut "develops normally in the absence of the head fold as well as in cases in which the nearby anterior [rostral] end of the neural primordium is defective by malformation or experiment" (Gruenwald, 1941a). In other words, the foregut "depends very little upon the condition of the surrounding structures and develops normally whenever there is no mechanical obstacle" (*ibid.*).

The foregut is intimately related dorsally to the floor of the neural groove. At first a shallow pocket (of 0.17 mm in Da 1), the recess soon attains a length of 0.5 mm (in No. 1878). Caudally, the foregut appears triangular or even T-shaped on cross section, and it presents internally a trough in its floor as well as a corresponding ventral keel externally. The keel is closely related to the developing heart, and the trough indicates the general site of the future respiratory groove. In some embryos (Da 1 and Prague No. 2008), however, the keel is scarcely developed and the foregut is oval or reniform (fig. 9-9) rather than triangular in cross section. The "earliest trace" of the first pharyngeal pouches (fig. 9-4) and perhaps an "early indication" of the first pharyngeal cleft have been detected in one specimen (Ingalls, 1920).

It is now nearly half a century since, in a discussion of "fishy nomenclature," it was proposed that the word "branchial" be dropped from mammalian embryology (Frazer,1923). The visceral pouches of embryonic reptiles, birds, and mammals "bear little resemblance to the gill-slits of the adult fish" but rather "resemble the visceral pouches which appear in the *embryonic* stages of fish" (de Beer, 1958). Indeed, "all that can be said is that the fish preserves its visceral pouches and elaborates them into its gill-slits, while reptiles, birds, and

mammals do not preserve them as such but convert them into other structures" (*ibid.*).

The oropharyngeal membrane is generally absent (e.g., in Da 1) but is quite well defined in one specimen (No. 1878) where it attains a width of about 0.05 mm (fig. 9-5). The stomodeum is beginning to form.

Although a pit in the ventral wall of the foregut has been claimed to represent the beginning of the thyroid gland (Wilson, 1914; Ingalls, 1920), it is likely that the thyroid primordium does not make its appearance until the following stage. Similarly, an indication of the liver is not found before stage 10.

In the chick embryo, the hindgut has been described as initially a hollowing out of the ventral portion of the "trunk-tail-node" and its "formation is not the result of a folding" of the blastoderm (Gruenwald, 1941a).

NERVOUS SYSTEM

Stage 9 heralds the onset of that developmental phase (largely stage 10) during which the neural folds dom-

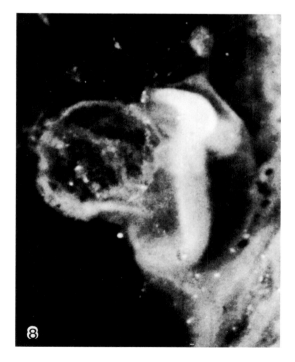

Fig. 9-8. Left lateral view of Prague embryo No. 2008, by courtesy of Dr. J. E. Jirásek. The gentle curvature of the body and the absence of kinking suggest the normal appearance to be expected at this stage. The umbilical vesicle is seen in the left-hand half of the photograph.

inate the external picture. The neural groove, which appeared during stage 8, is now quite deep although it is still open throughout its entire extent (fig. 9-3). About one-half of the longitudinal extent of the groove represents the future brain. The area of the forebrain is conspicuous, and its neural folds are separated rostrally from each other by the terminal notch, which leads to the oropharyngeal membrane.

In the more advanced specimens of stage 9, the neural axis, at the caudal end of the forebrain, changes its direction through an angle of about 115 degrees (in No. 1878). This alteration of axis constitutes the mesencephalic (or cranial) flexure, which, in this and subsequent stages, occurs at the midbrain (fig. 9-4). The flexure is probably the result of the more rapid growth of the dorsal, as compared with the ventral, lamina of the midbrain (Bartelmez and Evans, 1926).

A distinct isthmus rhombencephali separates the midbrain from the hindbrain. The latter comprises four rhombomeres (proneuromeres of Bergquist and Källén).

The interval between the summits of the neural folds is narrowest in the junctional region between hindbrain and future spinal cord, and it is here that closure of the neural groove will first take place during stage 10.

It is frequently not appreciated that the three major divisions of the brain appear before any portion of the neural tube is present as such. The correct interpretation was clearly implied in an important paper by Bartelmez (1923), as stressed by Streeter (1927b), who discussed the myth of the brain vesicles in mammals and pointed out that "the brain begins to build its definitive parts before the closure of the neural tube."

The division of the brain elaborated by Bartelmez (1923) is based on identification of (1) "the midbrain which is located by the cranial flexure," and (2) the otic segment of the hindbrain, which is in close relation to the otic plate. "The hindbrain is the dominant feature of the brain in early stages. It is subdivided into three segments (of which the middle is the otic): RhA, RhB, and RhC." However, in the opinion of the present writers, a fourth segment (RhD) should be included as part of the hindbrain because, being related to the rostralmost (i.e., occipital) somites, it must represent the hypoglossal region of the hindbrain (Müller and O'Rahilly, 1983, fig. 1).

Neural Crest

The head ectoderm is undergoing differentiation such that several areas (fig. 9-4) have been mapped out in one specimen (Bartelmez and Evans, 1926, plate 3, fig. 3): the otic disc (already mentioned), the trigeminal nerve area, the ectodermal area that will later cover the hyoid (second pharyngeal) arch, and the site of the first pharyngeal membrane (overlying the first pharyngeal pouch).

Although the neurosomatic junction is unclear at this stage, mitotic figures are more numerous at the presumed junction. This is especially marked in the mesencephalic region and to a lesser extent in the rhombencephalic area. These dividing cells are believed to be neural crest. Such areas are visible in at least two embryos (Vant and No. 7650) and represent probably the rostral crest and the facial crest. These two embryos are the earliest examples of the initial formation of neural crest, which is generally associated more with stage 10. Unfortunately the plane of section of No. 1878 is unsuitable for plotting the neural crest, which is probably present. A cellular collection near the otic disc has been claimed to be perhaps the primordium of the trigeminal ganglion (Ingalls, 1920).

Eye

Shaner (1945) believed that the "blunted tips" of the neural folds (his fig. 3) are the optic primordia. Although this is not impossible (see O'Rahilly, 1966, for discussion), it is generally maintained that the optic primordia appear first during stage 10.

Ear

The otic disc (or plate) makes its appearance during stage 9 (fig. 9-6). At first ill defined and merely suggested (Ludwig, 1928, fig. 9), it is soon (O'Rahilly, 1963) a better marked ectodermal thickening (in No. 1878; fig. 9-6) approximately opposite the middle of the rhombencephalic fold. The otic disc probably involves more ectoderm than is later incorporated into the otic vesicle (Bartelmez and Evans, 1926).

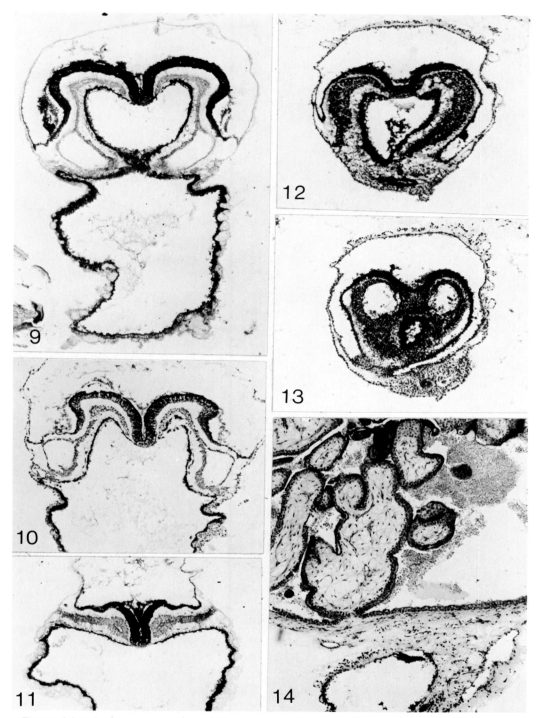

Figures 9-9 to 9-14 are sections through Prague embryo No. 2008, by courtesy of Dr. J. E. Jirásek.

Fig. 9-9. The amniotic cavity, neural groove, foregut, and umbilical vesicle are evident. The foregut, which appears reniform, has been sectioned immediately rostral to the rostral intestinal portal. The limbs of the pericardial cavity can be seen, one on each side, and the cardiogenic mesoderm is found on the ventral aspect of the cavity.

Fig. 9-10. A view of the neural groove and pericardioperitoneal canals in the region of the future midgut.

Fig. 9-11. Transverse section through one of the pairs of somites. So-called myocoeles are visible.

Fig. 9-12. Section through the hindgut.

Fig. 9-13. Section through the hindgut and caudally located, bilateral coelomic cavities. The allantoic primordium is visible in cross section in the lowermost portion of the photomicrograph.

Fig. 9-14. Section through the caudal end of the amniotic cavity (lower quarter of photomicrograph) to show the chorion and the chorionic villi (upper two-thirds of photomicrograph).

SPECIMENS OF STAGE 9 ALREADY DESCRIBED

(listed in order of number of pairs of somites)

1 somite, Carnegie No. 5080. Studied and illustrated by Davis (1927, figs. 2–5 and 39–42) and Severn (1971, figs. 1–4). First pair of somites not separate rostrally and contain no myocoeles (Arey, 1938). Chorion, 14.5 × 1.5 mm. Embryonic disc, 1.5 mm. Reconstructed by Müller and O'Rahilly (1983, fig. 2).

1 somite. A specimen described briefly by Bagiński and Borsuk (1967).

1–2 (or more?) somites, Carnegie No. 7650. Reconstructed by Müller and O'Rahilly (1983, fig. 5).

2 somites, Da 1 (Dann). An important specimen (fig. 9-2) possessing 2 pairs of somites (Studnička, 1929; Florian and Völker, 1929; Arey, 1938), although featured originally as having only one. Described and illustrated in detail by Ludwig (1928). Removed from uterus. Chorion, 12 mm. Embryo, 1.8 mm in a straight line, 2.4 mm by flexible scale. Sectioned transversely at 8 μm. Stained with alum cochineal. Neurenteric canal present. Sections are housed in the Anatomisches Institut, Basel. Photographs of sections are in Carnegie Collection under No. 5982. Presumed age, about 21 days. Dorsal and median projections published (*ibid.*, figs. 1 and 2; Florian and Völker, 1929, fig. 14). Reconstructed by Müller and O'Rahilly (1983, fig. 3).

2–3 somites, H3. Described by Wilson (1914), according to whom it "possessed probably two, possibly three, pairs of somites." Chorion, 8.5 × 5.7 × 5 mm. Embryo, 1.43 mm. Sectioned obliquely (transversely) at 10 μm. Stained with hematoxylin. Fixation not adequate for reconstruction. The relatively longer primitive streak suggests that this embryo may be less advanced than No. 1878. Prechordal plate, or at least prechordal mesoderm, figured (Hill and Florian, 1931b). Presumed age, 18–21 days.

2/3 somites, Carnegie No. 1878 (figs. 9-3 to 9-7). An important specimen possessing 2 somites on the right side and 3 on the left. Florian (1934b) had certain difficulties and considered the embryo to be too small. Curettage. Chorion,

12 × 10.5 × 7.5 mm. Embryonic disc, 1.38 mm in a straight line. Described in detail and illustrated by Ingalls (1920), who believed that "the earliest recognizable stage of dextrocardia" is present, "to which might have been added later a more or less complete situs inversum viscerum"; at any rate, Davis (1927), who studied and illustrated the heart, considered that "the cardiac area is distorted." Angiogenesis in chorion described by Hertig (1935). Primitive streak and node, 0.13 mm, according to Ingalls, but about 0.22 mm in fig. 15 of Florian and Völker (1929) and more than 0.3 mm in plate 5, fig. 9, of Bartelmez and Evans (1926). Neurenteric canal not patent but pit present (Bartelmez and Evans, 1926). Median projection published (*ibid.*, plate 5, fig. 9; Florian and Völker, 1929, fig. 15; Müller and O'Rahilly, 1983, fig. 1).

3 somites, T439 (Toronto). Possesses 3 pairs of somites (Arey, 1938), although considered originally as having only 2. Described by Piersol (1939). Embryo (along surface), 2.03 × 0.72 mm. Sectioned sagittally. Neurenteric canal closed but its remains are identifiable. Primordial germ cells near allantois. Embryonic disc rostral to somites, including cardiac area, is retarded. Said to contain no blood vessels in any part of the embryo itself.

3 somites, Vant embryo. Described by Shaner (1945), who found "two to three pairs of somites." Embryo (along curve), 1.5 mm. Thought to be 25 ± 2 days. Reconstructed again from original sections by Müller and O'Rahilly (1983, fig. 4).

3 somites, Gv (Madrid). Described by Jiménez Collado and Ruano Gil (1963). Heart described by Orts Llorca, Jiménez Collado, and Ruano Gil (1960). Tubal. Embryo, 1.81 mm. Sectioned at 7 μm. Stained with hematoxylin and eosin. Reconstructed. On the basis of its external characters, said to lie between stage 9 and stage 10. Presumed age, 21 ± 1 days.

3 somites, No. 2008 (Prague). Excellent specimen (figs. 9-8 to 9-14) belonging to Dr. J. E. Jirásek. Embryo, 1.73 mm. Fixed in calcium formol. Sectioned transversely at 10 μm. Various stains used, including histochemical procedures. Should be published.

3 somites (?), His embryo E. This 2.1-mm specimen is listed by Bartelmez and Evans (1926) between No. 1878 (2–3 somitic pairs) and No. 3709 (4 somitic pairs, stage 10).

STAGE 10

Approximately 1.5–3 mm in length
Approximately 22 ± 1 postovulatory days
Characteristic feature: 4–12 pairs of somites

SUMMARY

External: 4–12 pairs of somites; fusion of neural folds is imminent or in progress; the optic sulcus may have appeared; pharyngeal arch 1 begins to be visible on the surface.

Internal: the cardiac loop is appearing; the laryngeotracheal sulcus develops; the intermediate mesoderm becomes visible.

SIZE AND AGE

The chorion generally has a diameter of 8–15 mm. The greatest length of the embryo, although not of great informational value (Bartelmez and Evans, 1926), is usually 1.5–3 mm.

The age is approximately 22 postovulatory days.

A brief review of stage 10 was published by Heuser and Corner (1957), and a detailed investigation of this stage was undertaken by Müller and O'Rahilly (1985), who provided graphic reconstructions. Both of these publications contain an appropriate bibliography.

EXTERNAL FORM
(figs. 10-1 and 10-2)

The criterion for stage 10 is the presence of 4–12 pairs of somites. This stage is particularly important because, during it, the neural tube first begins to be formed from the neural folds and groove. In the less advanced specimens the neural groove is open throughout its whole length, whereas by the end of the stage the groove is closed from the rhombencephalon to below the level of the last somites present.

The embryo is becoming longer, and the umbilical vesicle continues to expand. The rostral portion of the neural folds becomes elevated, a caudal fold begins to appear, and the whole embryo comes to rise beyond the level of the umbilical vesicle (i.e., a variable degree of lordosis usually becomes evident). By the end of the stage the cardiac region has become a prominent feature of the external form (Boyden, 1940).

Representative specimens of this stage are illustrated in figures 10-3 and 10-4. These outlines, showing the dorsal aspect of a median section of each specimen, are enlarged to the same scale. As pointed out by Bartelmez and Evans (1926), the mesencephalic flexure is present in all embryos of this period. A dorsal flexure may or may not be found. The curvature of the dorsal profile varies from a gentle convexity through all degrees of concavity (lordosis) from the least possible curve to a deep, sharp kink. Bartelmez and Evans (1926) and Streeter (1942) have discussed the significance of this variation as seen in human and rhesus embryos of early somitic stages. On the whole, the evidence indicates that, whereas extreme dorsal flexion should be regarded as an artifact, anything from a gentle convexity to a moderate dorsal concavity can be considered normal.

The optic sulcus develops in the forebrain and, toward the end of the stage, an indication of invagination of the otic disc is found.

During stage 10, swellings begin to appear for the mandibular arch (Politzer, 1930, fig. 5), and the hyoid arch and probably the maxillary process become identifiable (Bartelmez and Evans, 1926, fig. 6). Pharyngeal cleft 1 becomes visible (Corner, 1929, figs. 4 and 10).

The future ectodermal ring (O'Rahilly and Müller, 1985) is beginning to form as a thick area overlying pharyngeal arch 1. An indication of an intermediate band is present and represents the future intermembral part of the ectodermal ring.

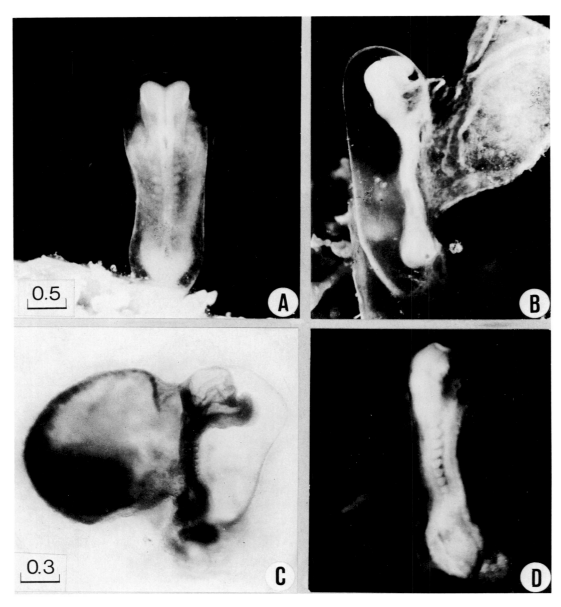

Fig. 10-1. Photographs of three embryos with 7–12 pairs of somites. (A) In the dorsal view of No. 6330 the neural folds are well shown both in the brain and in the spinal area. The folds are actually fused in a short region of the embryo, as indicated in the outline sketches of the same specimen (figs. 10-3 and 4). The amnion and amniotic cavity are distinguishable. (B) The mandibular arch is visible in the lateral view of No. 6330. (C) The 8-somite embryo, H 98 (Wilson, 1914) or No. 7251 has an unusually abrupt upward bending of the rostral third of the body. The relations of heart, umbilical vesicle, and other details are evident. (D) The somites and the caudal eminence are well shown in No. 3710. Photographs A–C are enlarged to the same scale.

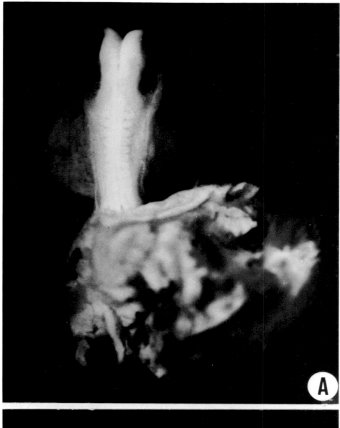

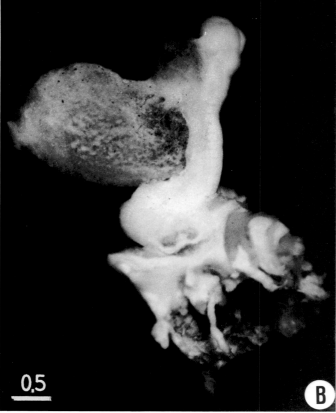

Fig. 10-2. Photographs of the 10-somite embryo No. 5074, made after most of the amnion had been removed. The general body form and structural details of the embryo are well shown in both the dorsal and lateral views. The neural closure extends a short distance caudal to the last somite, to the level of the otic segment of the hindbrain. The pericardial cavity is quite large in this specimen. In B the heart itself is faintly visible through the thin, translucent body wall.

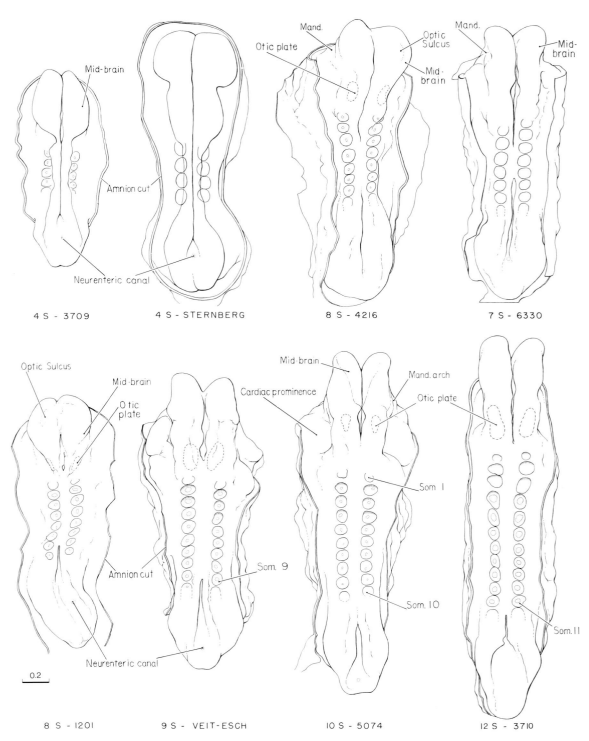

Fig. 10-3. Outline drawings showing, in dorsal view, eight embryos belonging to stage 10. The number of somitic pairs and the collection number are given for each specimen. The neural folds still gaping apart or separated from each other in the 4-somite specimens come together, and the fusion rapidly spreads rostrally into the region of the hindbrain and caudally about as far as the last somites formed; the rostral and caudal neuropores shrink, but they are still relatively large in the more advanced members of the group. The pericardial region, relatively small in the 4-somite embryos, is prominent in embryos of 10 or more somites. The tracing of one 4-somite embryo was made from figures by Sternberg. No. 6330 and Veit-Esch were drawn from Born reconstructions. The others are drawings based on reconstructions and figures by Bartelmez and Evans (1926), Payne (1925), and Corner (1929).

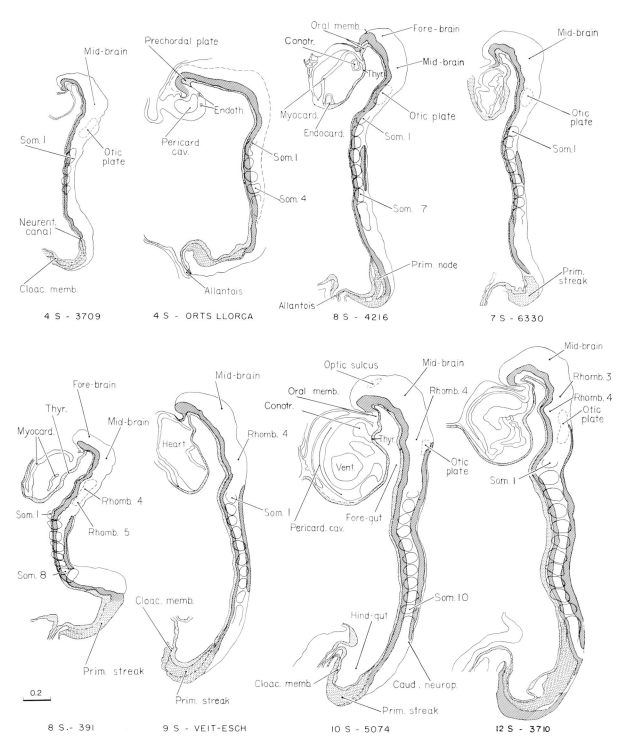

Fig. 10-4. Outline drawings of median sections of embryos belonging to stage 10. The head fold is prominent in all specimens shown, and the caudal fold is just beginning to appear in the 4-somite embryo; the hindgut shows the first sign of separating from the yolk sac. The line of fusion of the neural folds lengthens rapidly after 7 pairs of somites have appeared. In more-advanced embryos, the general form of the body is greatly influenced by the enlarging heart and pericardial cavity.

The drawing of one 4-somite embryo was slightly modified from a figure by Orts Llorca (1934). Data for the Veit-Esch embryo were obtained from a Born reconstruction and from a figure by Florian and Völker (1929). No. 6330 was drawn from a Born reconstruction. The others are drawings based on reconstructions and figures by Bartelmez and Evans (1926), Payne (1925), and Corner (1929).

HISTOLOGICAL FEATURES

Primitive streak. In stage 10 the primitive streak is limited to the caudal part of the body, an area that has been termed the caudal eminence (Müller and O'Rahilly, 1983) or future *Endwulst* (end bud). As illustrated in an informative scheme by Florian (1934b), the length of the primitive streak in relation to total embryonic length becomes smaller and smaller (Bartelmez and Evans, 1926; Müller and O'Rahilly, 1985). In stage 10 the primitive node "is about at the entrance of the hindgut" (Heuser and Corner, 1957).

Caudal to the neurenteric canal or its site (fig. 10-7a), dense axially located cells represent a part of the primitive streak. This area was formerly (Corner, 1929; Heuser and Corner, 1957) regarded as a portion of the notochord. The caudal end of the embryo consists of the hindgut and its thick endodermal lining, the primitive streak and an axial mesenchymal condensation adjacent to the site of the neurenteric canal, undifferentiated mesenchyme laterally, and, dorsally, an extension of the neural plate. A primitive groove is present only occasionally.

Somites. The number of somites increases during stages 10 and 11, and the rostralmost 4 are occipital. Somitocoeles are present but are no longer visible at stage 11. Sclerotomic cells are distinguishable at the ventromedial angle of the somite (Corner, 1929, fig. 25).

The average length of a somite is 80 μm (Müller and O'Rahilly, 1985). The number of presomitic spaces is 4–6.

It has been shown by Arey (1938, table 3) that the first somite is large (equals the second in size) in stages 9 and 10, up to 9 somites. From 10 somites to the end of stage 11, the first is generally much smaller than the second somite.

Notochordal plate. Although frequently referred to as the notochord, the axial cells caudal to the prechordal plate are still merely notochordal plate at this stage. The notochord *sensu stricto* is present only where notochordal cells have become completely separated from a continuous endodermal lining (Müller and O'Rahilly, 1985), and this does not occur until the next stage.

Rostral to the neurenteric canal, the notochordal plate is directly continuous with the endoderm and

still forms a portion of the roof of the gut. In transverse section the plate begins to project dorsally, and U-shaped areas become increasingly extensive. The notochordal plate is in contact with the basement membrane of the neural plate or tube. Relatively few mitotic figures are evident, and they are mostly near the neurenteric canal or its site.

Neurenteric canal. Although a neurenteric canal soon ceases to be evident, at least its site can be recognized in all embryos of this stage (Müller and O'Rahilly, 1985, figs. 1–3).

Prechordal plate. The prechordal plate, which is constantly present, lies under cover of the rostral part of the prosencephalon, being separated by only the basement membrane of the brain. The plate is generally regarded as a source of proliferation of prechordal mesoderm.

The migration of prechordal cells began in stage 9, and prechordal mesoderm continues to form in stage 10. The rotation from a position in the longitudinal axis to a right angle had also already begun in stage 9 (Müller and O'Rahilly, 1983). Gilbert (1957) believed on morphological grounds that the prechordal plate is the source of those extrinsic muscles that are innervated by the oculomotor nerve. His data have been confirmed and completed by experimental work and by electron microscopy in the chick embryo. In birds the muscle cells of all extrinsic ocular muscles develop probably from the prechordal plate rather than from somitomeres (i.e., from paraxial and not axial mesenchyme). The relationship of the prechordal plate to the foregut may vary with species.

Umbilical vesicle. From stage 7 onward, the external and internal strata of the bilaminar umbilical vesicle are referred to as the mesodermal and endodermal layers, respectively. Three layers can be distinguished by electron microscopy at stage 10: mesothelium, mesenchyme, and endodermal epithelium (Hesseldahl and Larsen, 1969, 1971). The chorionic villi have also been investigated by electron microscopy (Knoth, 1968).

CARDIOVASCULAR SYSTEM

The pericardial cavity is always present and, in the more advanced specimens, a passage connects the intra- and extra-embryonic coeloms (Dandy, 1910, fig. 11; Corner, 1929, fig. 7). It is probable that the coelom serves as a means for access of nutritive fluid to the embryonic tissues before blood vessels take over this function (Streeter, 1942).

In addition to such vessels as the umbilical arteries and veins, aortic arches 1 and 2 develop.

Heart
(figs. 10-5 and 10-6)

Cardiac contraction "is believed to commence at the beginning" of stage 10 (de Vries and Saunders, 1962) or at the end of stage 9.

The wall of the heart comprises a thin myocardial mantle, recticulum ("cardiac jelly"), and endocardium (Payne, 1925, fig. 10). A dorsal mesocardium is formed (Davis, 1927), and perforation of it may begin (Corner, 1929).

Three steps in the development of the heart can be recognized in stage 10 (fig. 10-6).

(1) The endocardial primordium is a plexus of delicate vessels lying on the foregut, and consists of two parallel channels interconnected by two or more small transverse vessels (Davis, 1927, fig. 12). The atria are widely separated from each other, and the more centrally placed cardiac elements (according to current interpretation) comprise, caudorostrally, the prospective left ventricle, prospective right ventricle, and conotruncus. The left interventricular sulcus is well marked on the surface of the heart (McBride, Moore, and Hutchins, 1981), so that the organ appears already to have lost its symmetry (de Vries, 1981).

(2) The two endocardial tubes become fused (Davis, 1927, fig. 22) so that a single tube now comprises caudorostrally, the left ventricle, right ventricle, and conotruncus. In addition, the cardiac loop forms when 7–20 pairs of somites are present. It is usually directed to the left and it includes ventral bowing and (when viewed from the front) counterclockwise rotation of

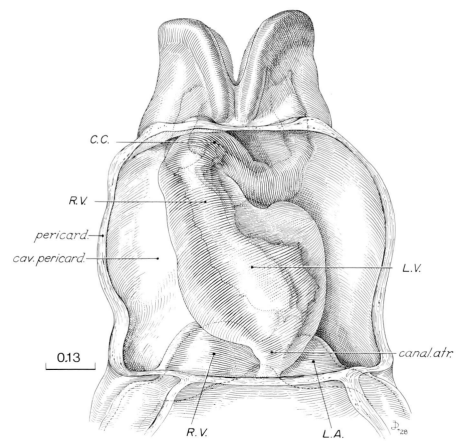

Fig. 10-5. The heart, ventral view, from a reconstruction in translucent material, showing pericardial cavity, myocardial mantle, and the endocardial tube. From Corner (1929). Labels modified according to current interpretation. *C.C.*, conus cordis.

the ventricular segments (de Vries and Saunders, 1962). Although a sinus venosus as such is not present until the next stage, left and right sinusal horns appear during stage 10.

(3) The endocardial tube adopts a definite S-curve, the middle portion of which is formed by the ventricular loop, and hence the organ is now markedly asymmetrical (Davis, 1927, fig. 24).

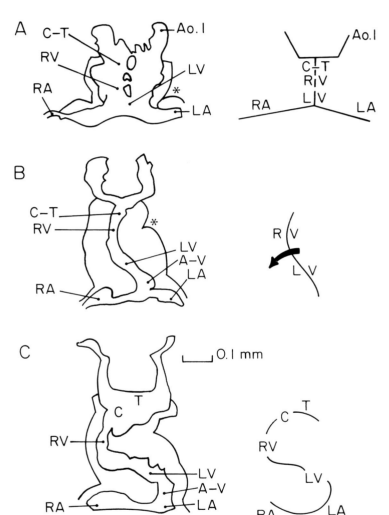

Fig. 10-6. Outlines of the myocardial mantle and endocardial tube showing three successive phases of cardiac development during stage 10. Schematic representations are shown on the right. A, plexiform phase (No. 3709). B, beginning cardiac loop (arrow)(No. 391). C, definite S-curve (No. 3707). The outlines are based on Davis (1927) with current (e.g., de Vries and Saunders, 1962) interpretation. Asterisk: left interventricular sulcus. *A-V*, atrioventricular junction. *Ao.1*, aortic arch 1. *C*, conus cordis. *C-T*, conotruncus. *T*, truncus arteriosus.

DIGESTIVE AND RESPIRATORY SYSTEMS

During stage 10, when mesenchymal cells are no longer found between the ectoderm and the endoderm at the summit of the foregut, an oropharyngeal membrane is present.

A small portion of the ectoderm adjacent to the summit (chiasmatic plate) of the neural plate is considered to be the primordium of the adenohypophysis.

Pharyngeal cleft 2 and pouch 2 are identifiable, and pharyngeal pouch 3 may be indicated. The thyroid primordium appears (O'Rahilly, 1983a). A median pharyngeal groove and ridge are present, and include the laryngotracheal sulcus. The pulmonary primordium appears at the caudal end of this sulcus, and the two constitute the respiratory primordium (O'Rahilly and Boyden, 1973). A transverse groove between the umbilical vesicle and the ventral surface of the pericardial cavity foreshadows the "cranial coelomic angle" (Gitlin, 1968). The hepatic plate has been identified as an endodermal thickening at the rostral intestinal portal, caudal and ventral to the heart (Severn, 1971, 1972). The caudal intestinal portal, and hence the midgut, is becoming delimited.

URINARY SYSTEM

The intermediate mesoderm becomes visible and, when 10 pairs of somites are present, the nephrogenic cord becomes differentiated from this mesoderm. However, "the concept of the pronephros does not apply to the human embryo" (Torrey, 1954).

NERVOUS SYSTEM
(fig. 10-7)

The rostral part of the neural plate is relatively flat at first but the neural folds soon become elevated, in association with the deepening neural groove. The elevation is related to (1) an increase in the amount of the underlying mesenchyme, caused by migration of mesencephalic crest and mitotic activity *in situ*, and (2) increasing size of the dorsal aortae and the aortic arches. The mesenchyme is believed to possess a supportive role during the initial phase of encephalic neurulation, and mesenchymal deficiency may prevent further neurulation.

The subdivisions of the rhombencephalon, which appear during stage 9, were clarified by Bartelmez (1923), whose system is followed here, with the addition of a more recently recognized segment D (Müller and O'Rahilly, 1983).

The terminal notch, which appears during stage 10 but is not always identifiable, indicates the telencephalic part of the forebrain (fig. 10-7b). This is the earliest stage at which the telencephalon has been identified. The telencephalic area represents the beginning of the lamina terminalis and therefore of the telencephalon medium (impar). The prosencephalic folds can be divided into an optic part (D1) and a postoptic part (D2). In the median plane, D1 is thicker than D2 and constitutes the primordium chiasmatis. In some embryos the optic sulcus continues medially and forms a slight indentation that indicates the future postoptic recess (primitive optic groove of Johnston, 1909). D1 shows many cellular inclusions. Parts D1 and D2 of the diencephalon are evident as "segments" (transverse partitions) up to stage 13 inclusive. In the median plane, D1 comprises the chiasmatic plate, D2 the area of the future neurohypophysis and the mamillary region. The mesencephalic flexure becomes reduced during stage 10, resulting in a ventral bending of the prosencephalon. The factors leading to flexure are believed to be intrinsic to the mesencephalon. The four divisions (A, B, C, D) of the rhombencephalic folds, first seen in the previous stage, are again distinguishable, and part D is the longest.

From stage 9 to stage 10 the prosencephalon increases in length, the mesencephalon remains the same, and the rhombencephalon decreases considerably. A correlation exists between the total length of the C.N.S. and the percentage of closed parts. Furthermore, rhombomere D and the spinal area grow relatively more, and these are the areas that close first. The spinal part of the neural plate increases fivefold in length. The elongation of the C.N.S. is related to the formation of new somites. Although this somite-related elongation is reflected chiefly in the spinal region, the cerebral portion lengthens also. The frequency of mitotic figures is highest in the spinal part of the neural plate and somewhat less in the rhombencephalon and prosencephalon.

Closure of the neural groove occurs first during stage 10, in embryos of approximately 5 paired som-

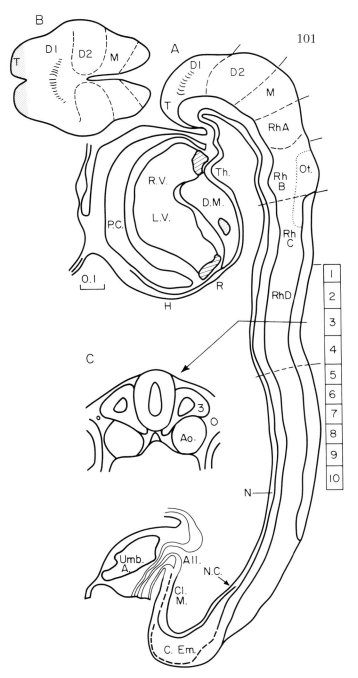

Fig. 10-7. (A) Median section of No. 5074 (10 pairs of somites, the levels of which are indicated by rectangles marked 1–10). Based partly on Corner (1929), with current (Müller and O'Rahilly, 1985) interpretation. (B) "Top" view of the rostral end of the embryo. The telencephalic portion is shaded and the optic sulci (in D1) are indicated. Based on Müller and O'Rahilly (1985). (C) Transverse section at the level of somites 3, showing neural tube, notochordal plate, dorsal aortae, and intermediate mesoderm.

Abbreviations. *All.*, Allantoic diverticulum. *Ao.*, Dorsal aorta. *C.Em.*, Caudal eminence. *Cl.M.*, Cloacal membrane. *D1 and D2*, Diencephalon. *D.M.*, Dorsal mesocardium. *H*, Hepatic primordium. *L.V.*, Left ventricle. *M.*, Mesencephalon. *N*, Notochordal plate. *Ot.*, Otic disc. *N.C.*, Site of neurenteric canal. *P.C.*, Pericardial cavity. *R*, Respiratory primordium. *RbA–RbD*, Rhombomeres. *R.V.*, Right ventricle. *T*, Telencephalon medium. *Tb.*, Thyroid area. *Umb.A.*, Umbilical artery.

ites. The site of initial closure appears to be rhomb-encephalic (part D) or upper cervical, or both. It seems that closure may soon occur in several places independently, so that the process is not entirely comparable to a zip fastener. The maximum limits of closure found are to rhombencephalon 1 rostrally and to the level of somites 15/16 caudally. The caudal extension of the closure proceeds at about the same rate as the formation of new somites (Bartelmez and Evans, 1926), so that the margin of the caudal neuropore is usually opposite the latest pair of somites. Rostrally, progress is slower and apparently more variable.

The neural plate in stage 9 extends caudally to the level of the neurenteric canal. In stage 10 differentiation into neural plate extends beyond that landmark, as indicated by a radial arrangement of cells and separation from the underlying primitive streak by a basement membrane. The transition to the more caudally situated, undifferentiated ectoderm is gradual.

Cytoplasmic inclusions in the developing nervous system have been noted by several authors and have frequently been considered to indicate degeneration. Such inclusions are found in a number of areas, including the apices of the neural folds, the primitive streak, and the prechordal plate.

The histological features of neurulation have been investigated (Müller and O'Rahilly, 1985). In the spinal region, the neural folds approach each other and the surface ectodermal cells of the two sides make contact while a gap remains between the neuro-ectodermal cells of the two sides. Where fusion of the surface ectoderm and of the neuro-ectoderm has occurred across the median plane, a wedge-shaped area of neural crest is present in the dorsalmost part of the neural tube. Protoplasmic processes then protrude, and crest cells emerge from the tube. A more or less similar appearance of wedge-shaped neural crest and migrating cells is found also in part D of the hindbrain. Further rostrally in the hindbrain, and also in the midbrain and the forebrain, at the apices of the open neural folds, neural crest cells are emerging from the neurosomatic junction and also from the adjacent neural ectoderm in areas where the basement membrane is deficient. At the mesencephalic level, preparation for fusion is occurring. The surface ectoderm protrudes more medially, thereby overhanging the neuro-ecto-

derm. Certain intermediate areas that are still open have been misinterpreted as neuroschisis. The neural folds show a high alkaline phosphatase activity (Mori, 1959a). It is important to note that differences in the process of neurulation have been recorded in various species.

Neural Crest

The neural crest continues to develop during stage 10 when, in the head, it probably reaches its peak. The rostral (mesencephalic) and facial portions are constantly present. The crest material for the superior ganglion of the vagus appears before that for the glossopharyngeal. The probable succession of appearance is: facial, rostral (mesencephalic), trigeminal, vagal, occipital, and glossopharyngeal. The facial crest is the most conspicuous. In the area of the vagal crest, the neural crest material is clearly joined by cells of the surface epithelium in some of the embryos. The otic plate, at least in some instances, may be seen to contribute cells to the facial (acousticofacial) crest. The cells of the neural crest appear to be derived from the open neural plate at the neurosomatic junction, mostly in areas where the neural tube has not yet formed. Apart from its formation of cranial ganglia, the neural crest migrates into the head mesenchyme and is believed to contribute to the skull and face. Illustrations purporting to show precisely the extent of the contributions in the human (based on the chick embryo) are quite unwarranted in the present state of knowledge.[1] The proposal of failure of crest cell formation as a facial pathogenetic mechanism has been disputed. Neural crest cells clearly leave the neural plate at areas where the basement membrane is interrupted. After closure of the neural groove in stage 10, neural crest still seems to be derived from the neural ectoderm, although a simultaneous origin from the surface ectoderm cannot be excluded.

---

[1]It has frequently been pointed out that the "static" appearances seen in serial sections cannot justifiably be used for the interpretation of "dynamic" processes. It has less frequently been emphasized that there are equally grave problems in assuming that the results of experimental embryology can be transferred without more ado to the human embryo.

Eye

By approximately 7–8 paired somites the neural folds of D1 consist of thick neural ectoderm that comprises the optic primordium. Identification of the optic primordium is difficult, and reconstructions are necessary. The thickened area, which contains many mitotic figures and cytoplasmic inclusions, continues across the median plane as the chiasmatic plate (primordium chiasmatis). A more or less indented area in D1 represents the optic sulcus (fig. 10-7). In contrast to the shallow ventricular surface in D1, the ventricular surface in D2 is convex and represents the future thalamic area of the diencephalon. The optic sulcus does not always reach the median plane, but, when it does so, it indicates the future postoptic recess (Johnston, 1909). The area rostral to the optic primordium on both sides of the terminal notch represents the telencephalic primordium (fig. 10-7B). Some of the earlier specimens in which an optic primordium or sulcus has been described are unfortunately not of sufficient histological quality to avoid the suspicion that artifacts are present. Moreover, the plane of section is of the utmost importance in the identification of the optic region. D2 gives rise later to the thalami, but it is not correct to state that "the entire dorsal thalamic wall... had originally been incorporated in the optic evagination" (Bartelmez and Blount, 1954). Careful plotting of the optic sulcus in the Payne embryo shows that it is confined to D1 and is transverse in direction, in contrast to the vertical markings shown by Payne (1925, fig. 2). Similarly in the Corner embryo, the optic sulci (which do not quite meet in the median plane) are limited to D1, and the optic primordia (i.e., the surrounding thickenings) occupy more or less the whole of D1. The lateral limit of each optic sulcus appears to be beginning to extend caudally. Corner (1929, fig. 1) plotted the sulcus more caudally, probably because of the influence of the early interpretations of Bartelmez (1922). An improved plotting of the Corner embryo was illustrated by Bartelmez and Dekaban (1962, fig. 67), although the midbrain was placed too far rostrally, thereby not allowing adequately for D2. By the end of stage 10, the optic sulci extend more caudally, as in the Litzenberg embryo (Boyden, 1940, fig. 13), in which the label superior colliculus should read thalamic primordium in D2.

Ear

The otic plate in at least one embryo contributes cells to the facial (or faciovestibular) neural crest. Such a contribution continues to at least stage 12 (O'Rahilly, 1963). It may be that the non-neuronal cells in the vestibular and cochlear ganglia are derived from the neural crest.

SPECIMENS OF STAGE 10 ALREADY DESCRIBED

4 somites, Carnegie No. 3709 (University of Chicago H 279). Characterized with outline sketches, by Bartelmez and Evans (1926).

4 somites, Histologisch-Embryologisches Institut, Embryo A, Vienna. Fully described by Sternberg (1927).

4 somites, Histologisch-Embryologisches Institut, Embryo Ca, Vienna. Fully described by Orts Llorca (1934).

4–5 somites, Florian's Embryo Bi II. The whereabouts of this, the following embryo, and the 10-somite Bi XI (see below) are not known; Florian's collection has not been found since his untimely death during World War II. The embryo Bi II was briefly characterized by Studnička (1929), cited and partly illustrated by Florian (1928, 1930a).

4–5 somites, Florian's Embryo Bi III. (See note on previous embryo.) Briefly characterized by Studnička (1929) and cited by Florian (1928).

4–5 somites, Carnegie No. 2795. Cited and briefly characterized by Bartelmez and Evans (1926). The specimen is distorted and somewhat macerated.

5 somites, Anatomisches Institut, Zürich, GM 1954. Described and illustrated by Schenck (1954).

5 somites, No. 103, Department of Anatomy, Tohoku University, Sendai. Distribution of alkaline phosphatase studied by Mori (1959a) in this and in another (No. 101), possibly 8-somite, embryo.

5–6 somites, Pfannenstiel "Klb" (originally at Giessen; was in Keibel's Institute at Freiburg i. Br. about 1911, may now be in Berlin). This well known embryo is No. 3 in the Keibel and Elze *Normentafel* (1908). Models by Kroemer (1903). A partial set of tracings made by H. M. Evans is in the Carnegie Collection, No. 5463.

6 somites, Carnegie No. 8244. Somewhat distorted; histologically fair.

6 somites, University of Michigan No. 71, Ann Arbor. Briefly described by Arey and Henderson (1943). A full description in an unpublished doctoral dissertation is in the files of L. B. Arey at Northwestern University, Chicago.

6 somites, Carnegie No. 8818 (University of Chicago H 338). Pathological; not used in present study. Listed here because cited by Bartelmez and Evans (1926).

6–7 somites, His's Embryo "SR." Cited by His (1880) and

by Bartelmez and Evans (1926). Has been studied only in the gross.

6–7 somites, Embryo LM (present location unknown). Cited here from manuscript notes at Carnegie laboratory, made from Russian text of Burow (1928). Condition said to be poor.

7 (?) somites, Embryo "Ludwig," Berlin. Described by Streiter (1951). This specimen, which is somewhat macerated, is in certain characteristics considerably in advance of others of similar somitic number.

7 somites, Carnegie No. 6330 (University of Chicago H 1404). Extensive manuscript notes on this specimen, made under the supervision of G. W. Bartelmez, are in the files of the Carnegie laboratory.

8 somites, Carnegie No. 4216. Described by Payne (1925), and very frequently cited.

8 somites, Dublin. Described by West (1930); see also Arey (1938). Photographs and models are in the Carnegie Collection, No. 4923. Bartelmez (personal communication) thinks that this distorted embryo had only 5–6 somites.

8 somites, Carnegie No. 391. Described by Dandy (1910) and frequently cited (cf. Bartelmez and Evans, 1926, with additional illustrations). There were neither camera drawings nor photographs of the intact specimen, and therefore the reconstructions are not entirely satisfactory. The plaster models now at the Carnegie laboratory were made by O. O. Heard under the supervision of Bartelmez for the paper by Bartelmez and Evans (1926). The apparent lack of fusion of the neural folds described by Dandy is an artifact produced by a crack.

8 somites, Carnegie No. 1201 (University of Chicago H 87). Described briefly by Evans and Bartelmez (1917); cited, with illustrations, by Bartelmez and Evans (1926).

8 somites, Embryologisches Institut, Embryo Ct, Vienna. Fully described by Politzer (1930). Arey (1938) counts 8 paired somites in this embryo instead of 7 as stated by Politzer.

8 somites, University of Cambridge, Department of Anatomy H 98. Photographs and models in Carnegie Collection, No. 7251. Described by J. T. Wilson (1914). Cited by Bartelmez and Evans (1926), who consider it slightly abnormal in form although good histologically.

9 somites, Embryo "Esch I," Marburg. Elaborately described by Veit and Esch (1922), and cited, with illustrations, by Bartelmez and Evans (1926), who count 9 somites instead of 8 as stated by the original authors. Chorionic villi studied in detail by Ortmann (1938). Photographs and models are in the Carnegie Collection, No. 4251.

9 somites, Embryo "Du Ga," Geneva. Described by Eternod (1896); models by Ziegler were distributed commercially. Cited by Bartelmez (1922) and Bartelmez and Evans (1926), with illustrations. Tracings made by H. M. Evans at Geneva and models are in the Carnegie Collection, No. 4439.

*About 9 somites, Embryo Unger, Keibel Collection, Frei-*burg i. Br., No. 4 of Keibel and Elze (1908). Listed by Bartelmez and Evans (1926).

9 somites, Embryo "Jacobsen," formerly at Kiel (Graf Spee's collection was destroyed in World War II). Described by von Spee (1887). Listed by Bartelmez and Evans (1926) as having "at least" 9 somites.

9 somites, Embryo Ca of Orts Llorca, Madrid. Various details described by Mari Martínez (1950) and Martínez Rovira (1953).

9–10 somites, Embryo R. Meyer 335. (Robert Meyer's collection was purchased by the late Hedwig Frey and bequeathed by him to the Anatomisches Institut, University of Zürich.) Listed by Bartelmez and Evans (1926), and cited by Felix (1912).

10 somites, Da2, Anatomical Institute, Basel. Described by Ludwig (1929). Plastic reconstructions. Neural groove closure extends rostral to otic discs.

10 somites, Carnegie No. 5074 (University of Rochester H 10). Fully described by Corner (1929), and subjected to volumetric analysis by Boyden (1940). Excellent specimen.

10 somites, Grosser's Embryo Schwz (present location unknown). Briefly described, without illustrations, by Treutler (1931). Preservation said to be not altogether satisfactory.

10 somites, Florian's Embryo Bi XI. (See note on Bi II above.) Briefly described, with illustrations, by Politzer and Sternberg (1930); cited and partly illustrated by Florian (1930a).

10 somites, Anatomy Department, University of South Wales, Cardiff. Partly described and illustrated by Baxter and Boyd (1939).

11 somites, Embryo T 152, University of Toronto, Department of Anatomy. Cited by Arey (1938).

11 somites, Embryo G-dt, Uppsala. Described by Holmdahl (1943) as having 11 well-differentiated pairs of somites, with beginning delimitation of 4 more.

11–12 somites, Carnegie No. 8970 (University of Chicago H 637). Somewhat damaged. Cited, with illustrations, by Bartelmez (1922) and Bartelmez and Evans (1926).

12 somites, Carnegie No. 3710 (University of Chicago H 392). Cited by Bartelmez (1922) and Bartelmez and Evans (1926).

12 somites, Carnegie No. 3707 (University of California H 197). "Legge embryo." Cited, with illustrations, by Bartelmez and Evans (1926). The coital history accompanying this specimen, which was declared to be reliable, would give it a postovulatory age of either 18 or 39 days; the former seems rather brief but the latter is much too long.

12 somites, Litzenberg embryo, University of Minnesota, Minneapolis. Briefly described by J. C. Litzenberg (1933); characterized and subjected to volumetric analysis by Boyden (1940), who counts 12 somites instead of 13–14 as in the original description. Photographs and model in Carnegie Collection, No. 6740.

12 somites, M. 24, University of Michigan, Ann Arbor. Cited by Arey (1938).

STAGE 11

Approximately 2.5–4.5 mm
Approximately 24 ± 1 postovulatory days
Characteristic feature: 13–20 pairs of somites

SUMMARY

External: the rostral neuropore is in the process of closing; the otic invagination is shallow or still widely open; pharyngeal arches 1 and 2 are evident.

Internal: the sinus venosus develops; the oropharyngeal membrane ruptures; the mesonephric duct and nephric tubules appear; the optic vesicle and otic pit develop.

SIZE AND AGE

As for the size of the chorion, out of eight specimens five had largest diameters between 20 and 25 mm, two had largest diameters between 17 and 18 mm, and one was 15 mm. In average diameter (i.e., the mean of the largest and smallest diameters) six of these eight chorions fall between 15 and 18 mm. One is smaller than this (14 mm) and one is larger (21 mm). The size of the embryo itself is also variable, depending on the amount of shrinkage, manner of handling, and straightness or curvature of the specimen. Moreover, the accuracy of the measurement has to be taken into account. At this early stage it is difficult to use calipers without injuring the specimen. The most satisfactory measurements are those taken on reconstructions based on serial sections. Here, of course, one must allow approximately 25 percent for shrinkage. Omitting the obviously long and short specimens, the lengths of the sectioned embryos of this stage fall between 2.5 and 3 mm. An exceptionally long one measured 3.3 mm and an exceptionally short one measured 2.2 mm in length. When measured in formalin or 80 percent alcohol before sectioning, the embryos varied from 3.0 to 4.5 mm. One stretched in the linear axis was 5 mm long. Neither the relative size of the chorion nor the size of the embryo is constant enough to determine the level of development within the stage, although

the embryo is the less variable of the two.

The age of embryos of this stage is believed to be approximately 24 ± 1 postovulatory days. The coital history in one instance (No. 1182b) gave an age of 26 days.

A detailed investigation of this stage, with particular reference to the nervous system, was published by Müller and O'Rahilly, 1986c, and similar studies of subsequent stages are in preparation.

EXTERNAL FORM
(fig. 11-1)

The criterion for stage 11 is the presence of 13–20 pairs of somites. This is the period of the delimitation and closure of the rostral neuropore. In the less advanced specimens of the group the fusion of the neural folds has extended rostrally to the region of the midbrain. In the more advanced specimens the neuropore is closing or has just completed its closure. An equally definite characteristic of the group is the presence of the mandibular and hyoid arches. The otic invagination can be recognized in most specimens as a slight depression, and in transparent specimens it can be clearly seen because of the refraction of its thick margins.

The general form of a less advanced member (13 somites) of the group is shown in figures 11-1 and 11-2A, B. A more advanced member (19 somites) is shown in figure 11-2E in profile view, revealing its widely open communication with the umbilical vesicle. In the latter specimen there is a marked dorsal flexure, which is exaggerated here but commonly occurs in some degree in the more advanced embryos of this stage. As was pointed out by Bartelmez and Evans (1926), the more precocious head end and the heart tend to elevate that end. Similarly the relatively larger mass of the caudal end raises it above the level of the flattened, thin umbilical region, and a moderate dorsal flexure should be regarded as normal (Orts-Llorca and Lopez Rodriguez, 1957). Later, as the spinal cord and body walls of this dorsal region take on more bulk, the flexure disappears, and a smooth, convex dorsal contour becomes permanently established.

The views shown in figure 11-2C, D illustrate details of the head and cardiac region, showing the appearance of the closure of the rostral neuropore and the form and relationships of the central nervous system. In formalin specimens the fifth and the acousticofacial nerves can usually be recognized. Although reconstructions have great value in reaching an understanding of the anatomy of young embryos, it is important also to form impressions of the character of the different tissues from study of the actual specimens and from good photographic reproductions, such as those shown in figure 11-2.

Drawings of eight representative specimens of this stage are shown in figure 11-3. These are enlarged to the same scale, so that the variations in size, posture, and proportions of the specimens can be observed. If it were not for the unavoidable handling of the specimens, it appears likely that there would be but slight variations in these respects. The neural tube is the chief determiner of the form of the embryo at this time. For that reason it is shown in median section, whereby its parts and topography are made more readily recognizable. It will be seen that the dorsal flexure occurs at the transition from the larger and more precocious rostral end of the neural tube to the smaller, newly closed tube that terminates in the caudal neuropore. This flexure can be seen in some degree in all specimens of 17–20 pairs of somites.

The surface ectoderm at stage 11 possesses areas of at least three different thicknesses, and the ectodermal ring begins to form as an inverted U (O'Rahilly and Müller, 1985).

HISTOLOGICAL FEATURES

Primitive streak. The caudal eminence, which lies between the cloacal membrane and the site of the neurenteric canal, represents the region of the former primitive streak. It contains dense axial material from which new parts of the notochord are added, and paraxial condensations from which the somites develop

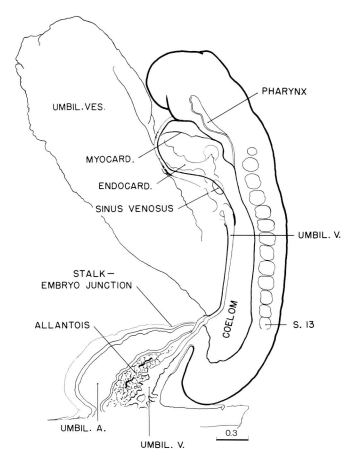

Fig. 11-1. Outline drawing of the left lateral view of No. 6344 (13 pairs of somites), showing the features that can be identified in the photograph of the right lateral view (fig. 11-2A).

(Müller and O'Rahilly, 1986c).

Somites. Four pairs of somites are considered to be occipital, although it is only in the next stage that the neural crest for the cervical region is clearly delineated and can be used as a criterion for distinguishing the occipital from the cervical region.

Somite 1 is small and makes almost no contact with the surface ectoderm. It is situated immediately caudal to the vagal-accessory neural crest. Numerous mitotic figures in its walls indicate the beginning of its transformation into material for the hypoglossal cord (O'Rahilly and Müller, 1984b). In general, the rostrocaudal extent of an individual somite is variable. Calculations show that a clear gradient in size between rostral and caudal regions is lacking. In most cases the rostral somites are larger in embryos with 13 as well as in

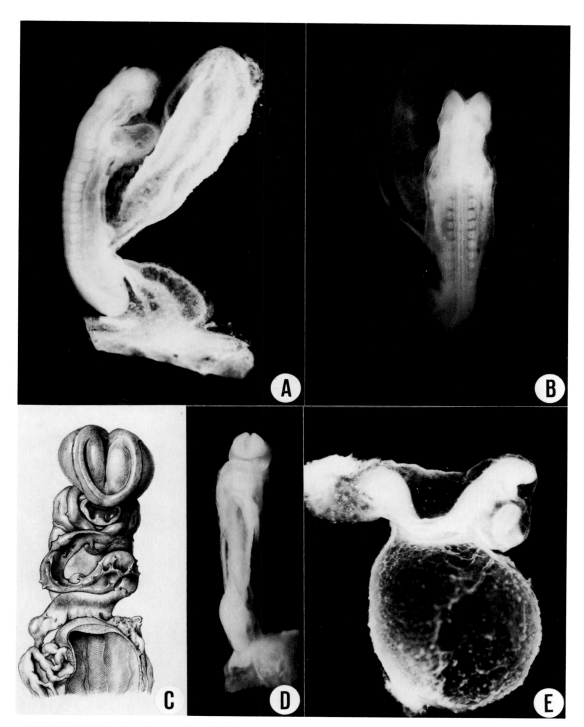

Fig. 11-2. (A) Right lateral view of No. 6344 (13 pairs of som-ites). (B) Dorsal view of the same embryo, showing that neural closure has advanced rostrally to the area of the trigeminal nerve. The somites and spinal cord are distinguishable. The median dark line that extends along the spinal cord is the transparent central canal. On each side of it is a narrow, white, opaque strip, which is the line of greatest thickness of neural tissue. Lateral to it the cord rounds off and to that extent is thinner. (C) No. 4529 (14 pairs of somites), based on a reconstruction by Osborne O. Heard. It shows how the neural lips begin to close rostrally and come to cover D2. (D) No. 6784 (17 pairs of somites), showing a later phase in the closure of the rostral neuropore, with the typical blunt end of the neural tube. (E) No. 6050 (19/21 pairs of somites), showing the umbilical vesicle. A dorsal curvature is common at this time. It is caused by the flexibility of the thin central part of the embryo as contrasted with the two ends, the bulbous caudal tip with connecting stalk at the rear, and the advanced head structures and heart rostrally. This specimen shows the entrance through which the coelomic fluid gains access to the mesoblast. By chance there was a break in the umbilical vein and some embryonic blood escaped into the cardiac region of the coelom, delineating its dorsal contours, as though injected. As is typical of this stage, the umbilical vesicle still opens widely into the gut.

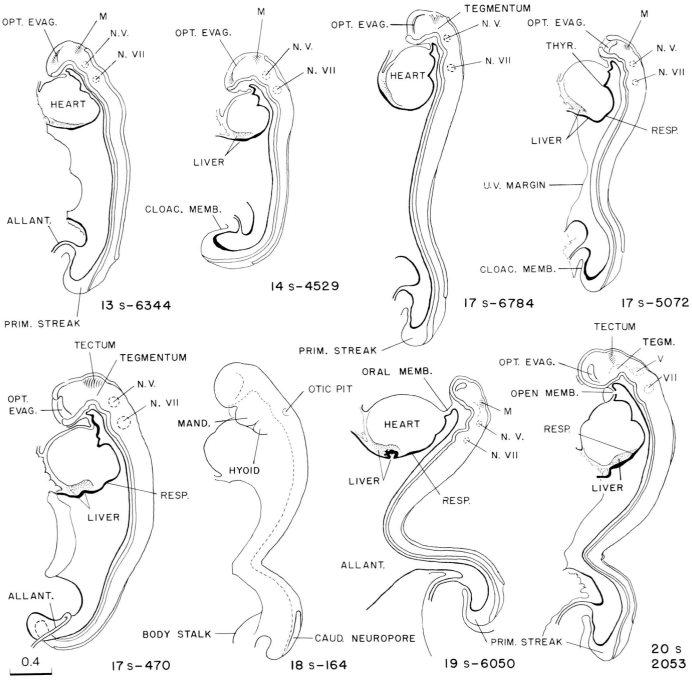

Fig. 11-3. Eight representative specimens of stage 11, enlarged to the same scale and hence directly comparable as to size, proportions, and posture. It will be noted that the neural tube appears to be the chief factor that determines form, and the primary neural parts are already distinct. The number of somitic pairs and the collection number of the embryo are given for each specimen. The tracing of the 18-somite embryo, No. 164, was made from a photograph. All the others are median-section drawings made from Born reconstructions. It will be seen that active proliferation in the hepatic region is beginning in the more advanced members of the group.

those with 20 somites. The mean time for the formation of one pair of somites during stages 9–12 inclusive is 6.6 hours (Müller and O'Rahilly, 1986c).

Coelom. Streeter, whose detailed description of the coelom follows, defined the term coelom as "any walled-off space or fluid reservoir uniformly present in the mesoblast" and "also any similar space formed in the extra-embryonic mesoblastic reticulum." Furthermore, under the term coelom "are to be included both the free passage for coelomic fluid and the enclosing walls that are irrigated by it." This idea has been explored further in the rat by Langemeijer (1976), who writes of a "coelomic organ," i.e., a single, tubular organ serving as the blastema of various thoracic organs and comparable to the neural tube in possessing a specific wall that encloses a cavity.

When mesoblastic cells become detached from the pluripotential cells of the primitive streak, they are advanced one degree in specialization, which means that they are therewith restricted to certain potentialities in respect to development; they no longer share with the epiblast the possibility of becoming skin ectoderm or neural ectoderm. They can still take on many forms, however. As they proliferate and spread out in the form of a reticular sheet, some of them can soon be recognized as vasoformative strands, representing the elements of the blood vascular system.

The first conspicuous event in mesoblastic organization, however, is the beginning bilateral segmentation of the medial part of the mesoblast along its longitudinal axis. On each side, along the neural tube, focal centers of active differentiation occur serially, and there are thereby produced the highly characteristic somites. In its more peripheral regions the mesoblastic sheet shows no trace of segmental development. Instead, the proliferation of mesoblastic cells produces a thickened marginal band in which the cells become arranged as coalescing vesicles, resulting in a continuous mesoblastic cavity or passage. This development first occurs in a crescentic field at the rostral end of the embryonic disc. Such a passage is already present in stage 9 and, in stage 10, it has extended caudad and opens freely on both sides into the extra-embryonic coelom. In this manner an advantageous arrangement is provided by which the more deeply lying mesoblastic parts of the embryo can be freely reached by the coelomic fluid, which at this time is the sole source

of nutriment. Although this is but a primitive type of circulation, it appears to serve that function adequately up to the time it is superseded by the blood vascular system. In other words, in the early organization of the mesoblastic tissue the first two major events are the differentiation of the medial part as segmental somites and the differentiation of the peripheral part as the non-segmental coelom. The coelomic walls respond with characteristic activity, and later give origin to various kinds of structures.

By stage 11 the coelom has become a conspicuous feature. Its distribution in a 13-somite embryo is shown in figure 11-4. In this drawing, slabs have been removed, exposing schematically three representative levels: upper cervical level, somite 4, and somite 8. It will be seen that below the level of somite 6 there is a free opening from the exocoelom into the intra-embryonic coelom in the cleft separating the umbilical vein and the primordium of the abdominal wall from the umbilical vesicle. Caudally, the coelom extends along the side of the intestinal epithelium and spreads caudad with it as the caudal bud continues its differentiation, always remaining widely open to the exocoelom and communicating with the opposite side across and caudal to the junction of the gut and umbilical vesicle. Above, at the level of somites 5 and 6, a trace of the multiple openings from the intra-embryonic coelom into the exocoelom, which originally characterized this system, still persists in the form of a partition marking off an upper opening from the main communication. In the more advanced specimens of this stage, this partition disappears, and there remains but one common opening. Following the coelom rostrally, it is seen again as a closed passage at the level of somite 4, and rostrally from there it soon widens out into the original coelomic space, which now invests the endothelial heart and its gelatinous envelope. It would seem that the first cardiac movements would tend to facilitate the flow of fluid through the coelomic passage.

Typical transverse sections through the same 13-somite embryo are shown in figure 11-5. It will be seen that everywhere along the margins of the coelom an active proliferation of cells is taking place, more active in some regions than in others. In addition to proliferating, these mesoblastic cells also are differentiating into special tissues that will constitute the connective tissues, muscle, and vasoformative elements of the heart, lungs, and alimentary canal. Thus in section *A*, through the rostral end of the heart, the visceral part of the coelomic wall is producing myocardium and the parietal part is shedding cells that will form various elements of the thoracic wall. The definitive pericardium will be formed by the residual coelomic cells after the more special cells are segregated out. As for the pleurae, they are even more remote. Photographs showing early histogenesis of the myocardium are reproduced as figure 11-6A, D. It will be seen that the visceral surface of the coelomic passage does not exist as a membrane, separate from the myocardium; instead, the surface cells merge directly into the more deeply lying cells. The surface cells are more-actively proliferating and remain more primitive than the deeper ones, whereas the deeper ones are on the way to specialization and to that extent have sacrificed their potentialities. The surface cells do not yet exist as a distinct and separate layer.

Proceeding to the level of somite 1, section *B* of figure 11-5 passes through the base of the heart and obliquely through the primordium of the liver. In respect to the heart, the section shows the sinus venosus and the area where the heart rests on the liver. It will be noted that the coelom is actively giving off cells that form a condensed mass constituting the early mesoblastic framework of the liver. Photographs illustrating this process under higher power in a slightly more advanced embryo are shown as figure 11-6A–C. Note is to be taken of the transition of the coelomic surface cells into the deeper cells and the phenomenon of angiogenesis that immediately begins in the latter (fig. 11-6B). The digestive epithelium lies under the more dorsal part of the hepatic primordium, and doubtless is playing a role in its development, but it is not until the next stage that a really distinct hepatic diverticulum and the origin of hepatic epithelial cords that penetrate the mesodermal framework provided by the coelomic wall become apparent. Figure 11-6B shows the digestive epithelium underlying the hepatic primordium shortly before the epithelial cords invade the liver. Thus, in the formation of the liver its mesodermal elements are supplied by the coelom, whereas its epithelial elements come from the opposite direction (i.e., from the gut).

At the level of somite 4 (fig. 11-5C), not only does

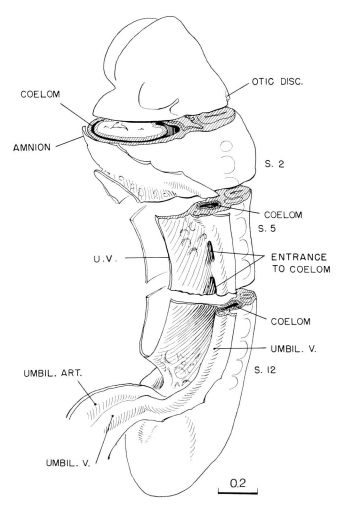

Fig. 11-4. The distribution of the coelom in a 13-somite embryo (No. 6344). At three representative levels the surfaces are exposed schematically, showing the relations of the coelomic channel to the mesoblast and to the heart. The first pulsations of the latter presumably aid in the movement of coelomic fluid, which at this time is the sole source of nutriment for these tissues.

the coelom provide a passage for its contained fluid, but also its walls are actively proliferating cells that are to take a large part in the formation of the gut wall, the adjacent vessels, and the body wall itself. Further caudally (section *D*) is shown the free communication of the intra-embryonic coelom with the exocoelom. It will be seen that coelomic proliferation is in general the same at all levels. The proliferation and accompanying specialization of these cells are roughly comparable to what is seen in the differentiation of the neural tube. There too the germinal cells lie near the

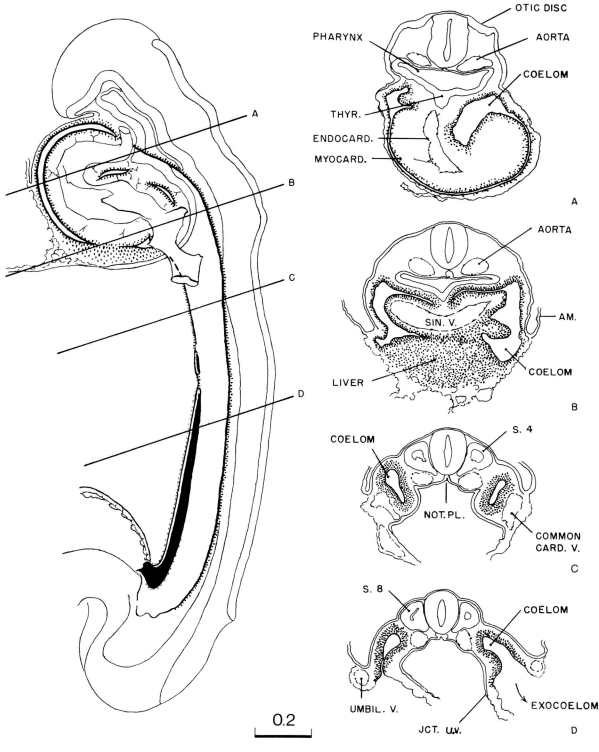

Fig. 11-5. Typical sections through the coelom of No. 6344. The mesoblastic surface bathed by the coelomic fluid is a locus of active cell proliferation. It is a germinal bed from which the specializing daughter cells move inward radially to form various structures according to the field from which they arise. Thus the coelomic walls give origin to such divergent tissues as myocardium, the framework of the liver, and the muscular coats, blood vessels, and connective tissue envelopes of the gut. The coelomic walls are demarcated at this stage into territories each of which has its own characteristics.

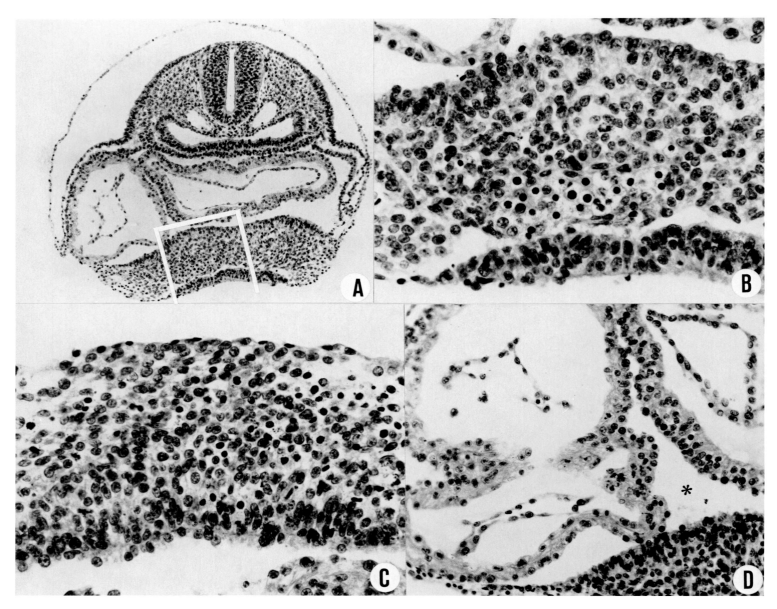

Fig. 11-6. (A) Section showing the hepatic and cardiac regions in a 16-somite embryo (No. 7611, section 3-4-1). (B) Same section, area enclosed by white line in A. This is the hepatic primordium. The cells that are to form the framework are proliferating at the coelomic surface and crowding downward. Some of them are already undergoing the first steps in angiogenesis. Below is the gut epithelium, which is not yet giving off epithelial cords. (C) Section at a more rostral level (3-2-6) of the same specimen. Framework cells are proliferating from the coelomic surface and show early angioblasts. This is just in front of the junction between the gut and umbilical vesicle, and no gut epithelium is included. (D) Detail of the myocardium in the same embryo (section 3-3-2). The coelomic fluid (asterisk) comes in contact with the hepatic region below, and it bathes the surface of the folded myocardium above. The surface cells of the myocardium constitute a germinal bed from which specialized myocardial cells are arising. Differentiation follows rapidly. Aside from the germinal bed, there is no surface membrane that can be designated as pericardium, which will appear later.

central canal, and the segregated special cells (mantle zone), produced in the course of proliferation, move away from the border of the lumen. It is also to be noted that certain fields of this coelomic proliferation are sharply marked off from one another.

After this orientation on the structure and topography of the coelom, it is easier to understand the surface anatomy of embryos of this stage as seen in photographs. Specimens at this time are quite transparent after formalin fixation, and by means of stereoscopic photographs much of the anatomy can be observed. A large part of the coelomic passage can be seen in the specimen shown in figure 11-2A. This is to be compared with the accompanying explanatory diagram (fig. 11-1). A more advanced specimen (19 somites) is illustrated in figure 11-2E. On each side of this embryo, a single and wider opening from the exocoelom into the intra-embryonic coelom can be plainly seen. By a fortunate accident, there was a slight extravasation of embryonic blood, apparently from a tear through the umbilical vein, and this blood found its way into the cardiac region of the coelomic passage in such a way as to outline the dorsal confines of the cavity as though it were injected. Such an opening into the coelomic passage provides ready access of the exocoelomic fluid to the deeper tissues of the embryo. In the next stage the opening is still larger.

The coelomic epithelium is exceptional during early development in its close structural and histogenetic relationships to the underlying mesenchyme. The capacity of embryonic coelomic cells to change from epithelial to mesenchymal, or vice versa, can be seen in the development of their derivatives. Thus, in the initial formation of the gonads (and the suprarenal cortex), the coelomic wall reverts to an early condition in which the surface lining acts as a germinal layer and produces mesenchymal cells, the basement membrane of the mesothelium being abolished (Gruenwald, 1942). The blastema thereby formed differentiates into the epithelial primary sex cords and the intervening mesenchyme (*ibid.*).

Notochordal plate and notochord. The development of the notochordal plate into notochord proceeds longitudinally from caudal to rostral, and the last areas to retain the plate are in the pharynx. The separation of the notochordal plate from the alimentary system involves the following: (1) the plate becomes U-shaped even in stage 10, (2) the vertical limbs of the U begin to move medially and touch each other, (3) the adjoining digestive epithelium begins to form a thin cytoplasmic bridge, and (4) mitotic figures appear and the still U-shaped notochord is cut off entirely (Müller and O'Rahilly, 1986c).

The part of the notochord that forms directly from the axial condensation in the caudal eminence is far thicker and more advanced in differentiation. The notochord has a dual mode of origin: (1) rostral to the neurenteric canal or its site, it develops from the notochordal plate, and (2) caudally it arises from the axial condensation.

The notochordal plate and notochord are still intimately related to the neural tube (and the notochord to the digestive epithelium), and their basement membranes are in contact.

Neurenteric canal. The former site of the canal can generally be determined but with much more difficulty than at the previous stage. The site moves caudad during stages 10 and 11.

Prechordal plate. The prechordal plate (Gilbert, 1957), which is more difficult to recognize than in previous stages, lies adjacent and rostral to the notochord, and caudal and lateral to the adenohypophysial area. Scant prechordal material is found in the median plane, most having migrated laterally to form the premandibular condensation.

CARDIOVASCULAR SYSTEM

Not only is the heart beating but "it is generally accepted that peristaltic flow begins" during stage 11 (de Vries and Saunders, 1962).

A description of the heart and blood vessels present in a 14-somite embryo has been given by Heuser (1930) and in a 20-somite specimen by Davis (1923). Here attention will be confined to the general characteristics of a vascular system that is adequate for an organism having the size and complexity found at this stage.

In figure 11-7 are shown in outline the endothelial vessels and plexuses that characterize the embryo at the time when its heart has begun to beat. The vascular apparatus still consists of simple endothelium. Only in the cardiac region have auxiliary tissues been differentiated. The endothelium of the heart is enclosed in a jelly-like envelope, as has been well described by

Davis. This cardiac jelly is in turn enclosed by a mantle of contractile tissue, the primordium of the myocardium. The character of this myocardium is shown in figure 11-6A, D. It is to be remembered that the myocardium is a specialization of the coelom, and its outer surface is bathed directly by the coelomic fluid. The immediate consequence of its specialization is its beginning pulsations.

Returning to figure 11-7, it will be seen that the vascular system of the caudal half of the embryo consists of a changing capillary plexus, which along with the laying down of the caudal end of the embryo spreads backward, always readjusting its communications with the large vascular channels of the connecting stalk. In the rostral and more advanced half of the embryo, the endothelial channels are attaining a more mature pattern. As would be expected, the endocardium and its associated coelomic derivatives, which originally were situated at the rostral end of the embryonic disc, show the most-advanced differentiation. The embryo is thereby provided at this time with a mechanism that serves to stir, and thereby aid the diffusion of, the substances contained both in the fluid of its endothelial plexus and in the coelomic fluid. Although it is too early to speak of a true circulation, under the conditions of an ebb and flow, there is a directional tendency from the heart to the aortae and from the umbilical vesicle to the heart. The capillaries of the rostral part of the umbilical vesicle, where it joins the gut endoderm, have already responded to the precocious endocardium by active growth and adjustment in the form of enlarged channels, which communicate with the heart. In a 16-somite embryo a sinus venosus is already present, and in more-advanced specimens of this stage a constriction begins to mark the boundary that separates it from the atrium proper. The cardiac pulsations may well be a factor in this endothelial adjustment. Although the plexus of the umbilical vesicle is not well advanced at this stage, one can distinguish at its rostral end the numerous communications that will later result in the omphalomesenteric veins, and likewise the mesh from the aorta that will produce the omphalomesenteric arteries. The umbilical veins and arteries are already formed; for this development, the connecting stalk and allantoic influences appear to have been responsible. The primary blood vessels of the central nervous system are more or less connected up

in the more advanced parts, but the cardinal veins and the segmental branches from the aorta and their spinal cord communications are incompletely connected. At the caudal end of the embryo, they are represented merely by isolated vesicles. The common cardinal veins do not yet bridge the interval to the atrial endocardium, and a true circulation must await that development.

The fluid throughout the endothelial system, during this ebb-and-flow period, contains relatively few cells. A survey was made by Streeter of serial sections of thirteen embryos of this stage. For the most part the vessels were free of cells in the rostral half of the embryo, including the atria, ventricles, aortae, and umbilical veins. Occasionally, a few scattered embryonic blood cells or small clumps of them could be seen. In the caudal half, the aortae and the umbilical arteries and veins of the connecting stalk either were empty or contained a few cells. In some, numerous cells or clumps of cells were noted. In two specimens both the caudal region of the aorta and the umbilical arteries were moderately distended with blood cells, as though the cells had backed in from the umbilical vesicle. In one specimen the umbilical vein on one side was moderately distended with blood cells. This does not signify that the blood had escaped from the embryo into the chorion, because the latter likewise was largely free of blood cells. The villi contained very few cells. The vessels of the chorionic membrane, usually the branches of the umbilical artery, contained a moderate number of cells, but none of them was distended. The umbilical vesicle showed uniformly the presence of active blood islands, close together in the collapsed sac and separated by intervals of tenuous wall when the vesicle was distended. In most regions of the umbilical vesicle, all capillaries were filled with blood cells. In the proximal part of the sac, where it is continuous with gut endoderm, one frequently finds large capillaries completely empty or nearly so. It is such connecting branches that open into the sinus venosus and the cardiac end of the umbilical vein.

In addition to the rather complicated vascular system described above, one finds a differentiation of many new foci of angiogenesis, particularly along the surface of the central nervous system and in other mesoblastic regions. In figure 11-6B is shown an early stage of angiogenesis in the coelomic mesoblast of the hepatic

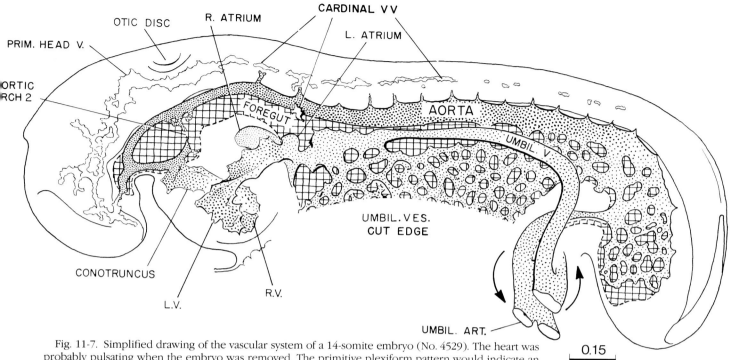

Fig. 11-7. Simplified drawing of the vascular system of a 14-somite embryo (No. 4529). The heart was probably pulsating when the embryo was removed. The primitive plexiform pattern would indicate an ebb-and-flow type of circulation. At the cardiac end of the plexus of the umbilical vesicle, the channels are beginning to be specialized into trunks characteristic of the venous end of the heart. The central nervous system, because of the widely open neuropores, is not yet dependent on a blood supply, and one can see only the first elements of a cardinal system. This drawing is based on the reconstruction published by Heuser (1930).

primordium. The segregation of specialization of these angioblastic cells apparently occurs during proliferation of the coelomic cells. Among these new cells are some that become blood-forming cells, and these become set apart from the less specialized embryonic connective tissue cells, all of which, however, are destined to form the final framework of the liver.

In short, one can say that at this stage the embryo is adequately maintained by a simple system of large endothelial channels that course through the deep tissues, and that in these channels an almost cell-free fluid ebbs and flows because of the action of the pulsations of the myocardium. What is necessary in the way of regulation of osmotic pressure and nutrient supply is provided in this manner, over and above the diffusion already secured by the services of the coelomic fluid that irrigates the various areas of the coelom.

By the end of stage 11 (fig. 15-5) the sequence of the cardiac chambers is: sinus venosus, right atrium, left atrium, atrioventricular canal, left ventricle, right ventricle, conotruncus, aortic arches. The "sinus venosus has almost completed its separation from the left side of the heart and opens into the dorsum of the right atrium, a fundamental relation which it ever after retains" (Davis, 1927). The ventricles have descended relative to the atria (Müller and O'Rahilly, 1986b), and the atrioventricular canal has changed from a vertical to a dorsoventral orientation (Davis, 1927). The ventricles have become trabeculated and the interventricular septum may have appeared (McBride, Moore, and Hutchins, 1981). The conus cordis has differentiated from the right ventricle (de Vries and Saunders, 1962), and the aortic sac (or sinus) develops as additional aortic arches form (de Vries, 1981). The dorsal mesocardium has ruptured.

DIGESTIVE AND RESPIRATORY SYSTEMS
(figs. 11-3 and 11-5)

Pharyngeal arch 2 develops and arch 3 may do so. Pharyngeal membrane 2 appears and pharyngeal pouch

4 may form. The thyroid primordium has been subject to varying interpretations (O'Rahilly, 1983a). The oropharyngeal membrane may have begun to rupture. Esophagorespiratory and hepatorespiratory grooves may be found, the hepatic diverticulum grows into the septum transversum, and the cystic primordium may become distinguishable.

The pulmonary primordium is more evident than previously and it shows a high alkaline phosphatase reaction (Mori, 1959b).

URINARY AND REPRODUCTIVE SYSTEMS

The mesonephric duct develops as a solid rod *in situ* from the nephrogenic cord (Torrey, 1954) or perhaps from ectodermal buds lateral to somites 8–13 (Jirásek, 1971). The nephrogenic tissue develops into nephric vesicles which are connected by (at first solid) tubules with the mesonephric duct.

The cloacal membrane is in a central, oval depression on the ventral surface of the caudal part of the body wall.

The primordial germ cells are migrating from the umbilical vesicle to the hindgut (Witschi, 1948).

NERVOUS SYSTEM
(figs. 11-8, 11-9, 11-10, and 13-10)

The brain at stage 11 has been described in detail by Müller and O'Rahilly (1986c).

The neural tube appears to be the chief factor that determines the form of the embryo at this time. All embryonic organs seem to be influenced in their form by their environment, but of them the central nervous system is perhaps the most nearly independent. Its form seems to be the unmixed expression of the proliferation and enlargement of the cells that compose its wall.

The closure of the rostral neuropore in stage 11 (figs. 11-3 and 11-8) is basically a bidirectional process: it continues from the rhombencephalon to the mesencephalon and proceeds from the optic chiasma toward the roof of D1, thereby forming the "adult" lamina terminalis and the future commissural plate. In embryos with 13 somites the rostrocaudal closure has scarcely begun, and hence the material of the future lamina terminalis still lies laterally. By 14 somites, clo-

sure at the level of the lamina terminalis has commenced. In embryos having about 20 pairs of somites, the forebrain is completely closed.

When the neural ectoderm becomes shut off from contact with the amniotic fluid, compensation is simultaneously made by the development and spread of blood capillaries, and these promptly invest the neural tube with a close-meshed network. Later, as the neural wall becomes thicker, this capillary network responds by sending in branches, thereby bringing the required service to the more deeply lying cells. The skin ectoderm continues to obtain what it needs from the amniotic fluid and for a long time requires no special provision in the way of capillaries.

A typical example of brain form in embryos of this stage is shown in figure 11-9. The drawing of a well-preserved 16-somite embryo should be compared with the dorsal view shown in figure 11-2B (See also fig. 13-10.) The forebrain, consisting of D1 and D2 (already present in stage 10, see fig. 10-7), is still relatively simple. Part D1 is largely the area of the optic primordium and, in the median plane, the chiasmatic plate. The caudal limit of the plate is sometimes indicated by a postoptic recess. The floor of D2 includes mamillary and neurohypophysial components, and the latter is recognizable indirectly by the primordium of the adenohypophysis, which is the ectodermal region at the summit of the oropharyngeal membrane. Part D2 still protrudes toward the median plane, and its right and left convexities almost touch each other in the least advanced embryos. As the optic primordia become more evaginated, the walls of D2 recede and the ventricular cavity begins to expand. The medial parts of the forebrain rostral to D1, which fuse during the closure of the rostral neuropore in stage 11, are telencephalic. They contribute to the formation of the embryonic lamina terminalis and commissural plate.

The most uncertain part to identify precisely is the mesencephalon (tectum and tegmentum in fig. 11-9) because its delineation toward both the diencephalon and the rhombencephalon is difficult. It appears to consist of only one segment at this stage.

Neuromeres, which are transverse swellings in the developing neural tube, can best be assessed by evaluating the three main planes of section. Swellings and grooves are best shown in reconstructions of sagittal sections, whereas transverse sections are preferable in

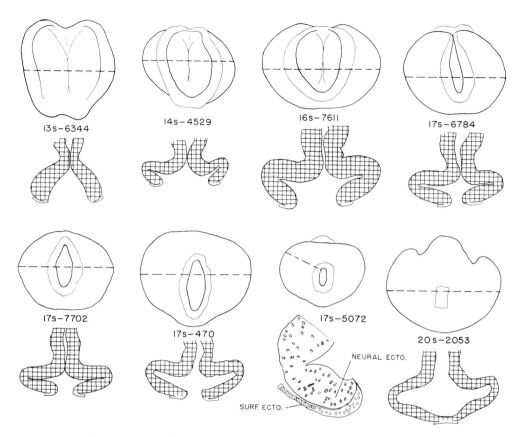

13s–6344   14s–4529   16s–7611   17s–6784

17s–7702   17s–470   17s–5072   20s–2053

NEURAL ECTO.

SURF ECTO.

Fig. 11-8. Outline drawings of the rostral end of the neural tube in a series of embryos, showing the steps in the closure of the rostral neuropore. Underneath each specimen is shown a horizontal section taken at the level indicated by the broken line. These show the extent of the optic evaginations. In the section of the 17-somite specimen (No. 5072) only the right side is drawn, showing the demarcation between neural and skin ectoderm. With the exception of No. 5072, all are drawn to the same scale.

determining the relationship to ganglia. Indications of neuromeres are already evident at stages 9 and 10. A combination of the various data shows two neuromeres in the forebrain (D1 and D2), one in the midbrain, and 6–7 in RhA–RhC. Part RhD, the area of somites 1–4 (the hypoglossal region), is clearly delineated neither by a groove nor by a deepening. D1 and D2 correspond to neuromeres a and b, M to proneuromere B, RhA, RhB, and RhC to proneuromeres C, D, and E of Bergquist and Källén (personal communication, 1969). Their inventory contains no equivalent for RhD of the present authors. RhA–RhC, as described by Bartelmez (1923) for stage 9, were termed proneuromeres by Bergquist (1952) because of their existence in the still open neural groove. Three-dimensional reconstructions demonstrate the neuromeres clearly to be serial swellings of the brain.

The rhombomeres can be distinguished comparatively easily by the developing ganglia (fig. 11-9). The trigeminal ganglion characterizes Rh2, the faciovestibulocochlear ganglion Rh4, the glossopharyngeal Rh6, and the vagal Rh7; Rh3 and Rh5 appear to have no neural crest. Somites 1–4 enable RhD, the region of the hypoglossal nerve, to be identified.

The picture presented by the walls of the spinal cord at this time reveals, by the frequency of mitotic figures, that the germinal bed of proliferating cells lies along the margin of the central canal. It is from the canal that nutriment still diffuses among the cells. From this germinal bed new cells move externally. Cell proliferation and the concomitant cell specialization is only in its early phases at this stage, and one cannot yet mark off ependymal and mantle zones, such as characterize later stages.

Neural Crest

Neural crest cells are still being given off at the site of Rh4, Rh6, and Rh7, all of which are now closed. Therefore, the same areas, open in stage 10 and producing neural crest already at this former stage, continue the production of neural crest material when closed. What is the same in both modes is the fact that the neural crest cells are clearly derived from the neural ectoderm.

Neural crest cells contribute to the formation of head mesenchyme together with the material from the prechordal plate. The mesencephalic neural crest is still being produced and spreads toward the optic evagination, and, in more-advanced embryos, mixes with optic crest cells thereby forming the sheath of the optic vesicle. The trigeminal neural crest is more condensed than in stage 10. A condensation of cells is visible within the mandibular arch, but it is not possible to decide whether it is neural crest material deposited there during stage 10, or paraxial mesenchyme, or

both. Also in pharyngeal arch 2, two different groups of cells seem to be present, the first clearly representing ganglion 7/8, and the second, also slightly more condensed, forming a prolongation within the arch. Prechordal mesenchyme was spreading out laterally in the premandibular area and ventrally to the heart in stage 10; it is now limited to the premandibular area.

The nasal plate is one of the ectodermal areas giving rise to neural crest. Although it does so only in later stages, the plate becomes apparent in stage 11 and lies on both sides of the neuropore (O'Rahilly and Müller, 1985).

The histological character of the neural tube in a 17-somite embryo is shown in figure 11-10. The sections A and B are taken at two different regions. The upper is at the level of somite 5, cutting obliquely through the spinal cord and thereby exaggerating its ventrodorsal diameter. Compared with the section through the lower level (somite 16), it is larger; its walls are thicker and contain more cells, and the central canal is correspondingly compressed. Another fea-

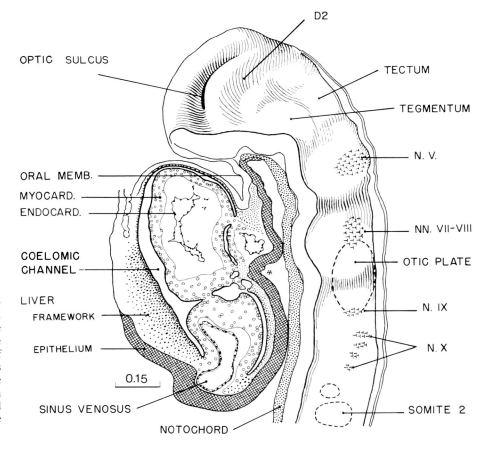

Fig. 11-9. Median view of the rostral half of a 16-somite embryo (No. 7611), showing segmental structures in the forebrain (D1 and D2) and in the hindbrain. The area of ganglion 5 is rhombomere A, the area of ganglion 7/8 is RhB, and the area of ganglia 9 and 10 is RhC. The adjacent structures that participate in giving form to this part of the embryo are shown in the drawing. The median ventral pocket of pharyngeal epithelium, marked with an asterisk, indicates the beginning of the thyroid gland.

ture showing advance in maturity is the migration of the neural crest cells, which have detached themselves from the cells of the dorsal lips at the closure line. At the more caudal level the neural crest cells have not started their migration, and because of their presence the dorsal seam has the gross appearance of a keystone closing in the arched lateral walls. These crest cells do not appear to be proliferating as actively as the other cells of the neural wall, and the wedge-shaped area formed by them is correspondingly paler. It is after their migration that the active proliferation of the crest cells occurs. The progress of neural crest formation has been plotted for stage 11 by Bartelmez and Evans (1926) and by Heuser (1930).

Eye

The right and left optic primordia meet at the optic chiasma and, together with the latter, form a U-shaped rim in the least developed embryos of stage 11 (fig. 11-2C).

The optic evagination is produced at the optic sulcus when about 14 pairs of somites are present, and the optic ventricle is continuous with that of the forebrain (O'Rahilly, 1966, 1983b). The optic evagination constitutes the optic vesicle when approximately 17–19 pairs of somites are visible (fig. 11-8).

The wall of the optic evagination contributes neural crest to its mesenchymal sheath from about 14–16 pairs of somites onward (Bartelmez and Blount, 1954). The sheath probably also acquires cells from the mesencephalic neural crest (Müller and O'Rahilly, 1986c). The sheath then separates the evagination from the overlying ectoderm. A caudal, limiting sulcus develops between the optic evagination and the forebrain.

Ear

The invaginating otic disc is already a sharply demarcated structure, and with suitable illumination it can be seen in a gross specimen. It is seen to best advantage, however, in stained sections. A series of such sections is shown in figure 11-11, and they cover the range of development that characterizes this stage. The definite line that marks the junction of the disc with the skin ectoderm is characteristic of this stage. It is to be noted that this feature is acquired before a

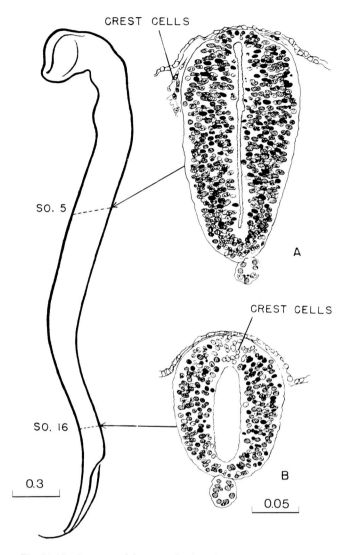

Fig. 11-10. Contour of the neural tube of a 17-somite embryo (No. 6784). The upper two-thirds is definitely more advanced than the recently closed lower third. Thus section A, through the level of somite 5, is more mature than section B, through somite 16. In the former the neural crest cells have migrated ventrally, whereas at the more caudal level they are still incorporated in the neural wall.

distinct pit appears. The disc may be regarded as an island of neural tissue that has the appearance of having floated away from the main neuroectodermal mass and is now separated from it by the intervening skin ectoderm. During its proliferative period, this disc of specialized neural ectoderm closely resembles the parent neural tube. To go further back, it is to be remem-

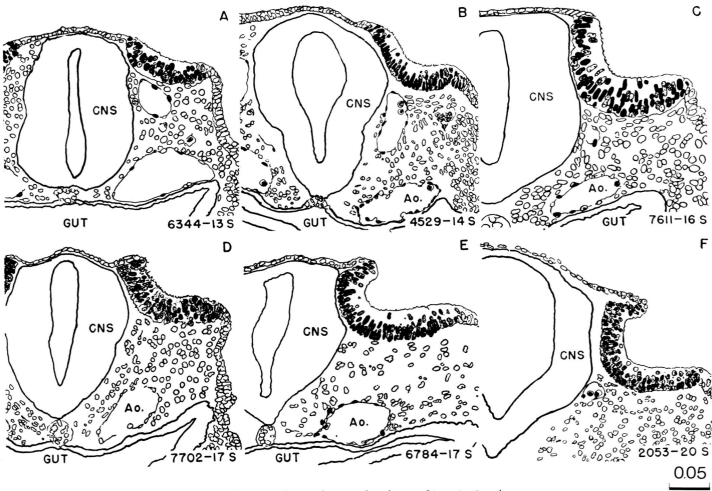

Fig. 11-11. Sections of the otic plate in selected embryos, showing the phases of invagination that characterize this stage. The serial number of the embryo and the number of somites are given in each case. All are enlarged to the same scale.

bered that the neural ectoderm is a product of the proliferation of the pluripotential mother cells of the epiblast. The neural ectoderm becomes segregated by stage 8 and becomes one of the primary embryonic tissues. As it does so, the central strip laid down becomes the neural tube with its particular potentialities. It is possible that at the same time some of the marginal neuroectodermal cells are specialized in the direction of forming various plates and neural crest masses. These become detached, some earlier and some later, from the main neural plate, and it is possible that the otic disc is an example of such a detached island of specialized neuroectodermal material. It can be readily understood, from examination of the sections in

figure 11-11, that operative removal of this specialized otic plate would result in complete absence of an otic vesicle on that side of the head, and that the adjacent skin ectoderm, being different in composition, would not have the requisite potentialities to repair the loss. This has become a familiar experiment.

The specimens selected for illustration in figure 11-11 are especially well preserved and may be accepted as presenting the normal form. In macerated embryos the marked histological difference between skin ectoderm and the neural ectoderm of the otic disc is easily overlooked. In such material the otic plate may be thinned out and its outlines distorted.

In stage 11 it is possible to see cells leaving the otic

epithelium even more clearly than in stage 10. The basement membrane is disrupted at those sites. Ventral to the otic pit the migrating cells form a characteristic cellular sheath, and they still have the appearance of neural crest cells.

SPECIMENS OF STAGE 11 ALREADY DESCRIBED

13–14 somites, University of Chicago collection, No. H 8. A macerated and damaged specimen. Described by Bartelmez (1922) and also included in the study by Bartelmez and Evans (1926).

13–14 somites, No. 121, Department of Anatomy, Tohoku University, Sendai. Distribution of alkaline phosphatase studied by Mori (1959b).

14 somites, Carnegie No. 12. A pioneer specimen sectioned under poor technical facilities. Described by Mall (1897).

14 somites, Pfannenstiel III, Giessen. Described as embryo No. 6 in the *Normentafeln* by Keibel and Elze (1908). Representative sections schematically shown in text figure 6, *a–w*. External form of embryo pictured on plate 5 as figures *Vr.* and *Vv.* Embryo described in monograph form by Low (1908). Plastic models are shown by him of external form, central nervous system, digestive system, heart and large vessels. The specimen has two pharyngeal arches, clearly marked. The neural lips are closed rostrally as far as the collicular region.

14 somites, Carnegie No. 4529. A well-preserved specimen, well described by Heuser (1930). More monographs of this standard are needed.

14 somites, embryo von Bulle, Anatomical Collection, Basel. Described by Kollman (1889). Also pictured by Kollman in his *Handatlas* (1907). Described in the Keibel and Elze *Normentafeln* as No. 5, and external form pictured on plate 1 as figure IV. Kollman originally reported that there were 13 somites, but his figures show 14 distinct elevations. The closure of the neural tube was probably further rostralward than is shown.

14 somites, Cano embryo, Madrid. Described by Orts-Llorca, Lopez Rodriguez, and Cano Monasterio (1958). Histological condition only fair.

14 somites, Carnegie No. 779. This highly abnormal embryo is included because of the detailed account that has been published of its complete dysraphia (Dekaban, 1963; Dekaban and Bartelmez, 1964).

Approximately 15 somites, collection of First Anatomical Institute of Vienna, embryo Hal. 2. Heart described by Tandler and pharynx by Grosser in Keibel and Mall (1912). Embryo reported as swollen and not suited for cytological studies (Politzer, 1928a).

15 somites, von Spee collection, No. 52, Kiel. Camera lucida drawing by Graf Spee before treatment with alcohol, showing right profile of embryo, umbilical vesicle, and connecting stalk. There are 15 discernible somites (Döderlein, 1915, fig. 37). Sections reveal good histological condition of tissues. Used by Evans in Keibel and Mall (1912, fig. 411).

15 somites, University of Chicago collection, No. H 810 (Carnegie No. 8962). Series incomplete, histology fair. Described by Dorland and Bartelmez (1922).

17 somites, Carnegie No. 470. Description, chiefly of central nervous system, published by Bartelmez and Evans (1926).

17 somites, Carnegie No. 4315 (University of Chicago No. H951). Described by Wen (1928) with particular reference to the nervous system. Possibly 18 somites but probably not (Arey, 1938).

17 somites, Carnegie No. 5072. Monographic description, based on three-dimensional reconstructions in addition to the study of the serial sections, published by Atwell (1930).

17 and 19 somites, twins, Toronto collection, No. V and No. VI. Described by Watt (1915).

18 somites, Giglio-Tos, embryo A. Description published by Giglio-Tos (1902). Embryo reported to have 15 segments, but from other evidence it is probably more advanced. The author notes that the caudal neuropore is open, and the reader must infer that the rostral neuropore is closed. The otic invagination appears to be well advanced, although still open. There should therefore be 18 or more somites. The cytological description of the neural tube indicates good preservation. There are no drawings to portray the form of the embryo and the status of organogenesis.

18 somites, Embryological Institute, Vienna, embryo B. Described in part by Sternberg (1927) in a study of the closure of the rostral neuropore. A monographic description of this embryo was published by Politzer (1928a), which establishes it as one of the best representatives of this stage. Unfortunately destroyed.

18 somites, von Spee, Kiel. Only drawings of the external form, right profile and dorsal views, and a sketch showing perforation of the oropharyngeal membrane, are available. The rostral neuropore appears closed. These drawings seem to have been made by Graf Spee and constitute figures 38, 39, and 42 in Döderlein's *Handbuch* (1915). Apparently the embryo has never been sectioned or studied in detail.

20 somites, Embryological Laboratory of Geneva, embryo Eternod-Delaf. Described in monographic form by Bujard (1913–1914). A well-preserved normal embryo. Description given of its external form. Carefully made plastic and graphic reconstructions reveal the form of the central nervous system, digestive system, coelom, vascular system, and somites. The rostral neuropore is almost closed; there are two pharyngeal arches. It is probable, therefore, that the somitic count is correct.

20 somites, Carnegie No. 2053. A notable description of this embryo was published by Davis (1923). Because of its histological excellence and the care with which it has been studied, this specimen deserves a position of distinction.

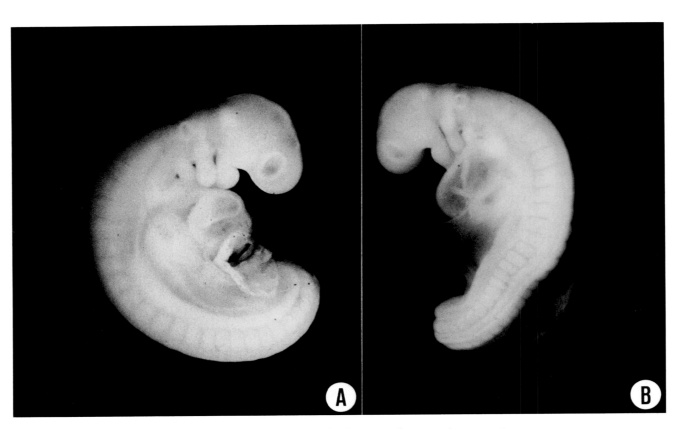

Fig. 12-1. (A) Right lateral view of No. 5923 (28 somites). See also fig. 12-2E. The internal structure is shown in figs. 12-4, 12-6, and 12-9. (B) Left lateral view of No. 6097 (25 somites). From somite 14 caudalward the body is smaller and less mature. Hence the contour is deflected. See also fig. 12-2B.

STAGE 12

Approximately 3–5 mm
Approximately 26 ± 1 postovulatory days
Characteristic feature: 21–29 pairs of somites

SUMMARY

External: three pharyngeal arches are visible; the dorsal curvature of the body is becoming filled out into a smooth convexity; the caudal neuropore is closing or closed; the otic vesicles are almost closed but not detached; the upper limb buds are appearing.

Internal: the interventricular septum has begun; the cystic primordium and the dorsal pancreas are becoming distinguishable; the lung bud appears.

SIZE AND AGE

The greatest length of the specimens of stage 12 is conditioned by the curved posture that is common among them, caused by the rounding out of the thoracolumbar region. In the preceding stage the specimens were characterized by a relatively straight linear axis. The curved axis that is characteristic of stage 12 reduces their length to that extent. The result is that of seventeen specimens, measured in 80 percent alcohol, all but two have a greatest length of 3–4 mm inclusive. The two exceptions were artificially elongated and measured 4.5 and 5.3 mm, respectively. When corrected for posture, the length of each is 4.1 mm. Nine of the seventeen specimens fall between 3.2 and 3.8 mm. Thus the length of the embryo at this time is misleading as an indication of growth, because these measurements are about the same as those of the previous stage.

As for the size of the chorion, one must omit tubal specimens, which are usually undersized. Moreover, some uterine specimens are too large. In the latter cases the chorion appears to have grown after arrest of development of the embryo. Not counting the tubal specimens, out of ten examples studied in which the size of the chorion was recorded, eight had a greatest diameter of 20–25 mm. Two were over 30 mm. If the mean of the greatest and least diameters be taken as the average diameter, eight of the ten specimens showed an average diameter of 15–20 mm, whereas two had average diameters of 20–25 mm.

The age of embryos of stage 12 is believed to be approximately 26 postovulatory days.

EXTERNAL FORM
(figs. 12-1 to 12-3, 12-6, and 12-9)

When the number of somites in a given embryo is known, it can be decided immediately whether or not it belongs to this stage. The number is not known precisely, however, until the embryo has been cleared or has been sectioned serially. Furthermore, it should be kept in mind that, from 10 somitic pairs to the end of stage 11, somite 1 is generally much smaller than somite 2. In stages 12 and 13, somite 1 is contributing to the hypoglossal cord (O'Rahilly and Müller, 1984b) and hence, "in embryos with more than 20 somites" (i.e., from the beginning of stage 12), the first ones visible "actually are second somites" (Arey, 1938).

Four occipital somites are present, as determined by their relationships to (1) the concentrations of the cervical neural crest (which are caudal to the occipital region), and (2) the primordia of the hypoglossal nerve.

An apparent rotation of the somites takes place between stages 11 and 12 (O'Rahilly and Müller, 1984b). The longitudinal axis of the dermatomyotome, as seen in cross section, comes to make a more acute angle with the median plane. Associated with this, the dorsal surface of the body, as seen in cross section, is changing from a gentle to a steeper curvature.

Among the several features that are characteristic, a prominent one is the presence of three pharyngeal arches, in contrast with the two of the preceding stage. There are now three bars and three membranes where skin and gut epithelia come in contact, and furthermore the pharyngeal arches are subdivided into dorsal and ventral parts. In exceptional cases in later stages, a fourth pharyngeal arch may appear, but three are the usual final complement seen externally. Caudal to the third there is a depression consisting of the condensed mass that is to form the mesoblastic elements of the larynx, and it is in this mass that the superior laryngeal nerve terminates. This is the region of the cervical sinus, which will be considered with the next two stages.

The previous stage was characterized by successive steps in the closure of the rostral neuropore. Stage 12 is similarly marked by the gradual closing of the caudal neuropore, which process is completed in the more advanced members of the group. With the increase in bulk of the spinal cord, somites, and surrounding mesoblast, the back of the embryo becomes filled out and takes a characteristic C-shaped form, eliminating the easily flexed region at the levels of somites 10–18, which so commonly results in a dorsal kink in stage 11.

Other features defining the group include the near closure of the otocyst, a slight opening or pore being still recognizable in the more advanced members in at least one of the vesicles. Also, what had been a wide opening between gut and umbilical vesicle now begins to narrow down so that an umbilical stalk is taking form. Finally, in distinction from the next stage, there is no really conspicuous upper limb bud. In the less advanced embryos none can be seen. In more-advanced specimens a condensation representing the primordium of the upper limb bud can be fairly well outlined. It is centered opposite somites 8–10 and merges caudally with the lateral unsegmented strip of mesoblast that is to form the ventrolateral body wall.

The ectodermal ring, described by Schmitt in 1898 and named by Blechschmidt in 1948, is complete at stage 12 (O'Rahilly and Müller, 1985). The ring, which may well be an important example of epithelial-mesenchymal interaction, comprises six parts: (1) the rostral part, containing the situs neuroporicus, and nasal and lens discs, (2) the pharyngeal part, the covering of the pharyngeal arches, (3) the occipital and cervicothoracic parts, related at first to the four occipital somites and later to the cervicothoracic junction, (4) the membral part, represented by a preliminary ectodermal thickening, followed within 2 days by the apical ectodermal ridge, (5) the intermembral part, related at first to the underlying coelom, and mesonephric duct and ridge, and (6) the caudal part, containing the cloacal membrane and a temporary "caudal ectodermal ridge." It is stressed that the incorrectly named *Milchstreifen* is merely the intermembral part, in which the mammary crest (*Milchlinie* or *Milchleiste*) appears one week later.

CARDIOVASCULAR SYSTEM

In stage 11 the coelom provides a means by which the exocoelomic fluid is brought into direct contact with the deeply lying mesoblast. By such a system of irrigation the increasing amount of embryonic tissue is insured an adequate supply of nutriment. At its best, the coelom provides only an elementary type of circulation. It is certainly an improvement on the tissue-culture mechanisms of the presomitic period, but it will not prove adequate for the larger and more elaborate organism that is to follow. Already in stage 12, the principal solution of this problem, in the form of a blood vascular system, is well under way.

The coelomic channel is part and parcel of the mesoblast, and as late as 30 somites is still meeting most of the circulatory requirements of the mesoblastic derivatives. The brain and spinal cord, however, which together constitute the largest and most compact tissue

Fig. 12-2 (facing page). (A) Dorsal view of No. 7852 (25 somites). The fourth ventricle is evident and the trigeminal ganglia can be distinguished. See also fig. 12-2C. (B) Ventral view of No. 6097 (25 somites). The remains of the oropharyngeal membrane can be seen. The right and left mandibular arches are partially united in front. See also fig. 12-1B. (C) Left lateral view of No. 7852 (25 somites). The otocyst, trigeminal ganglion, and vestibulofacial complex are distinguishable. The cardiac and hepatic regions are translucent. See also fig. 12-2A. (D) Left ventrolateral view of No. 6488 (28 somites), showing junction of umbilical vesicle and intestine. Here one can speak of an umbilical stalk. Note the free opening to the coelom. (E) Ventral view of No. 5923 (28 somites), showing the umbilical vesicle. The neural walls are visible in the head, and the optic vesicles can be distinguished. See also fig. 12-1A.

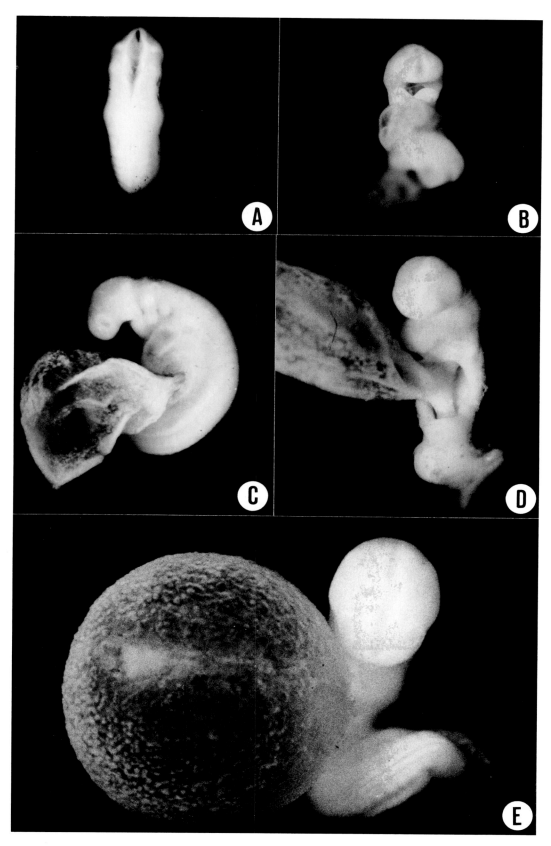

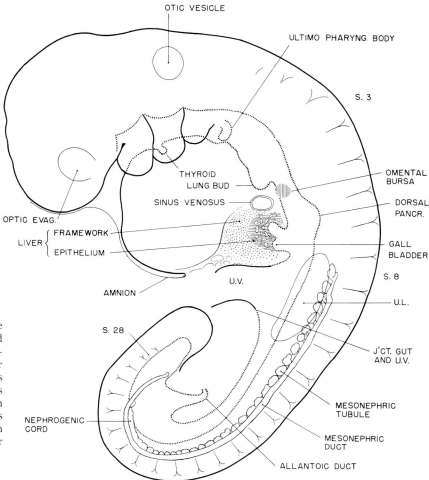

Fig. 12-3. Profile reconstruction of the digestive system in a 29-somite embryo (No. 1062), based on a photograph. Several of the primary endodermal derivatives are sharply delimited, and their topography relative to the body of the embryo is indicated. The omental bursa is shown because this marks the region that is to form the stomach. In reality the bursa lies to the right of the gut, as shown in section *C*, figure 12-4. The urinary system included in the figure was drawn from a plaster reconstruction.

mass in embryos of stage 12, do not share in its services. Earlier the neural tissue, in the form of a plate, is exposed directly to amniotic fluid, which at that time appears to differ but little from the general exocoelomic fluid. The proliferating neuroectodermal cells are thereby just as well supplied as the cells of the skin ectoderm. But when the neural plate becomes the neural tube and becomes separated from the surface by the overlying skin ectoderm, its cells are deprived of their previous source of nutrient fluid. Their protoplasmic requirements call for some new provision, and this is supplied by the blood vascular system. As soon as the margins of the neural folds begin to fuse across the median plane, which occurs during stage 10, one finds endothelial sprouts extending dorsally from the aortae toward the neural tissue. These sprouts are found in the spaces that intervene between the somites, and are designated the dorsal segmental arteries. The sprouts soon anastomose and spread as a capillary plexus, closely investing the surface of the neural tube.

At the same time, superficial to and connected with the capillary sheet of the neural tube, a loose plexus is laid down in the mesoblast lateral to the neural tube, including the brain. It is evident that throughout the early mesoblast there are many cells having the potentiality of becoming blood capillaries, and needing only an appropriate stimulus. In the plexus that is forming about the brain and spinal cord, one cannot always be sure whether a given vessel is a sprout from the aortic branches or a new structure differentiated *in loco*. Judging from the detached way in which its units make their appearance, it is probable that the superficial lateral plexus here referred to is differentiated *in loco*. The early steps in the formation of this plexus can be seen in stage 11, as shown schematically in figure 11-7. The more advanced phases are in the cranial region, and are particularly associated with the

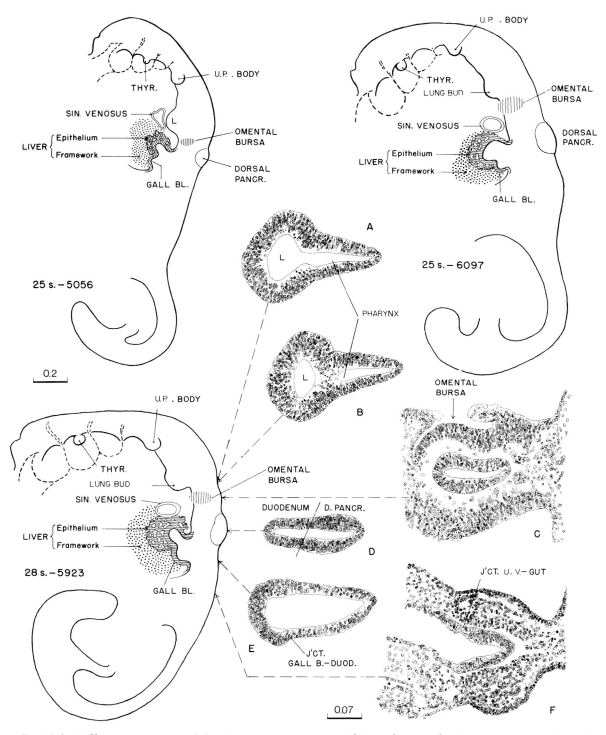

Fig. 12-4. Profile reconstructions of the digestive system in three embryos (No. 5056, 25 somites; No. 6097, 25 somites; and No. 5923, 28 somites). All three are based on sections enlarged to the same scale. A–F, detailed sections of the 28-somite specimen. For their position in the embryo these drawings can be compared with figure 12-3. The sections show the degree of specialization of the gut epithelium at six levels. In sections C and F, similar specializations are present in the coelomic wall, the cells of which will compose the connective tissue, muscle, and blood vessels that are to combine with the epithelium to constitute the wall and mesenteries of the gut. The residual coelomic surface cells will form the peritoneum, which is antedated by the omental bursa.

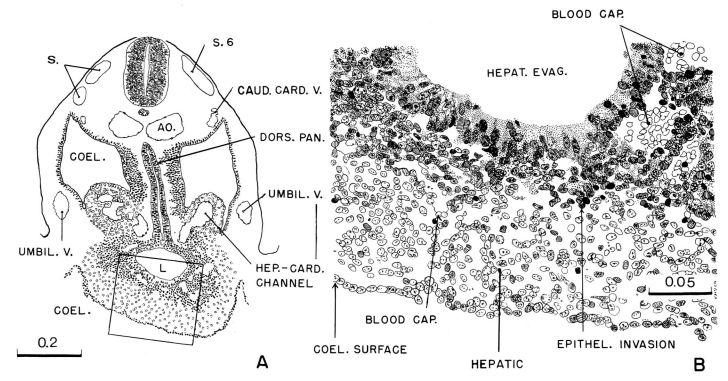

Fig. 12-5. (A) Section through the hepatic region of a 25-somite embryo (No. 7852), showing the invasion of the stroma of the liver by the hepatic epithelium. (B) Part of the same section.

cranial ganglia and neural crest cells, which may well be the stimulus to endothelial differentiation. Main channels soon make their appearance so that one can speak of a primary head vein, and along the spinal cord one can soon recognize the cardinal veins. In stage 12 the rostral and caudal cardinal veins flow together bilaterally as the right and left common cardinal veins, which in turn empty into the sinus venosus. By that time the blood flow has a definite direction, and the central nervous system can be said to have at least a surface blood supply and drainage. In this respect it is somewhat in advance of any other of the permanent organs.

In embryos of 14 paired somites the blood circulation is largely limited to an ebb and flow in the wall of the umbilical vesicle, produced by the early pulsations of the heart. In general, the flow is toward the heart from the rostral region of the umbilical vesicle, and toward the caudal part of the umbilical vesicle from the aorta. Annexed to this system is the connecting stalk. This is primarily associated with the allantoic diverticulum, and its large vessels are to be converted into the umbilical veins and arteries. These vessels will constitute the highway to the stroma of the placental villi, the stroma being separated from the maternal blood by the villous epithelium. Such is the picture in stage 11. In stage 12 one encounters several modifications and adaptations that produce for the first time a simple but connected circulatory system. A profile reconstruction of the larger elements of the vascular system of one of the more advanced embryos is shown in figure 12-6, and this should be compared with figure 11-7 of the preceding stage. A list of the principal items in vascular specialization found at this stage would include: (1) changes at the venous end of the heart, (2) vascularization of the central nervous system, (3) establishment of the cardinal venous drainage, (4) the hepatic plexus, and (5) alterations in the vitelline plexus resulting in main trunks, representing vitelline arteries and veins.

The changes at the venous end of the heart during stages 10–13 are shown in figure 12-7. One can see how enlarged parts of the vitelline plexus become the right and left atria, and how on each side an enlarged

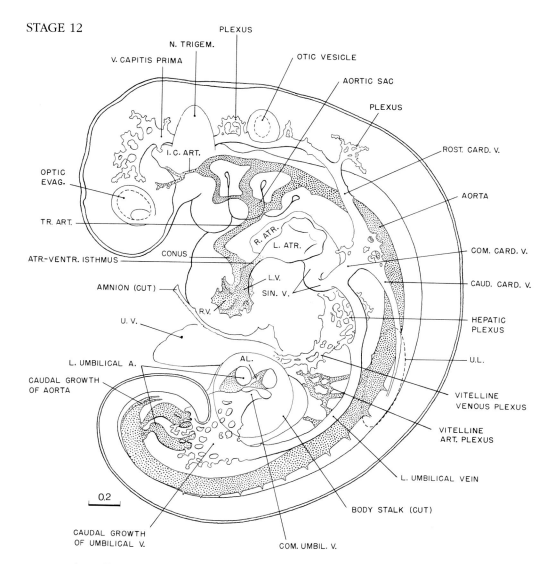

Fig. 12-6. Profile reconstruction of the blood vascular system in a 28-somite embryo (No. 5923). The liver, the umbilical vesicle, the cranial ganglia, and the surface of the central nervous system have a good blood supply, whereas the caudal end of the embryo is less advanced. The plexiform pattern is characteristic of rapid transformations and provides the means for caudal migration of the communications of the umbilical arteries and veins. The smaller capillaries are not shown, although they can be seen in the sections.

sac of the plexus becomes the point of outlet for the common cardinal vein. As part of the latter transformation, the left atrium becomes cut off from the channel that is to form the sinus venosus. The sinus venosus at this stage serves as a terminal venous reservoir into which blood from all parts of the embryo is emptied. It is separated from the right atrium by a narrow passage, the sinu-atrial foramen, which, reinforced by the enclosing myocardium and gelatinous cushions, appears to have the effect of hindering a backflow of blood on contraction of the atrial myocardium (fig. 12-

8). In other words, it could be regarded as a provisional element in the mechanism that directs the blood flow during the period before true valves have formed. The formation of atrial chambers and the atrioventricular canal, combined with proper synchronization of the myocardium, also serves the same end. At any rate, the heart is now capable of maintaining some circulation of blood around the surface of the central nervous system, throughout the wall of the umbilical vesicle, and through the chorion and its villi. Compared with the later placenta, this circulation is elementary, and

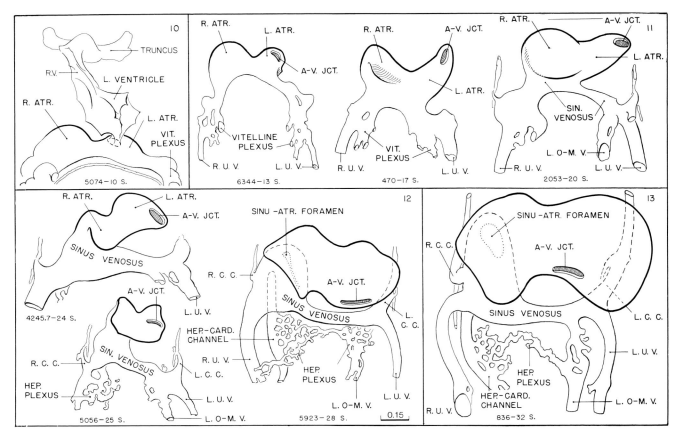

Fig. 12-7. Drawings made from reconstructions showing the venous end of the heart viewed from the front. The series includes four stages (10–13), and represents embryos having 10–32 somites. The collection number of the embryo and number of somites are indicated in each case. All are enlarged to the same scale. Except in the least advanced specimen, the ventricular part of the heart is removed at the atrioventricular junction. It can be seen that the atria are new formations, superimposed on the vitelline plexus. The sinus venosus retains more definitely its identity with the vitelline plexus, taking on the character of a reservoir into which all the veins of the embryo empty their contents. It, in turn, discharges its contents through the sinu-atrial foramen into the right atrium. This foramen, therefore, marks the boundary between veins and heart proper. The marked expansion of the atria in the 28- and 30-somite embryos is coincident with the specialization of the coelomic wall of the hepatocardiac channel, by which it appears to become more permeable to coelomic fluid. Compare figure 12-10. Abbreviations: *A–V. JCT.*, atrioventricular junction; *L.C.C.*, left common cardinal vein; *R.C.C.*, right common cardinal vein; *L.U.V.*, left umbilical vein; *R.U.V.*, right umbilical vein; *L.O-M.V.*, left omphalomesenteric vein.

in the early villi the interchange must be scant between the embryonic blood and the maternal blood of the intervillous space.

The blood supply of the central nervous system and the establishment of the cardinal veins have already been mentioned. The specialization of the vessels in the hepatic region (item 4 in the above list) needs special attention. It is best seen from the right side. Already marked differences have developed between the two sides, an asymmetry that dates back to at least stage 10, when the lower end of the ventricular region,

in its elongation, first becomes deflected to the left. The asymmetry is more pronounced in the atria and sinus venosus than in most of the tributary vessels. The vessels of the hepatic region are an exception. They become right- and left-sided very early, as is shown in figure 12-7. The relationships of this region are shown in figure 12-9, which is based on a right-profile reconstruction of the embryo shown in figure 12-6. The heart proper may be said to start at the sinu-atrial foramen, whereas the sinus venosus serves as a common channel into which all the afferent veins empty. The com-

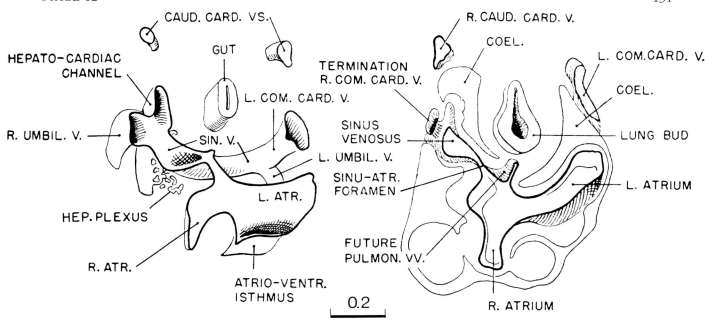

Fig. 12-8. Simplified drawings to show the communications at the venous end of the heart in a 28-somite embryo (No. 5923). The drawings represent two slabs. The caudal one (left) shows the relations of the sinus venosus beyond the level of the atria. The other slab is to be thought of as fitting directly over the caudal one. It shows the top of the sinus venosus and its communications through the sinu-atrial foramen with the right atrium. In this slab the coelomic contours are shown by a thin line. One can see the area of specialized coelomic wall over the hepato- cardiac channel and the communication of the latter with the sinus venosus. The device would appear to facilitate the passage of coelomic fluid into the blood stream. Compare with figure 12-10. These sketches were drawn from a transparent model of the heart made by Osborne O. Heard. Tracings of the sections were made and oriented on transparent films (cellulose acetate) and the whole series superimposed for study with illumination coming from below. The heart of this embryo was reconstructed anew by de Vries and Saunders (1962, plate 5).

mon cardinal and the umbilical veins terminate in about the same way on the two sides. The hepatic plexus is less symmetrical. The main part of the plexus is derived from the newly formed capillaries in the hepatic primordium. Anastomosing with the hepatic plexus on each side are the vitelline veins, which are transformed and enlarged elements of the vascular plexus of the umbilical vesicle. Dorsally the hepatic plexus empties by multiple anastomoses into an enlarged passage, the hepatocardiac channel, which leads to the sinus venosus and thereby to the heart. This channel is either single or multiple. It reaches its full expression on the right side (fig. 12-9). The tributary channel from the left side is more plexiform, and its communication with the sinus venosus is transitory. By virtue of the plexus and these channels, the precocious primordium of the liver is highly vascularized and is in free communication with the plexus of the umbilical vesicle on the one hand and the heart on the other. This is in contrast with the remainder of the digestive system,

which thus far shows scant evidence of activity.

A special feature that characterizes the right hepatocardiac channel, and to a lesser extent the left, is a specialization of the coelomic wall, illustrated in figure 12-10. It is a provision by which a section of the large hepatocardiac channel is immersed in the coelomic channel. It is separated from the coelomic fluid by only the sharply marked-off specialized area of what is apparently easily permeable coelomic tissue. It consists of a thinned-out vesicular covering, the large spaces of which are filled with clear fluid. Embryos at this time are doubtless to some degree permeable through all surfaces, but there are some areas which, judging from their histological appearance, are more permeable than others. The areolar character of the connecting stalk indicates that it and its contained large vascular channels must be readily permeable to coelomic fluid. This condition goes back to presomitic embryos, in which the foamy character of the connecting stalk was pointed out and illustrated by Heuser

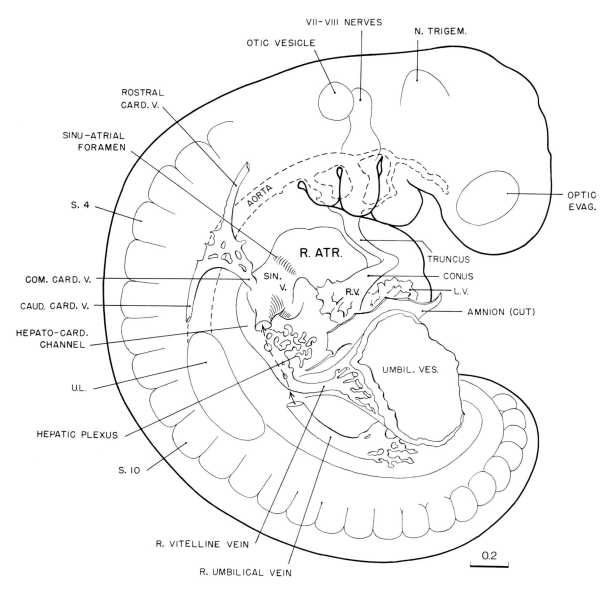

Fig. 12-9. Profile reconstructions of the right side of a 28-somite embryo (No. 5923). From this view one can see the formation of the hepatocardiac channel and its termination in the sinus venosus, and also the termination of the latter in the right atrium. It is over the rostral part of the hepatocardiac channel that the coelomic wall is structurally modified with respect to permeability, apparently facilitating exchange between the coelomic fluid and the blood stream. Compare figure 12-10.

Fig. 12-10 (facing page). Four sections at the same scale, showing the specialization of the coelomic wall over the large venous channels opening into the sinus venosus. These are from four different embryos and represent four different degrees of specialization. The effect appears to be an increase of permeability, facilitating exchange of fluid between the coelomic cavity and the bloodstream at the strategic point just where the blood enters the heart. (A) 28-somite embryo (No. 7999, section 2-5-7), showing right hepatocardiac channel opening (below) into sinus venosus. Where the channel projects into the coelomic passage (above), the wall is specialized as a fluid-filled reticular tissue. Droplets of fluid can be seen in the coelomic surface cells. The medial coelomic wall is characterized by a thick zone of pro-liferating cells that are becoming differentiated and detached to form the mesoblastic wall and enveloping tissues of the gut epithelium, the edge of which can be seen on the right side. (B) Left hepatocardiac channel of a 25-somite embryo (No. 7852, section 2-3-4). The coelomic wall is less advanced in its specialization than in A. (C) Section through the right hepatocardiac channel of a 28-somite embryo (No. 5923, section 2-1-9). The channel opens widely into the sinus venosus, essentially like that in A. Asterisk: coelomic cavity. (D) Left hepatocardiac channel in a 25-somite embryo (No. 6097, section 2-3-8). As is common on the left side, this channel is plexiform. The coelomic wall is the most advanced in its specialization of the four examples shown here.

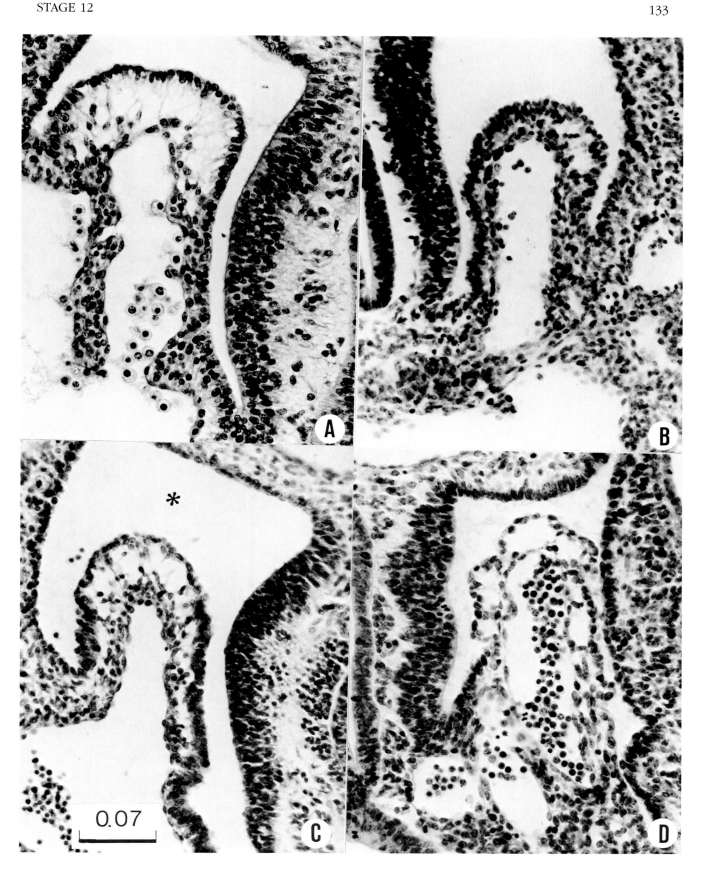

(1932b). The specialized area, where the large hepatocardiac channel projects into the coelom, appears to be even more favorable than the connecting stalk to the give and take between the coelomic fluid and the blood stream. It would seem that it is this kind of mechanism that provides the large amount of plasma necessary to fill the endothelial system, which at this time is so rapidly enlarging. This finding is supported by the fact that the filling out and expansion of the right and left atria follow promptly the differentiation of this particular coelomic area. Later, when the villous circulation becomes efficient and interchange is inaugurated between embryonic and maternal blood, the need for this device will have passed.

In stage 12 the right venous valve and the atrioventricular canal develop, and septum primum and foramen primum may appear (McBride, Moore, and Hutchins, 1981).

The circulatory system, which is now connected for the first time, comprises the following sequence: umbilical (and hepatocardiac and common cardinal) veins, sinus venosus, sinu-atrial foramen, right atrium, left atrium, atrioventricular canal, left ventricle, right ventricle, conus cordis, truncus arteriosus, aortic arches, aorta, and umbilical arteries.

The four main portions of the primary cardiac tube are the trabeculated part of the left ventricle, the trabeculated part of the right ventricle, the conus cordis, and the truncus arteriosus (O'Rahilly, 1971, in whose table 1 synonyms are given). The last two segments compose the outflow tract. These features are well seen in the heart illustrated by Rosenbauer (1955).

A historical review of the nomenclature of the embryonic heart has been published, but the conclusion that the term truncus arteriosus be used for the entire "arterial pole" from the ventricle to the origin of the aortic arches (Laane, 1974) seems to be highly inadvisable and is not followed here.

DIGESTIVE AND RESPIRATORY SYSTEMS

One of the major differences between stages 11 and 12 is the marked advance in the differentiation of the alimentary epithelium in the latter. Sharply outlined fields of epithelial proliferative activity mark the location of such primary organs as liver, lung, stomach, and dorsal pancreas. This occurs with such uniformity in the various members of the group that aside from their other characteristics it serves as a useful test of their eligibility for the group.

The position of the gut in relation to the embryo as a whole is shown in figure 12-3. This has been plotted for one of the more advanced embryos (29 somites). The digestive systems of three other embryos (25, 25, and 28 somites) are shown in figure 12-4. These plots are based on profile reconstructions, and show topographically the distribution and relative sizes of the early centers of epithelial proliferation.

In the pharyngeal region the more active proliferation is in the floor, in contrast with the roof, which is relatively thin. Similarly, the alimentary epithelium is thin as compared with that of the respiratory diverticulum. Among the earliest of the pharyngeal proliferative centers is the unilateral median thyroid, which projects ventrally into the concavity of the truncus arteriosus, and the telopharyngeal bodies, which proliferate bilaterally to constitute, according to Weller (1933), the lateral components of the thyroid and parathyroid glands. These particular fields of pharyngeal epithelium are already specialized and definitive, and thus far no environmental stimulus has been identified as a cause of their differentiation. Until such a stimulus is discovered we must conclude that this primary proliferation is inherent in the genic constitution of the cells. It is subsequent to this that we find the environment playing a part in the development of these structures. That the components of the thyroid are so precocious is an indication of the basic importance of this gland in development and growth.

Similarly, the greater proliferation shown by the respiratory as compared to the adjacent alimentary epithelium would seem not to be environmental in origin. Histological pictures of sections through the level of the lung bud are shown in figure 12-4A, B. These are adjacent sections and they illustrate the greater precocity of the respiratory epithelium as compared with that of the adjacent alimentary canal, which forms the dorsal half of the digestive tube. The only difference in environment, ventrally and dorsally, is the presence of a few capillaries from the sinus venosus which at this time extend toward the pulmonary evagination and are the precursors of the pulmonary veins (compare fig. 12-8). It would appear likely that the capillaries are a response to the pulmonary evagination rather than the reverse, in view of the sensitivity of capillaries to stimuli. The sections A and B indicate a specialized pulmonary epithelium.

A section immediately below the level of the lung bud is shown in figure 12-4C. The presence of the beginning omental bursa marks this part of the gut as the location of the stomach. It is at this time, between 25 and 28 pairs of somites, that the gastric part of the canal becomes elongated, increasing the distance between the lung bud and the hepatic diverticulum. It is not until the next stage that it undergoes the fusiform enlargement that is characteristic of the stomach. A transverse section through the gastric region (fig. 12-4C) reveals a very active proliferation of the coelomic cells, which are moving in to form, in course of time, the connective tissue coats and muscular wall of the stomach together with its rich supply of blood vessels.

Caudal to the stomach, one encounters an area of proliferation in the dorsal half of the intestinal epithelium that is to become the dorsal pancreas. This is sharply marked off from the adjacent intestinal wall, as can be seen in section D, figure 12-4. A little more caudally and on the opposite side is the hepatic diverticulum, which because of its special precocity will be described in a separate section. At the level where the gut opens into the umbilical vesicle, one can recognize a sharp transition from intestinal epithelium to the inner layer of the umbilical vesicle, although the two are continuous. This is true also of the enclosing coelomic tissues. By comparing 25-somite specimens with those having 28–30 somites, it will be seen that the opening between gut and umbilical vesicle becomes constricted. This constriction comprises not only a craniocaudal flattening but also an actual decrease in size of cross section. With this, there is a corresponding elongation of the umbilical vesicle, and in the 30-somite specimen one can speak of a vitelline duct, which is associated with the diverticulum ilei. In this way, a landmark indicates the junction of foregut and hindgut, cranial to which all of the small intestine is derived save the terminal third of the ileum, and caudal to which the remaining third of the ileum and the large intestine take origin. Certainty for this landmark, however, would require ruling out the occurrence of caudal migration of the point of attachment of the vitelline duct. The hindgut during this period is in an elementary state of organization, particularly

toward the caudal end. Comparison of the reconstructions shown in figure 12-4 reveals an elongation of the interval between the junction of the umbilical vesicle and the junction with the allantoic duct.

Additional features of the digestive and respiratory systems at stage 12 include the following: remains of the ruptured oropharyngeal membrane, the cervical sinus caudal to pharyngeal arch 3, the telopharyngeal body being separated from the caudal pharyngeal complex (pouches 3 and 4), and the tracheo-esophageal septum (O'Rahilly and Müller, 1984c), but no common esophagotrachea.

Liver

Of the different organs that compose the digestive system, the liver is by far the most precocious. Whether this is because it lies at an active center of angiogenesis or whether the development of the liver is the cause of the surrounding vascular activity is an open question. In the preceding stage it was seen that proliferation of the hepatic epithelium was accompanied by the formation of blood islands among the adjacent cells, evidently stimulated by the epithelium. In general, the embryonic endothelial apparatus is responsive to the stimulation (i.e., the requirements) of the surrounding structures. Hence it seems likely that the precocity of the liver is caused by the inherent constitution of its component cells. In consequence, the liver becomes established as a functioning organ early in development.

It has been shown in stage 11 that the stroma, or framework, of the liver is derived from proliferating mesoblastic cells that become detached from the surface germinal bed of the coelom in the cardiac region, whereas the parenchyma of the liver is derived from a specific area of alimentary epithelium that shapes itself as the hepatic diverticulum. The advance that is characteristic of stage 12 consists in the spread of the epithelium of the diverticulum outward into the stroma as a fringe of epithelial trabeculae, as is shown in figure 12-5. It will be seen that the digestive epithelium, because of its irregular foci of proliferation, loses the smooth contour of its outer surface and merges into the columnar extensions. In making this invasion the epithelial trabeculae enmesh the newly formed stromal capillaries. New stimulation is thereby given

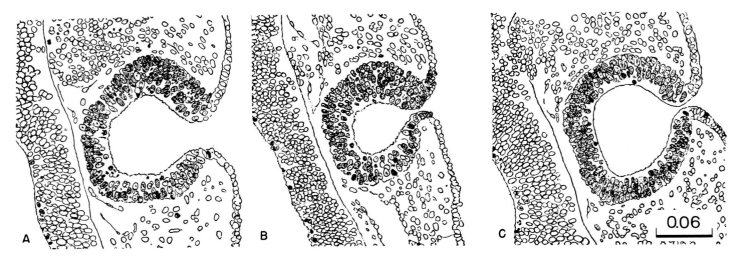

Fig. 12-11. Three phases in the development of the otocyst during stage 12. (A) 25-somite embryo (No. 6097, section 1-3-1). (B) 25-somite embryo (No. 7852, section 1-2-9). (C) 28-somite embryo (No. 5923, section 1-2-11). The ectoderm of the otocyst resembles that of the brain wall and is highly specialized compared with the simpler skin ectoderm, from which it is sharply demarcated. The three drawings are enlarged to the same scale.

to angiogenesis, and a large part of the stroma is converted into capillaries and blood cells. A relatively small part is required for capsule and interlobular connective tissue. In the less advanced members of the stage the epithelial invasion is just starting, and in the more advanced members it has spread through about one-half of the hepatic primordium. The invasion is completed in stage 13.

The caudal part of the hepatic diverticulum becomes set off from the start, forming a subdivision that constitutes the primordium of the cystic duct and gall bladder. This part does not participate in the formation of epithelial columns or in the invasion of the hepatic stroma. A typical section through this region is shown in figure 12-4, section *E*. Thus, this area of digestive epithelium is already specialized, having been assigned to the liver, and the part that will form hepatic cells and biliary ducts has already been distinguished from the parts that will form gall bladder and cystic duct.

Intervening between the liver and the heart is a conspicuous plexus of blood capillaries. During this period these vessels are rapidly becoming enmeshed by the proliferating hepatic epithelium, and it is quite likely that they are a response to its presence. The more ventrally lying capillaries are differentiated *in situ* in the primordial stroma of the liver. The larger

dorsal channels are enlargements and anastomosing extensions of the network of the umbilical vesicle. It is not accurate, however, to speak of the latter as the omphalomesenteric veins, which will make their appearance later as derivatives of part of the umbilical plexus. During the period under consideration these venous channels serve to drain the liver into the sinus venosus and through it into the venous end of the heart. A special function appears to be assigned to the large, sinus-like channels of the plexus, which occur bilaterally along its dorsal margins. For convenience these will be spoken of as the hepatocardiac channels. These passages and the mesoblastic cells surrounding them apparently correspond to what is spoken of by some writers as the right and left horns of the liver.

Two embryos of stage 12 were included in Lipp's (1952) study of the liver, and further details in staged embryos have been provided by Severn (1971, 1972).

URINARY AND REPRODUCTIVE SYSTEMS

The varied and highly specialized mesoblastic tissues that are derived from various areas of the coelom have already been noted. The mesonephros and its duct constitute another example of such specialization. In figure 12-3 is shown a profile view of the mesonephros as found in a 29-somite embryo, one of the more advanced members of stage 12. It is slightly less advanced than the first of those described by Shikinami (1926). The tubules begin at the level of somite 8 and are distinct as far caudally as somite 20, whence they extend as a continuous nephrogenic cord to the level of somite 24. Opposite each somite there are two or more tubules. Thus they are not metameric, any more than the mesonephric duct is metameric, or the umbilical vein.

The number of nephric vesicles is being increased by progressive differentiation caudally from the nephrogenic cord (Torrey, 1954). The mesonephric duct at first ends blindly immediately short of the cloaca, but soon becomes attached to the cloaca (i.e., to the terminal part of the hindgut) and acquires a lumen.

The primordial germ cells are in the wall of the hindgut (Witschi, 1948). Details of the arrangement of the germ cells in an embryo of 26–27 pairs of somites have been provided by Politzer (1928b).

Nervous System
(figs. 12-6 and 13-10)

The form of the central nervous system is shown in figure 12-6. It can be seen that the relatively large and compact neural tube is in large part responsible for the C-shaped outline that is characteristic of the embryo at this time. With the closure of the caudal neuropore, the caudal end of the tube becomes defined, and further elongation of the body is attained more by interstitial growth and less by segregation of neural ectoderm and mesoblastic somitic material, as is characteristic of the preceding stages. The part of the neural tube caudal to somite 24 is still undifferentiated and small, and conversely the hindbrain and cervical-cord regions are large and advanced in their differentiation. Perhaps the most notable improvement to be seen in the neural tube is the provision of a blood supply to its surface.

At stage 12 the first phase in the formation of the neural tube (primary neurulation) ends. Further elongation is caused by a poorly understood process termed secondary neurulation, in which neural ectoderm is not involved (Lemire et al., 1975).

The roof of the rhombencephalon is becoming thin. Eight rhombomeres can be distinguished. A sheet of motor neurons is present in the basal plate of the rhombencephalon, and is particularly clear in those embryos in which the roots of the hypoglossal nerve begin to differentiate (O'Rahilly and Müller, 1984b). Neurofibrils begin to form for the first time in the rhombencephalic wall, and in most embryos a marginal layer begins to develop. The cells constituting the superior ganglia of cranial nerves 9 and 10 are present as neural crest material.

The telencephalon enlarges and includes the embryonic lamina terminalis and the telencephalon medium rostral to the optic vesicles (fig. 13-10). The area adjacent to the closed, former rostral neuropore is the embryonic commissural plate. Thickenings in the diencephalon indicate the primordia of the ventral thalamus and the subthalamus. The diencephalic ventral thickening is continuous with a thickening in the midbrain that constitutes the tegmentum; the latter is clearly set off by the sulcus limitans, which at this time continues into the diencephalon. The mesencephalon has grown considerably and comprises two segments (M1, M2).

The nasal discs become thicker and form a portion of the ectodermal ring on both sides of the closed neuropore (O'Rahilly and Müller, 1985). The olfactory area of the brain is also becoming thicker, and mitotic figures become more numerous (Bossy, 1980a).

Eye

At stage 12 the optic neural crest reaches its maximum extent and the optic vesicle becomes covered by a complete sheath, giving the appearance of a "frightened hedgehog" (Bartelmez and Blount, 1954).

Ear

The otocyst in embryos possessing 21–29 pairs of somites is one of the most reliable characteristics for determining the degree of development. In the less advanced specimens the otocysts are conspicuously open to the surface, whereas in the more advanced members of the group the closure is nearly complete and detachment from the skin ectoderm is imminent. In the gross specimen the pore may be so small that it escapes attention and is not found until seen in sections. Three typical specimens are shown in figure 12-11. These are selected from well-preserved embryos, and their histology and general form can be relied upon. It is to be noted that the epithelium of the otocyst is highly specialized compared with the simpler skin ectoderm, from which it is sharply demarcated. The fact that from the outset it can be traced as a specialized area is good evidence that it is not to be regarded as modified skin, but rather as a detached island of neural ectoderm, related to but not identical with the ectoderm of the brain wall. It is to be added that in poorly preserved and in macerated embryos the otocyst may show distortions and abnormalities in form. It may be collapsed or distended. Distortions are commonly seen at the junction of the otocyst with the skin ectoderm. Thus there may be an unduly wide opening to the surface, but more frequently the open rim of the otocyst is stretched into a duct-like stalk by which the otocyst retains its attachment to the surface. This should not be confused with an endolymphatic appendage.

Vestibular neural crest is still forming from the wall of the otic pit and developing vesicle.

SPECIMENS OF STAGE 12 ALREADY DESCRIBED

22 somites, Girgis embryo, Royal School of Medicine, Cairo. Apparently a normal embryo, studied and reconstructed by the wax-plate method at the Institute of Anatomy, University College, London by Girgis (1926). Otic vesicle and caudal neuropore both still open. Three pharyngeal arches are present. Umbilical vesicle opens rather widely into gut. Morphology of central nervous system, digestive system, vascular system, and excretory system described in detail. The specimen had been kept in alcohol for a prolonged period, and apparently is not suitable for cytological minutiae.

22 somites, Carnegie No. 8963 (University of Chicago No. H 1093). Described by Wen (1928) with particular reference to the nervous system.

23 somites, Van den Broek embryo "A," Zentral-Institut für Hirnforschung, Amsterdam. Two similar embryos are described together by Van den Broek (1911). The description refers almost entirely to "A," which is the better preserved of the two. It is evidently normal, and judging from the form of the brain, open otocyst, and liver it corresponds to about a 23-somite embryo, although it is said to have 21–22 somites.

23 somites, R. Meyer, No. 300. The Meyer collection was transferred from Berlin to the University of Zürich in 1922, and placed in charge of H. Frey. This valuable specimen was described in monographic form by Thompson (1907, 1908). Also described and figured in the Keibel and Elze *Normentafeln* (1908). It constitutes a type specimen.

23 somites, Hertwig embryo "Wolff II," Anatomisches-biol-

ogisches Institut, Berlin. Normal, well-preserved specimen, having three pharyngeal arches and no trace of rostral neuropore. Described by Keibel and Elze (1908). Specimen has been reconstructed.

23 somites, Carnegie No. 8964 (University of Chicago No. H 984). Described by Wen (1928) with particular reference to the nervous system.

24 somites, Johnson, Harvard Collection, Boston. Complete description, based on many models and histological study, published in monographic form by Johnson (1917). Rostral and caudal neuropores closed. Otic vesicle retains a narrow opening to surface. Three pharyngeal arches are present. Hepatic trabeculae invading framework of liver. Umbilical vesicle is compressed rostrocaudally, i.e., early umbilical stalk. Probably originally 25 somites (Arey, 1938).

24 somites, Homo Nürnberger, Anatomisches Institut, Universität Köln. Described in detail and excellently illustrated by Rosenbauer (1955), with particular reference to the cardiovascular system.

25 somites, West embryo, University College, Cardiff. A 3-mm embryo much like the Johnson specimen and a good representative of the middle period of this stage (West, 1937). By means of profile and wax reconstructions the main organ systems are outlined, including an excellent study of the nephric system. The success attained by West in the orientation of his sections and the consequent accuracy in profile outlines is explained by the stained margins of the squarely trimmed paraffin block, which served as guides.

25 somites, Carnegie No. 6097. A graphic reconstruction was published by Müller and O'Rahilly (1980a).

26 somites, His embryo M, Basel, H. b. 1. One of the group of embryos carefully studied by His for surface anatomy, and then cut in serial sections for microscopical examination, setting a new standard in human embryology (His, 1880–1885). From the development of the liver, lungs, heart, brain, and otocysts, and the absence of upper limb buds, it is estimated that it belongs in the 26-somite group.

28 somites, His embryo Lr., Leipzig No. 67. Although used to good purpose by His, this specimen is probably not entirely normal (His, 1880–1885). The estimate of 28 somites is based on the narrowed umbilical stalk and the beginning upper limb buds.

28 somites, Hammar embryo (Nystroem), Anatomisches Institut, Uppsala. Described by Hammar in Keibel and Elze (1908). Digestive system described by Forssner (1907). The number of somites given above is estimated on the basis of three pharyngeal arches, full convex back, small opening in otic vesicles to surface, hepatic trabeculae, and appearance of section through cardiac region. Central nervous system shows folding of wall which characterizes imperfect preservation. External form appears normal.

28 somites, von Spee collection, Kiel. Sketches published in Döderlein's *Handbuch* (1915). Reported to have 31 somites, but absence of upper limb buds and the fact that the otic vesicles are still open to the surface makes it probable that an estimate of 28 somites is more nearly correct.

28–29 somites, Carnegie No. 148. Described by Gage (1905). Perhaps 29–30 somites (Arey, 1938).

29 somites, 20–21-day Coste embryo. Specimen not sectioned, but the exquisite drawings contained in Coste's atlas, *Développement des corps organisés,* Paris (1849), reveal many details of the surface form of this well-preserved embryo. In form it resembles closely Carnegie No. 1062, 29 somites, including rounded back curve, trace of upper limb buds, compressed gut-umbilical vesicle junction, size of hepatic area, form of cardiac tube, presence of otic pore, and outlines of head. Four pharyngeal arches are shown, but the fourth may have been an exaggeration of the depression lying caudal to the third bar. Also the somitic count seems to exceed the 29 estimated, but this may be caused by overemphasis on partial divisions of the terminal somitic ridge. In size its greatest length is about 4 mm. If it were straightened out as much as No. 1062, it would probably be close to 4.5 mm, like the latter.

29 somites, Janošík, Royal Bohemian University, Prague. Somitic count estimated on the following characteristics: three pharyngeal arches, closure of rostral and caudal neuropores, detachment of otocyst from surface, definite lung bud, elongated hepatic diverticulum with gut epithelium proliferating into adjacent tissue, narrowed umbilical stalk, and well-developed mesonephric duct and tubules. The main features of the vascular system are clearly shown. There were two embryos in this case, one of which was definitely stunted. The above description refers to the normal embryo (Janošík, 1887).

29 somites, Waterston, University of St. Andrews, Fife. Specimen reported as having 27 paired somites (Waterston, 1914). In several characteristics it appears to be transitional between stages 12 and 13. Probably more than 27 somites, perhaps 28 (Arey, 1938) or 29. Among its advanced structures are prominent lung buds, large primordium of liver with extensive invasion by gut epithelium, narrow umbilical stalk, elongated median thyroid, and advanced ear vesicles. The upper limb buds were not prominent on the surface but stand out clearly in the sections. The blood vessels are everywhere greatly distended with blood cells, which is probably a peculiarity of this particular specimen.

The somitic count for the following embryos is not available.

Harvard No. 714, 4-mm embryo. Described in detail by Bremer (1906). Probably belongs to stage 12 rather than stage 11 or stage 13. It shows some unusual features, such as arrested or delayed closure of the rostral neuropore.

No. 102 and No. 126, Department of Anatomy, Tohoku University, Sendai. These two embryos were assigned to stage 12 but the somitic count is not given. Distribution of alkaline phosphatase was studied by Mori (1965).

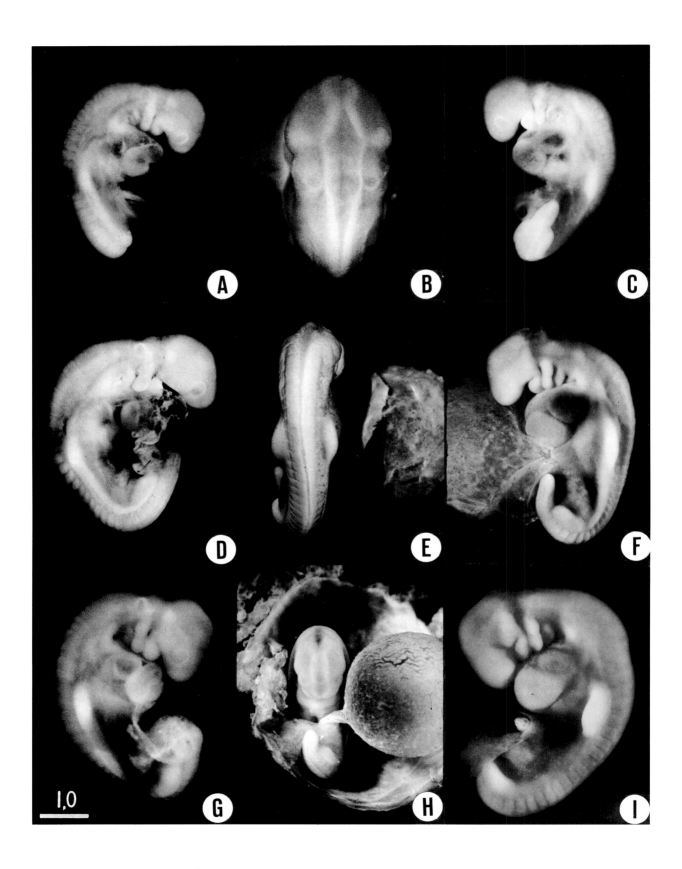

STAGE 13

Approximately 4–6 mm
Approximately 28 postovulatory days
Characteristic feature: 30 or more pairs of somites

SUMMARY

External: all four limb buds are usually visible; the otic vesicle is closed; the lens disc is generally not yet indented.

Internal: septum primum and foramen primum appear in the heart; right and left lung buds are recognizable, and the trachea begins its development; retinal and lens discs appear; the endolymphatic appendage becomes distinguishable by the end of the stage.

SIZE AND AGE

The overall size of the chorion in stage 13 commonly ranges between 19 and 30 mm (eleven specimens out of nineteen from which accurate measurements were available). The mean of largest and smallest diameters in the same eleven specimens ranges from 16.5 to 22.5 mm. The smallest diameter is less easily measured and introduces various inaccuracies. If we accept the greatest diameter as the most practicable measurement, we can then say that in the majority of specimens of this group it is between 20 and 30 mm. There is a minority group (four specimens) having somewhat smaller chorions 17–19 mm in largest diameter. In addition, two exceptionally small specimens and three exceptionally large ones have been noted.

The length of the embryos as given in Appendix I is based on their greatest length, measured in formalin solution or in some instances in 80 percent alcohol following fixation in another fluid. In the latter cases an 0.8 percent allowance was made for the shrinkage after alcohol. This allowance is based on observed shrinkage of similar material in similar fixatives. The measurements given are the corrected ones (i.e., greatest length after fixation). Of the 26 specimens, half are 4.5–5.8 mm long. About one-third of the 26 specimens are smaller and range from 3.9 to 4.3 mm in length. Thus 80 percent (21) of the specimens are found to be about 4–5 mm long. The remainder comprises two poorly preserved specimens of 3.0 and 3.5 mm, and three exceptionally large and borderline specimens each of 6 mm.

The age of embryos of stage 13 is believed to be approximately 28 postovulatory days.

Fig. 13-1 (facing page). (A–C) Embryo No. 6473 is among the less advanced embryos of the group and is on the borderline of the preceding stage. Because of the translucency of its tissues, much of the internal structure can be seen, particularly the details of the cardiac and hepatic regions. Aortic arches 2 and 3 course obliquely through their respective pharyngeal arches, and it can be seen that the form of the latter is not simply caused by the presence of the arches. The trigeminal and vestibulofacial ganglia, as well as the otic vesicle, can be seen in A. B is a "top" view showing the high degree of specialization of the different parts of the brain wall, and also the attachment of the trigeminal and vestibulofacial ganglia, along with the otic vesicle. Cavity of fourth ventricle is deeper and narrower than appears in the photograph. (D) Embryo No. 6469, showing especially well the optic evagination, the otic vesicle, and the condensed unsegmented mesenchymal strip, extending caudalward from the upper limb bud and probably supplying the body wall musculature. (E,F) Embryo No. 8066, showing a straighter posture than usual. The form of the upper limb buds is seen particularly well in E. (G) Embryo No. 7433. The roof of the fourth ventricle is thinner in two areas, which are separated by a strip of more-opaque tissue which crosses transversely from the region of one vestibulofacial ganglion to the other. (H) Embryo No. 7433 photographed *in situ*, showing the character of the umbilical vesicle and its relations to the connecting stalk. (I) Embryo No. 8119. An opaque Bouin specimen in an excellent state of preservation. Belongs to the second half of this stage. With the exception of B and H, all photographs are enlarged to the same scale.

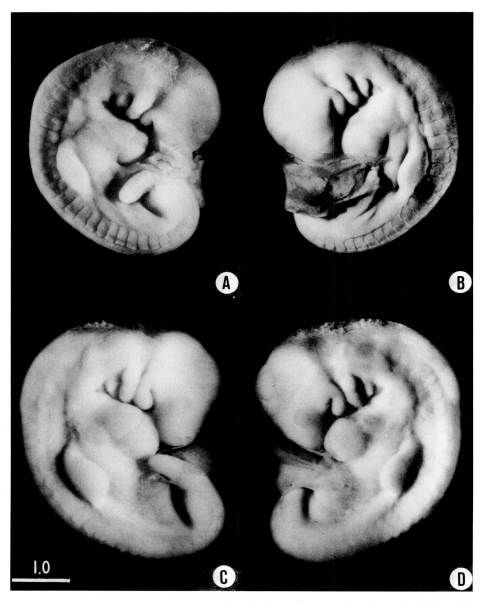

Fig. 13-2. (A–D) Two well-preserved embryos fixed in Bouin's fluid. Because of the opacity of the tissues, the surface details are well shown. Most of the photographs used in this study were made by Chester F. Reather. (A,B) Embryo No. 7889, belonging to the first half of stage 13. It is coiled more closely than usual, and this explains its measurement of 4.2 mm. In B the outlines of the nasal plate are distinguishable. (C,D) Embryo No. 7618, belonging to the more advanced members of the group and showing development of the upper limb buds. The pharyngeal arches in both embryos show individual and detailed characteristics which appear to be unrelated to the aortic arches that pass obliquely through them. Transmitting vascular channels would seem to be no more than a passing and minor function of the conspicuous structures. All photographs are enlarged to the same scale.

EXTERNAL FORM
(figs. 13-1 to 13-3, and 15-3)

After stage 12 the number of pairs of somites becomes increasingly difficult to determine and is no longer used in staging. Various numbers have been given for certain embryos. For example, No. 836 has sometimes been stated to possess 30 pairs, whereas the present authors believe that 32 pairs are present.

This is the stage when one can first see both upper and lower limb buds. As was true in stage 12, the central nervous system seems to be the chief factor in determining the form of the embryo, because the external contour of the neural tube is the same as that of the embryo. Otherwise the most prominent surface characteristics of the group are supplied by the series of bulging condensed masses, the pharyngeal arches, and the similarly appearing whitish opaque limb buds. To the rear of the hyoid mass lies the glossopharyngeal arch, and through it courses the large third aortic arch. Caudal to it is the depressed triangular area where the surface ectoderm sinks in to come in contact with the pharyngeal endoderm. As the surrounding parts increase in size, the floor of this triangular area becomes partly covered over, and the depression is known as the cervical sinus. In stage 13 the floor is still plainly visible. It is less so in the next stage. This is the region through which a new blood channel is forming, to become the fourth aortic arch. Also underlying this area is the telopharyngeal body.

In stage 12 there is either no upper limb bud at all, or in the oldest members of the group a representative of it in the form of a slight elevation. In stage 13 the upper limb buds consist of definite ridges, and there are also beginning lower limb buds. The cardiac chambers are now distended with fluid, making them and the heart as a whole more prominent. The hepatic mass is also larger. The combined volume of the heart and liver has become about equal to that of the overlying head. The communication between the umbilical vesicle and the gut cavity has been transformed from a wide space or, in some cases, a compressed slit-like passage to a slender, vascularized stalk. Its junction with the gut endoderm is sharply marked. The transformation from a spacious communication between the gut and umbilical vesicle to a slender stalk combines actual decrease in the transverse diameters with elongation of the structure: i.e., it is brought about by adaptation in shape, and no tissue appears to be wasted in the process. As this takes place, the amnion closes in and ensheathes the connecting stalk, the coelomic cavity, and the stalk of the umbilical vesicle. This marks the beginning of the umbilical cord.

In formalin-fixed specimens the major outlines of the brain and optic vesicle can be seen. The otocyst is completely closed off from the surface. In front of the otocyst is the vestibulofacial ganglion streaming down to the dorsal segment of the hyoid arch. The large trigeminal ganglion, connecting the maxillary and mandibular processes with the lateral pontine angle of the neural wall, is conspicuous, both in dorsal and profile views.

Four pairs of occipital somites are found in the human embryo at stage 13 (O'Rahilly and Müller, 1984b).

CARDIOVASCULAR SYSTEM
(figs. 13-3 to 13-5)

Even in the less advanced members of this group the blood circulation is well established. The current flows out through the arterial system supplying, notably, the massive central nervous system through capillaries that invest it as a surface network and from which drainage vessels lead back into the venous system. Numerous small arteries are also present throughout the mesoderm that will later constitute the walls of the lungs and intestine. At the rapidly extending caudal end of the embryo is a vascular plexus in which the channels progressively shift in adaptation to successive segments laid down by the active caudal bud. Out of this plexus stem the umbilical arteries, which join through the connecting stalk with the chorionic plexus and end in the terminal capillaries that are forming *in situ* in the chorionic villi. A moderate amount of plasma and numerous blood cells are seen throughout the villous network. The structural basis is now established for interchange between the maternal blood of the intervillous space and the embryonic blood in the capillaries of the villi. The venous return through the connecting stalk is made through a coarse venous plexus, which on reaching the body of the embryo terminates symmetrically in the right and left umbilical veins; these in turn empty into the sinus venosus at

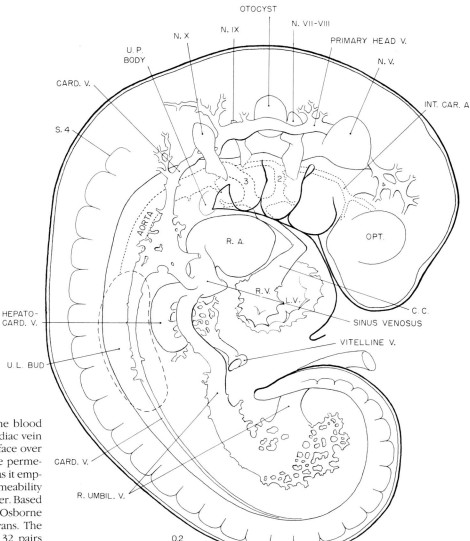

Fig. 13-3. The main channels by which the blood is returned to the heart. The right hepatocardiac vein is shown particularly well. The coelomic surface over it is modified in a manner that increases the permeability between the coelom and this channel as it empties into the sinus venosus. This greater permeability is most marked at this stage and disappears later. Based on Born reconstructions of No. 836, made by Osborne O. Heard under the supervision of H. M. Evans. The number of somites is now believed to be 32 pairs rather than 30.

the base of the heart. In addition, the specialized umbilical vesicle and the associated sinusoidal plexus of the liver possess a circulation. The communications between the vitelline plexus and the blood vessels of the body proper become limited to a vitelline artery arising in plexiform manner from the splanchnic branches of the aorta, and the right and left vitelline veins, which terminate in the vascular plexus that enmeshes the epithelial trabeculae of the liver (fig. 13-5). The hepatic plexus in turn empties into the sinus venosus, and thus this umbilical vesicle–hepatic circulation terminates at the heart. Mention will be made later of the special vascular communications that char-

acterize the liver in the period before the organization of the intestinal circulation and the portal vein.

The form and relations of the vascular pattern outlined can be best shown by drawings (see figs. 13-3 and 13-4). In figure 13-4 are illustrated the principal arteries and their distribution with reference to the alimentary canal. Only the larger arteries are shown. It is to be understood that these give off smaller arteries that terminate in various capillary networks; these in turn are drained into the venous system, and the blood is thereby brought back to the heart. The main channels of the venous return are shown in figure 13-3. In such a right profile view one sees how the sinus ven-

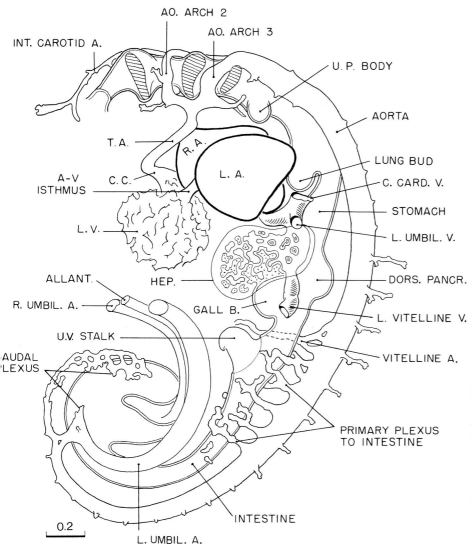

INT. CAROTID A.

AO. ARCH 2

AO. ARCH 3

U. P. BODY

AORTA

T. A.

R. A.

L. A.

LUNG BUD

A-V ISTHMUS

C. C.

C. CARD. V.

STOMACH

L. V.

L. UMBIL. V.

ALLANT.

HEP.

DORS. PANCR.

R. UMBIL. A.

GALL B.

L. VITELLINE V.

U.V. STALK

AUDAL LEXUS

VITELLINE A.

PRIMARY PLEXUS TO INTESTINE

0.2

INTESTINE

L. UMBIL. A.

Fig. 13-4. The endocardium and the endothelium of the large arteries. The angiogenesis of the capillary networks throughout the embryo would seem to be a response to their immediate environment. Although the heart and the aortae begin as capillary networks, they soon show individualities that indicate a higher order of specialization. Their form is controlled by a number of factors, including their response to the rapid accumulation of blood plasma, and the hydrostatic effects consequent on the specialization of the cardiac wall, which seems to be limited normally to a defined area of coelomic mesenchyme. Based on Born reconstructions of No. 836, made by Osborne O. Heard.

osus serves as a common antechamber to the heart, into which empty the cardinal system of veins draining the main axis of the embryo, the umbilical veins from the connecting stalk and chorionic villi, and the hepatic system from the umbilical vesicle. It is to be noted that, in addition to the blood from the umbilical vesicle and hepatic plexus, the portal system at this time includes a large channel (hepatocardiac vein) that projects into the coelom. Overlying this, the coelomic covering is specialized in a manner that makes it easily permeable to the coelomic fluid. The venous pattern is in general bilaterally symmetrical. The sinus venosus, however, is already asymmetrical, and the hepatic plexus becomes more and more so in adaptation to

the establishment of the one-sided pattern of the definitive portal system.

Aortic arches 4 and 6 develop (Congdon, 1922), and a fifth aortic arch can be found in at least some instances.

Many other, isolated features have been described at this important stage but the sources are difficult to locate. It is difficult to believe that in the foreseeable future it will be possible to enter in a computer such a question as "What does the venous system at stage 13 look like?" and be given the answer "A reconstruction of No. 588 was published by C. F. W. McClure and E. G. Butler in fig. 2, p. 339 of the *American Journal of Anatomy*, 35, 1925!"

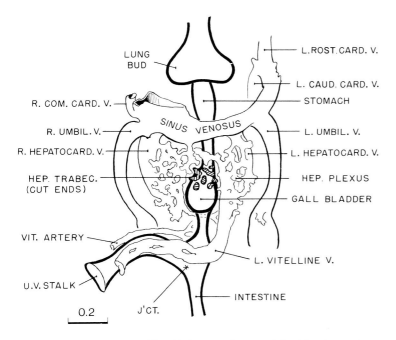

Fig. 13-5. Ventral view of the blood vessels of the hepatic region and their communications at the venous end of the heart. The umbilical veins still empty bilaterally into the sinus venosus. Based on Born reconstructions and serial tracings of No. 836.

Heart
(fig. 13-5)

It is convenient to follow Streeter's restriction of the term primary cardiac tube to the arterial part of the heart (i.e., distal to the atrioventricular junction). It should be appreciated, however, that the cardiac jelly is not confined to this tube but extends partly into the atria (de Vries and Saunders, 1962).

The four principal subdivisions of the primary cardiac tube are visible: (1) and (2) the trabeculated portions of the left and right ventricles, respectively, (3) the conus cordis, and (4) the truncus arteriosus (O'Rahilly, 1971, fig. 1). The last two (3 and 4) compose the outflow tract. Together with the sinus venosus and the atria, "these parts of the developing heart should not be simplistically identified with the components of the full-term heart" (Los, 1978).

The conus cordis is believed to give rise later to the conus arteriosus (of the right ventricle) and the aortic vestibule of the left ventricle. The truncus arteriosus is a feature of normal development and should not be confused with the anomaly known as truncus arteriosus communis. Los (1978) maintains that the truncus arteriosus "participates in the development of the outflow tracts of the ventricles . . . but not of the ascending aorta and the pulmonary trunk," both of which are stated to be derivatives of the aortic arches.

The first steps in the partitioning of separate right and left circulations begin already in stage 12, and "functional septation begins . . . in stage 13," whereby "the ventricular pumps now operate in parallel" instead of in series (McBride, Moore, and Hutchins, 1981). The "ejection stream from the left ventricle is dorsal to that of the right," a relationship that, according to de Vries and Saunders (1962), accounts for clockwise-spiralling streams.

Other features found at stage 13 are the left venous valve, septum primum and foramen primum (stages 12 and 13), the first indication of the common pulmonary vein (Neill, 1956, fig. 2), rostroventral and caudodorsal atrioventricular cushions (fig. 13-6), and the atrioventricular bundle (stages 13–16: Magovern, Moore, and Hutchins, 1986).

The motive force that propels the blood through the various channels is provided by a heart that still lacks true valves. The heart at stage 13 is shown in simplified form in figure 13-6. It will be seen that a considerable contractile force can be provided by the rapidly differentiating atrial and ventricular walls (myocardium), each having its own characteristics. From observations on early stages in animals, it is known that the rhythmic contractions of the myocardium and their coordination in contractile waves that progress from the sinus through the atrium, ventricle, and outflow tract to the aortic sac is a function of the myocardial cells. This myogenic period of the cardiac pulsations extends to the time of invasion by nerves. The establishment of neurogenic control probably occurs subsequent to stages 13 and 14, and it does not take place until after an active circulation is well in operation.

A summary of the histogenesis of the wall of the heart in stages 11–14 is shown in figure 13-7. In the least developed specimen the visceral coelomic wall is not distinguishable from the primordium of the myocardium. The latter should be regarded as a specialized part of the former, and its histological character can be seen in the photomicrograph. In a similar way, that part of the opposite parietal coelomic wall is producing the cells that are to become the framework and blood vessels of the liver. The coelomic primordium of the myocardium is separated from the partially distended endocardium by the myoendocardial interval throughout the whole length of the cardiac tube. This gap, at first with few or no reticular cells, is filled with a homogeneous transparent jelly which intervenes between the myocardium and the endocardium. This gelatinous layer is an incompressible elastic cushion by means of which the contractions of the myocardium produce obliteration of the lumen of the endocardium.

In stage 12 the myocardium has become three or four cells thick. One can distinguish the coelomic surface cells as the germinal basis from which more-specialized cells are crowding toward the endocardium as definitive myocardial cells. The residual cells at the surface will perhaps form the epicardium, but the latter is not defined until the delamination of myocardial cells is completed. Reticular cells now appear in the myoendocardial interval, and one may speak of a gelatinous reticulum or cardiac mesenchyme. The coelomic channel surrounding the heart is reduced to a thin space, outside which is a simple single-layered parietal coelomic membrane covered in turn by a thin surface ectoderm.

In stage 13 the cardiac chambers are distended with plasma and blood cells. It will be seen that those myocardial cells most advanced in their differentiation lie toward the cavity of the heart. Loops and strands of these cells extend inward, indenting and interlocking with the endocardium and thereby producing the trabecular character that so early distinguishes the ventricle from the atria. The trabecular arrangement of the wall requires a corresponding growth and elaboration of the endocardium.

In stage 14, the most advanced in the series illustrated, the wall is considerably thicker; passing from the surface to the cavity of the heart one can recognize the successive steps in the differentiation of the myocardial cells. Outermost is a compact wall or cortex of less-differentiated cells. Extending inward is the trabecular zone, consisting of loops or columns of elongating cells; these are the ones that first acquire fibrillae and striations. On the surface toward the narrow coelomic cleft, one can begin to recognize a thin layer of residual cells that appear to constitute the epicardium.

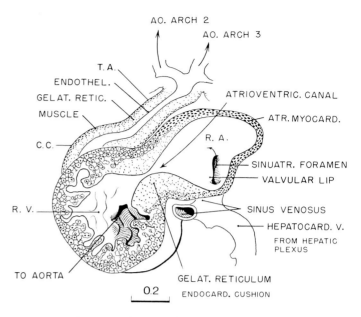

Fig. 13-6. A sagittal section through the heart, in the plane of the atrioventricular canal. The drawing shows in simplified form the character of the cardiac wall and the difference between the atria and the ventricles. The cardiac mesenchyme ("jelly") in the myoendocardial interval persists as endocardial cushions that serve as an atrioventricular valve. Similarly it persists in the conus cordis and truncus arteriosus, aiding in preventing backflow from the aortic arches. Based on serial sections and a Born reconstruction of No. 836.

By this time the cardiac wall is actively pulsating with rhythmic and coordinated contractions, progressing from the sinus to the outflow tract. The propulsion of the contained blood toward the aorta is in part aided by the virtually valve-like character of the cardiac tube at critical places. First of all, the fold of the atrial wall at the narrow opening of the sinus venosus into the atrium, the sinu-atrial foramen, serves as a valvular lip which, when the atrium contracts, tends to prevent the blood from escaping backward into the sinus (fig. 13-6). The next check to regurgitation is at the atrioventricular canal, where the so-called endocardial cushions reduce the passage from the atria to the ventricle to a narrow canal. Because of the gelatinous nature of the tissue of the cushions, the canal can be effectively closed by myocardial contraction. The third site of constriction of the cardiac tube is at the outflow tract and along the aortic trunk, stopping abruptly at the

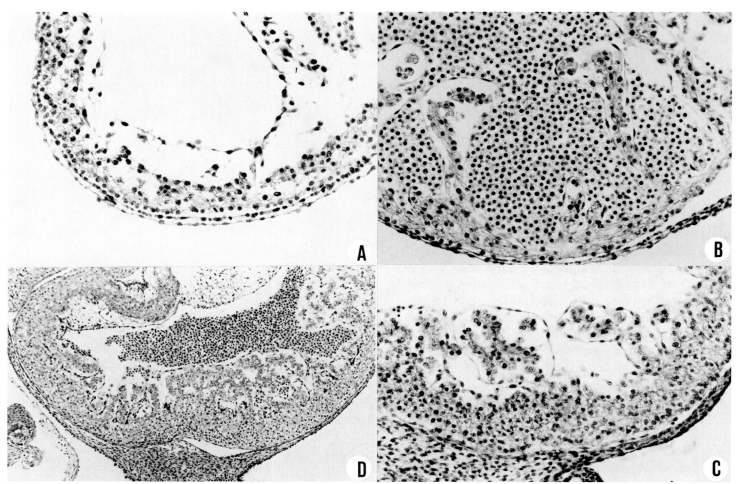

Fig. 13-7. (A–D) The histogenesis of the ventricular wall of the heart during stages 12–14. The myocardium begins as a specialized area of the visceral coelomic wall and is two or three cells in thickness. The surface cells are the less specialized germinal cells (A) No. 6079, stage 12. The myocardium is now four or five cells in thickness and constitutes a muscular plate that is separated by cardiac jelly from the endocardium. (B) No. 8066, stage 13. The internally situated myocardial cells have differentiated rapidly and form loops and strands that indent the endocardium. (C) No. 7618, advanced stage 13. The myocardial plate is well defined. (D) No. 6830, stage 14. Residual germinal cells are at the surface, covering the myocardial plate, deep to which is the trabecular layer, which will be the first to acquire fibrillae and striations.

aortic sac. This prevents regurgitation from the aortic arches. Also along this site there is found a zone or cushion of gelatinous reticulum, similar in character to the endocardial cushion at the atrioventricular canal. Both of these regions are to be regarded as parts of the cardiac tube where the myoendocardial interval with its gelatinous reticulum persists and where a valvelike function is being performed. Instead of extending the whole length of the tube, this cardiac mesenchyme is now limited to the particular areas where support against backflow is needed (fig. 13-6). Even in the absence of true valves, such a heart is capable of actively propelling the blood to the chorionic villi and back, through the umbilical vesicle and throughout the tissues of the embryo.

Blood Vessels of the Liver

In stages 11 and 12 the sinus venosus and the atria, if they are not enlarged specialized parts of the vitelline plexus, are at least intimately related to it. Multiple drainage channels from the plexus (fig. 13-5) converge at the caudal end of the heart and empty into the venous antechamber which lies rostrally athwart the umbilical vesicle near its junction with the intestine. This antechamber soon resolves itself into the right and left atria and the sinus venosus (fig. 13-3). In that transformation the atria become more specialized and are soon incorporated in the heart, whereas the sinus venosus retains its venous character and serves as the place of terminal confluence of all the large veins of the body, namely, the cardinal veins from the whole trunk, the umbilical veins from the connecting stalk and chorionic villi, and the vitelline veins from the umbilical vesicle. This is the vascular pattern one finds in the hepatic region at stage 13.

The section in figure 13-8 passes transversely through the central part of the liver and shows the typical appearance under low magnification of the epithelial trabeculae spreading outward and enmeshing the hepatic plexus, as is characteristic of this stage. This figure should be compared with figure 13-3, which is at the same magnification. One thereby recognizes the increase in size of the liver and its advance in complexity. Growth is particularly active dorsalward, producing right and left horns in which are found the hepatocardiac veins. From this time on, the area pre-empted by the vascular plexus in such a section of the liver increases in proportion to the amount of epithelial parenchyma. In more-advanced specimens of this group they are present in about equal proportion. The hepatic epithelium finally spreads close to the coelomic surface of the cardiac chamber, leaving but a thin rim to represent the location of the future diaphragm.

The large channels marked right and left hepatocardiac veins in figure 13-8 empty into the sinus venosus (compare fig. 13-5). It is through these that the main drainage of the hepatic plexus flows into the sinus venosus, at first through both right and left veins. Later the right vein enlarges and the left closes off (Ingalls, 1908, fig. 12). The right is finally transformed to become the terminal segment of the inferior vena cava. But in the present group, both of the hepatocardiac veins appear to be functioning chiefly in connection with the specialized coelomic walls separating them from the coelomic fluid. This relation is shown in figure 13-8. It can be seen that the permeable character of the tissue overlying the hepatocardiac veins would facilitate the passage of fluid from the coelomic cavity to these large veins just as they are about to enter the heart. At this time the chorionic circulation is but poorly established, and therefore the main source of water and food substances for the embryonic tissues must still be the fluid circulating in the coelomic channel. The areas covering the hepatocardiac veins shown in figure 13-5 appear to be the histological expression of that activity. A similar specialization of the coelomic surface is found in the region of the connecting stalk and on the inner surface of the body wall over the sac-like distention of the umbilical veins. Certainly such areas would be more permeable than those surfaces of the body covered with surface ectoderm.

For the purpose of determining the communications of the hepatic vessels, the view shown in figure 13-5 was made from reconstructions and serial tracings of one of the less developed embryos of this group. It will be seen that the hepatic plexus intervenes as a filtration, or perhaps an absorption, network between that of the umbilical vesicle and the general blood stream (sinus venosus). It foreshadows the portal circulation of later development, when the mesenteric blood from the digestive canal is passed through the hepatic parenchyma before reaching the heart. At any rate, in stage 13 all the blood from the umbilical vesicle passes through the hepatic plexus, and it is this blood alone that the liver receives. This is a temporary arrangement that coexists with the maximum development of the umbilical vesicle, and one might speak of it as a preportal system, pending further information on its functional activities.

It will be noted that the blood from the chorionic villi coming in through the umbilical veins bypasses the liver and is poured into the sinus venosus directly. Subsequently the terminal section of the umbilical veins becomes closed off, and the blood is rerouted through an anastomosis that is established between the left umbilical vein and some of the peripheral loops of the hepatic plexus. In this way a new channel, the ductus venosus, is established ventral to the liver, carrying the blood from the placenta directly to the base of the heart.

It can be concluded, first, that the blood vessels of the liver include the intrinsic hepatic plexus that arises *in situ* from cells of the coelomic mesoderm, apparently stimulated by the epithelium of the hepatic diverticulum. Secondly, the plexus of the umbilical vesicle empties into this intrinsic network through the vitelline veins. Thirdly, the left umbilical vein anastomoses with some of the peripheral loops of the hepatic plexus to form a direct channel, the ductus venosus, across the base of the liver, emptying into the inferior vena cava. Finally, there are the large hepatocardiac veins that drain the hepatic plexus into the sinus venosus, and that also appear to serve temporarily as permeable organs by means of which coelomic fluid gains ready access to the blood stream where it enters the heart.

DIGESTIVE SYSTEM
(fig. 13-9)

In stage 12 it can be seen that certain endodermal areas are at that time definitely allotted to the lung bud, dorsal pancreas, and liver. In stage 11 it is possible to recognize the pulmonary primordium and hepatic area. It can be concluded that long before that time (i.e., in the presomitic period), definitive areas of the endoderm are limited in their potentialities to the making of specific primary organs, although their outlines are not yet recognizable. It is also in those early periods that the primary induction of axial relationships with bilateral symmetries and asymmetries occurs (O'Rahilly, 1970). Although at first undetermined and uni-

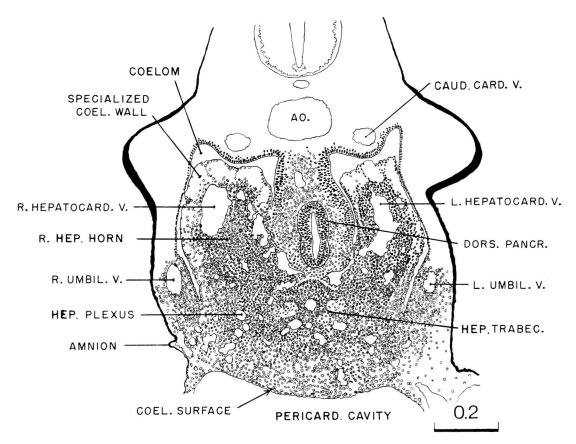

Fig. 13-8. Section through the liver, showing its blood vessels and the spreading of the hepatic trabeculae. The specialization of the hepatocardiac veins and the overlying coelomic wall is now at its height. In this less advanced embryo (No. 836) the umbilical veins still pass around the liver to reach the sinus venosus. Section 8-3-3.

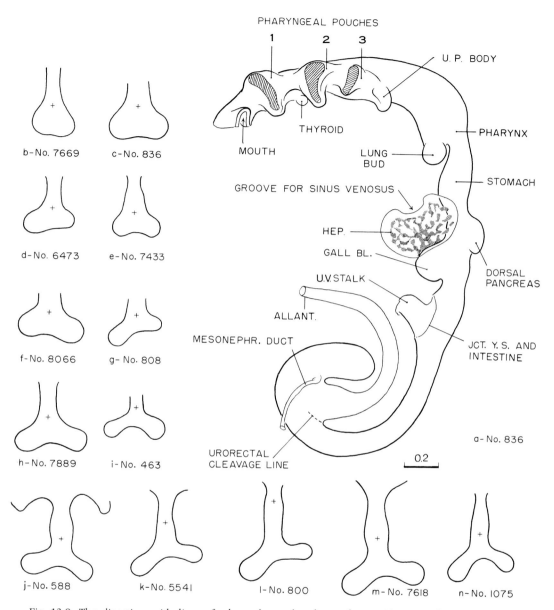

Fig. 13-9. The digestive epithelium of a less advanced embryo of stage 13. As yet the surrounding mesenchyme shows little change beyond a moderate cellular proliferation. Caudal to the stalk of the umbilical vesicle the intestine is less advanced, thereby participating in the rostrocaudal gradient of differentiation that characterizes the embryo as a whole. Based on Born reconstructions of No. 836, made by Osborne O. Heard under the supervision of H. M. Evans.

The small drawings show the progressive development of the right and left lung buds during stage 13. In each case a cross indicates the separation point between the respiratory and digestive tubes (i.e., between the beginning trachea, clearly visible in No. 800, and the esophagus).

form in their potentialities, subsequent proliferation of the endodermal cells provides them with a mechanism for segregation into groups having diverse constitutions. The consequent arrangement in organ territories is thus understandable, especially when account is taken of the directive influences of the overlying embryonic disc and its primitive node and notochordal process. These diverse fields of endoderm become the dominant tissues in the organogenesis of the structures composing the digestive system.

Some of the component organs of the digestive system are acquiring definite outlines, at least in their primary tissue, the epithelium (fig. 13-9). The roof of the pharyngeal region shows little activity, but the cellular proliferation of the floor and lateral margins is producing characteristic plates and folds that foreshadow the various derivatives that originate in this region. The bilobed median thyroid primordium and the telopharyngeal body are conspicuous (Weller, 1933). In addition, the thymic primordium of pharyngeal pouch 3 becomes distinguishable (*ibid.*). It will be noted that one of the factors in producing the pharyngeal pouches is the necessity of sparing spaces for the passage of large communicating channels from the aortic sac to the large dorsal aortae (figs. 13-4 and 13-9). These channels serve as functioning elements for the maintenance of the embryo. For each of these aortic arches there is produced a ridge on the surface and an indentation of the lateral margin of the pharynx. The surface ridges, or pharyngeal arches, are further conditioned by the precocious mesenchymal masses of the mandibular, hyoid, and other primordia. All these are to be considered in addition to the proliferative parts of the pharyngeal epithelium.

A Born reconstruction of the pharynx of No. 836 has been illustrated by Weller (1933, fig. 1).

The stomach now is definitely spindle-shaped. The dorsal pancreas is beginning its visible constriction from the intestinal tube. The ventral pancreas may perhaps be distinguishable. The epithelial trabeculae of the liver have spread almost to the ventral periphery of this organ. The stalk of the umbilical vesicle has become slender and longer, and retains its sharp demarcation from the intestinal epithelium. The intestinal system is larger, as is shown by comparison of figure 13-9 with figure 12-4, both drawn to the same scale. Further elongation of the intestine and the corresponding body axis is by interstitial growth.

The beginning of the omental bursa may be visible at stage 12 and is constant by stage 13 (McBride, Moore, and Hutchins, 1981). Pleuroperitoneal canals are becoming defined and the diaphragmatic primordium can be followed (Wells, 1954).

A "splenic primordium" has been identified as early as stage 13 (Gasser, 1975).

RESPIRATORY SYSTEM
(figs. 13-9 and 15-6)

The right and left lung buds with their characteristic diverging axial growth are the index of the advancement of growth of the lung. In figure 13-9 is shown the range included in this stage. A cross in each instance marks the level below which the respiratory diverticulum possesses an independent lumen. A trachea is present in the more advanced specimens. With few exceptions, the right primary bronchus, as soon as it acquires appreciable length, is directed more caudally, whereas the left bronchus is more nearly transverse. In this, the bilateral bronchial asymmetry existing in the maturer state is anticipated.

URINARY SYSTEM

Glomeruli begin to develop in the mesonephros, and nephric tubules become S-shaped (Shikinami, 1926). A ureteric bud may possibly be present in some specimens (Wells, 1954, fig. 4), although further confirmation is needed. The mesonephric duct, which becomes separated from the surface ectoderm except in its caudal portion, is fused to the cloaca, into which it may open (fig. 13-9). A urorectal cleavage line is apparent.

REPRODUCTIVE SYSTEM

The primordial germ cells migrate from the hindgut to the mesonephric ridges, and several hundred of them are present in the embryo (Witschi, 1948).

NERVOUS SYSTEM
(fig. 13-10)

The central nervous system is still a tubular structure, and from the midbrain region caudalward it presents the classic arrangement of basal and alar plates,

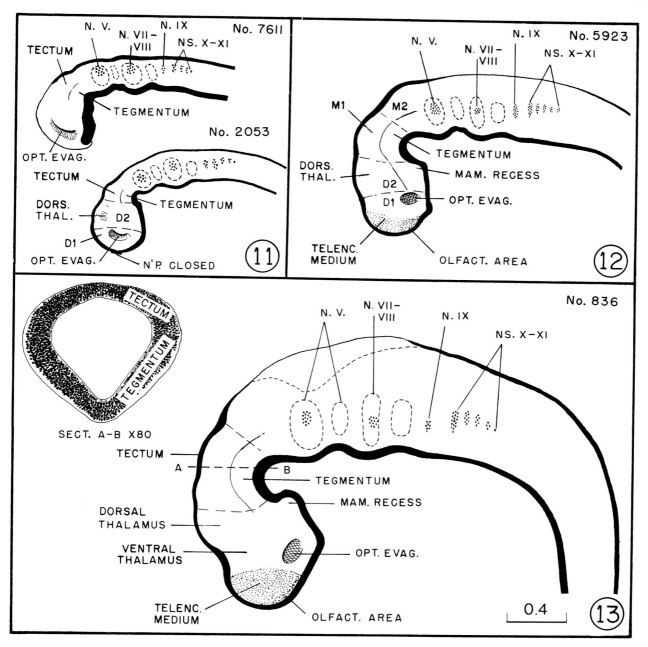

Fig. 13-10. Form and size of the brain at stages 11–13, drawn to the same scale. Various neural areas are indicated according to current interpretation. A section (at higher magnification) through the mid-brain at stage 13 (the level marked *A–B*) shows the appearance of the neural wall at this time. Based on reconstructions by Osborne O. Heard.

demarcated by a sulcus limitans. Transverse sections through the cervical levels of the tube show a narrow marginal layer. The remaining wall is made up of the undifferentiated ependymal zone, except for a beginning mantle zone in the region that is to form the ventral horn of gray matter. This nuclear zone in more-advanced specimens of the group shows early neurons, the processes of which can be seen emerging as ventral roots. Ventral root fibers are present as far caudally as the upper thoracic segments. The dorsal roots of the spinal nerves consist of a few fibers at the more rostral levels.

A marginal layer begins to appear also in the rhombencephalon and the mesencephalon in the area ventral to the sulcus limitans. The most differentiated part of the brain is still the rhombencephalon. Rhombomere 1 can be distinguished, and hence eight rhombomeres can be counted. In addition to the lateral bulges of the areas of the trigeminal and facial nerves, there are also dips in the floor in the median plane at corresponding levels. The trigeminal and facial dips are constantly present in this stage and constitute reliable landmarks. From the single sheet of motor cells present already in stage 12, two columns of motor nuclei begin to form in the midbrain and hindbrain: the ventromedial column contains the cells for nerves 4, 5, 7/8, 9, 10, and 11, the ventrolateral column the nuclei for nerves 3, 6, and 12. The motor nuclei of the spinal nerves are in continuity with the hypoglossal nucleus. The motor roots for nerves 5, 6, 9, 10, and 11 are present in most embryos. The hypoglossal nerve consists of several roots. The geniculate and vestibular ganglia form a unity; in the more advanced embryos, nerve fibers begin to develop in the vestibular part. The sulcus limitans terminates at the rostral end of the mesencephalon and hence does not continue into the diencephalon. Several afferent tracts are appearing in the hindbrain, as detailed by O'Rahilly *et al.* (1984). The cervical flexure is appearing.

Two segments can still be distinguished in the midbrain. The tegmental area is indicated by an internal swelling. The term synencephalon is sometimes used for an area that is transitional between midbrain and forebrain. Two segments are still identifiable in the diencephalon. Segment 2 contains the future thalamus. Segment 1 gave rise to the optic evagination. The telencephalon medium (impar) is adjacent to the nasal plate.

Outline drawings of reconstructions of typical brains from stages 11–13 are shown in figure 13-10. All are at the same enlargement. A less advanced and a more advanced specimen of stage 11 are illustrated to cover the transformation incident to the closure of the rostral neuropore.

Eye
(fig. 13-11)

In embryos belonging to stage 13 the optic evagination has grown and advanced in differentiation sufficiently to enable one to outline its parts, namely, optic part of retina, future pigmented layer of retina, and optic stalk. Four examples showing the range in development are shown in figure 13-11. These were selected from embryos all sectioned coronally. In such sections the evagination appears less rounded than when it is cut through its long axis, as in transverse series, and appears smaller. It is the better plane, however, in which to see the outline of the retina. The latter is still largely a flat disc, and its proliferating cells cause it to bulge inward. On the outer surface of the retinal disc, a marginal zone free of nuclei can be distinguished. This is the beginning of the framework through which the retinal fibers will pass on their way to the optic nerve. An abrupt transition occurs from the retinal disc to the thinner adjoining segment of the evagination, the part that is to become the pigmented layer of the retina. This latter, in turn, is indistinctly set off from the part that is to form the stalk—a thick, short segment at the junction with the brain wall. The optic vesicle is covered by a basement membrane, and the surface ectoderm is lined by a basement membrane (O'Rahilly, 1966, fig. 10). In the mesoderm adjoining the optic evagination, early stages of angiogenesis can be noted.

The retinal disc presses outward and is in contact with the overlying surface ectoderm, with little or no mesoderm between them. In response to this contact the ectoderm proliferates and forms the lens disc. This has been shown to be an inductive phenomenon. Although when the lens plate begins to invaginate the specimen is generally allotted to the next stage, the beginning of an optic cup can be seen in a few embryos of stage 13 (O'Rahilly, 1966, fig. 22).

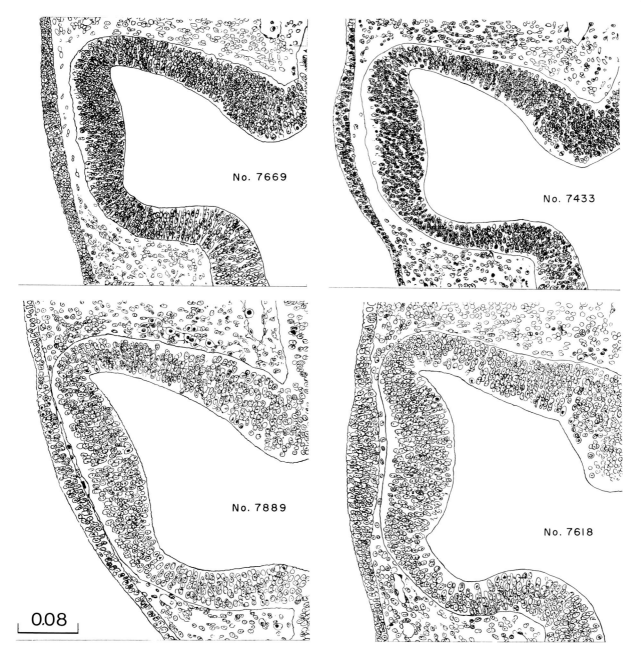

No. 7669

No. 7433

No. 7889

0.08

No. 7618

Fig. 13-11. Sections through the optic vesicle in four embryos, selected to show the range of development in stage 13. The major parts of the evaginated wall are already determined and, of these, the retina is the most advanced. The proliferation of its cells results in its bulging into the lumen of the evagination, and its outer surface is marked by its widening nucleus-free marginal zone. Where the retinal disc is in contact with the skin ectoderm, the latter has been stimulated to form the lens disc, which will become indented in the next stage. The angioblastic activity preceding the formation of the vascular coat can be seen in No. 7889. All drawings are at the same scale.

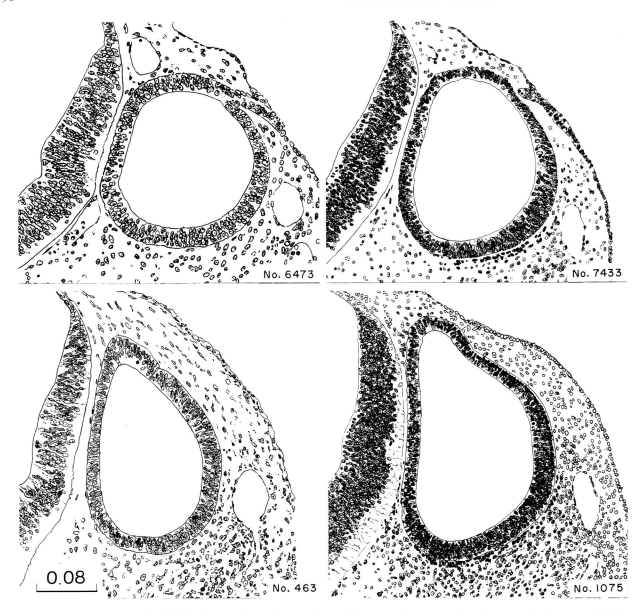

Fig. 13-12. Otic vesicles of four embryos, illustrating the range of development during stage 13. The vesicle is now closed, but the less advanced members still have some remnant of the ectodermal stalk. In the more advanced specimens the stalk has disappeared and the endolymphatic appendage is marked off as a recess from the main cavity of the vesicle. The endolymphatic appendage is apparently determined even before the vesicle is closed. In the more advanced specimens the surrounding mesenchyme is reacting by exhibiting the first steps in the formation of the otic capsule. All drawings are at the same scale.

Ear

(fig. 13-12)

For illustration of the range of development of the otic vesicle in stage 13, four specimens were selected in which the serial sections pass approximately through the long axis of the vesicle. Drawings of these, arranged in order of development, are shown in figure 13-12. It is to be pointed out that they are now all closed vesicles (Anson and Black, 1934). In the less developed specimens of the group a stalk of tissue may still attach the vesicle to the surface ectoderm, or the stalk may be detached from the vesicle but still be present as a tag or thickening of the overlying ectoderm. The cells included in this temporary stalk appear to be surface ectoderm stimulated to this activity by the adjacent neural ectoderm. At any rate, the stalk phenomenon has disappeared completely in the more advanced members of the group. Apparently the cells spread out in adaptation to the surface and resume their activity as ordinary surface ectoderm.

The otic vesicle is surrounded by the basement membrane of the otic disc (O'Rahilly, 1963).

Stage 13 covers the period of demarcation of the endolymphatic appendage. In the less developed specimens one can begin to recognize the segment of the vesicular wall that is going to form it. The cells of the appropriate region are characterized by a relatively greater amount of cytoplasm, meaning that this region is slightly further advanced in its differentiation. In macerated specimens these cells are more stable than those in the other parts of the vesicular wall, and they retain their form when the latter may have become completely disassociated. All the evidence points to a very early specialization of the potentialities of the several parts of the vesicular wall. In the more advanced specimens of the group the appendage projects dorsalward as a definite recess. By that time, when the tissues are sufficiently transparent, one can see it in a gross specimen as a distinct part of the vesicle.

This stage is further characterized by the reaction of the surrounding mesoderm to the growing vesicle. The first notable reaction is angiogenesis among the cells near the vesicle, producing a capillary network that closely invests it. This is followed by a proliferation of mesenchymal cells, which is greatest in the regions ventral and lateral to the vesicle. The vestibular part of the vestibulocochlear ganglion and vestibular nerve fibers can be distinguished.

Specimens of Stage 13 Already Described

His embryo (a), 4 mm. Described in detail by His (1880).

Fischel embryo, 4.2 mm, Hochstetter Atlas. This embryo is sharply and spirally curved, and the length given is approximate. Its place in stage 13 is verified by the form of the limb buds.

Keibel embryo No. 112, 5.3 mm. Described in the Keibel and Elze *Normentafeln* (1908). The lens is a flat, slightly thickened disc. The otic vesicle is detached, but a remnant of the stalk is still present; there is some indication of the endolymphatic appendage. There are 36 pairs of somites.

R. Meyer, 5-mm embryo, No. 318, Anatomisches Institut, Zürich. This embryo is a more advanced example of stage 13. The epithelium of the lens disc begins to indent. There are 38 pairs of somites. The embryo is referred to in the Keibel and Elze *Normentafeln.*

C. Rabl, 4-mm embryo. The specimen closely resembles the Fol 5.6-mm embryo and the Hertwig G 31 embryo. It was used by Rabl in his study of the face (1902).

Broman, embryo Lf., 3 mm, Anatomisches Institut, Lund. This embryo was described systematically by Broman (1896). He made revisions for the Keibel and Elze *Normentafeln.* Broman reports that it has 30 pairs of somites. Regarding its relatively small size, it is to be noted that it was fixed in absolute alcohol and then preserved for two years in weak spirits. This embryo is a less advanced example of stage 13.

Carnegie No. 148, 4.3 mm. A monographic description of this embryo was published by Gage (1905).

Fol, 5.6-mm embryo. This well-preserved embryo is a more advanced example. It was carefully described and illustrated by Fol (1884).

Hertwig, 4.9-mm embryo, G 31, Anatomisches-biologisches Institut, Berlin. This well-preserved embryo, a typical representative of stage 13, was first described in a study of the development of the pancreas by Jankelowitz (1895). An excellent systematic study followed later (Ingalls, 1907, 1908). The embryo was considered also in the Keibel and Elze *Normentafeln.* There are 35 pairs of somites.

4-mm and 5-mm twin embryos, University of Basel. A graphic reconstruction of the normal specimen was issued by Müller and O'Rahilly (1980a), and reconstructions, with particular reference to the nervous system, were published by Müller and O'Rahilly (1984), who described the cerebral dysraphia (future anencephaly) present in one twin.

Free Hospital for Women, Brookline, Massachusetts, No. 5, 5 mm. The histochemistry of this embryo was studied by McKay *et al.* (1955).

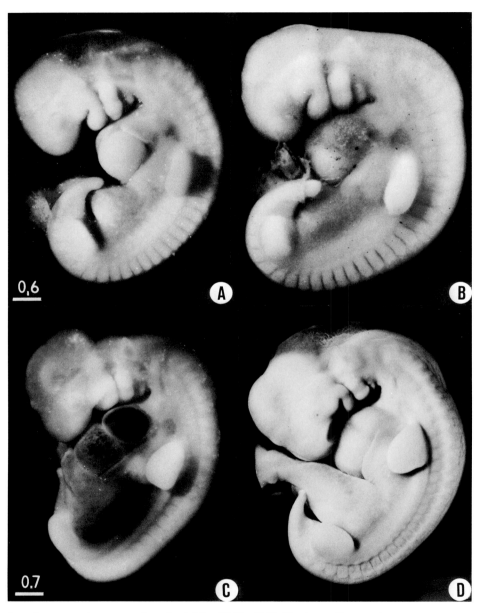

Fig. 14-1, A–D. Four embryos selected to cover the range of development included in stage 14. In the more translucent examples (A,C) much of the internal structure can be seen, whereas in the more opaque specimens (B,D) the surface features are more distinct. (A) No. 6830. The upper limb bud is beginning to elongate and curve ventrally, and the lower limb bud forms a distinct ridge. The spinal ganglia stand out clearly and are partly covered by the muscular plates. Various cranial ganglia (5, 7/8, 10) can be distinguished. (B) No. 1380. A right lateral view, reversed for comparison with the others. The flattening of the top of the head is caused by shrinkage. A *Nackengrube* is visible. (C) No. 7333. The heart, liver, and sinus venosus are evident ventral to the upper limb bud. A slender, tapering strip of mesenchyme extends between the upper and lower limb buds, and is thought to participate possibly in the formation of the muscles of the abdominal wall. The mesonephros lies ventral to it. The otic vesicle and its endolymphatic appendage can be discerned. (D) No. 6502. This embryo is on the borderline of the next stage. The lens pit, however, is still open to the surface. The nasal plate is evident. The roof of the fourth ventricle is well shown. A and B are at the same enlargement, as are also C and D.

STAGE 14

Approximately 5–7 mm
Approximately 32 postovulatory days

SUMMARY

External: invagination of the lens disc but with an open lens pit; a well-defined endolymphatic appendage; elongated and tapering upper limb buds.

Internal: the ventral pancreas (if not detectable earlier) is distinguishable at stages 14 and 15; right and left lung sacs grow dorsad; the ureteric bud acquires a metanephrogenic cap; future cerebral hemispheres and cerebellar plates begin to be visible.

SIZE AND AGE

Approximately 70 percent of the embryos after fixation range from 5.5 to 7 mm in length, and most of these are 6–7 mm. A few, however, are only 5 mm and some are 7.2–8.2 mm. The longer specimens can be accounted for in part by the fact that they were fixed in an exceptionally straight posture. Their organs (eye, ear, and lung) have the degree of development characteristic of the group. It happens that the least advanced specimen of the stage is found among the exceptionally small ones, and the most advanced is among the largest ones. When the embryos are arranged in order of their size, however, their sequence departs considerably from one based on the advancement of their organogenesis.

There is a greater range of variation in the size of the chorion for a given stage than in the size of the embryo. That the growth of the chorion is much influenced by environmental nourishment is indicated by its poor performance in tubal pregnancies, where it is likely to become isolated in stagnant blood. A small chorion is to be expected in a tubal specimen. Omitting three such cases in the present group, most specimens for which records are available fall into three groups: small, average (about 70 percent), and large.

These have overall largest diameters (1) between 20 and 25 mm, (2) between 30 and 38 mm, and (3) between 40 and 47 mm, respectively.

The age of the embryos of stage 14 is believed to be approximately 32 postovulatory days.

EXTERNAL FORM
(figs. 14-1 to 14-3)

The contour of the embryo appears still to be determined largely by that of the central nervous system. Here also there are long specimens and short curved ones but, as they acquire more mass, the embryos have become more uniform in shape. In most of them there is a depression in the dorsal contour at the level of sclerotomes 5 and 6. This is the *Nackengrube* of His. This cervical bend began to appear in the more advanced members of the preceding stage, but from now on it is a characteristic feature of embryos up to 30 mm. It is a ventral offset to the dorsal convexity of the precocious hindbrain above and the dorsal curve of the thoracic levels of the spinal cord below. It is apparently the forerunner of the flexure sequence of the primate vertebral column, although it so far antedates the latter that one hesitates to attribute to the central nervous system the entire determination of the flexures of the vertebral column.

The upper limb buds are no longer the simple ridges that were found in 4- and 5-mm embryos. Instead they are rounded, projecting appendages curving ventrally. They taper toward the tip, the terminal rim of which will form the hand plate, although the latter is not yet demarcated. In some of the specimens, however, a beginning marginal blood vessel can be recognized. The lower limb buds do not repeat the form of the upper buds. Extending from the upper bud to the lower bud are muscular plates that apparently give

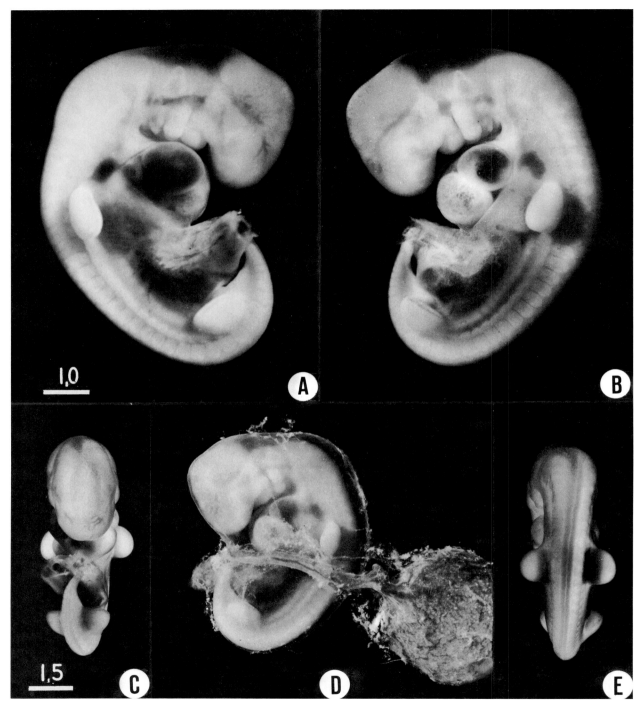

Fig. 14-2. Various views of No. 8141, which lent itself partic- ularly well to photography. (A) The opaque unsegmented band of mesenchyme between the upper and lower limb buds is evident. The mesonephros lies directly ventral to it. The otic vesicle is clearly visible, as is also a *Nackengrube*. (B) The opaque band and the mesonephros are separated from each other by the much darker caudal cardinal vein, the intersegmental tri- butaries of which lend an appearance of segmentation to the mesenchymal band. (C) Ventral view. The fourth ventricle is visible above (cf. O'Rahilly, Müller, and Bossy, 1982, fig. 8).

(D) Relations of the embryo to the umbilical vesicle. The vesicle is immersed in coelomic fluid, and embryonic blood is pumped through its highly vascular wall. The sparse, amniochorionic reticular strands that characterize the exocoelom have been re- tained, and the amnion is still intact. The caudal end of the embryo is more slender than in the preceding stage. (E) Dorsal view showing, particularly on the right side, the spinal ganglia lateral to the (darker) spinal cord. A and B are at the same enlargement, as are C–E.

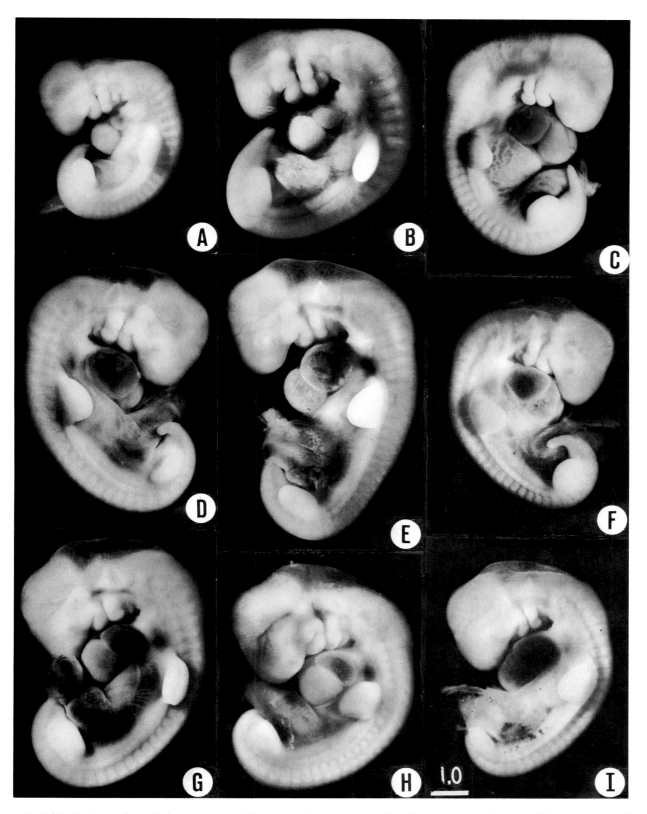

Fig. 14-3. Various embryos belonging to stage 14, to show the range of variation in size (all are at the same magnification), posture, and detailed form. (A) No. 5654, a less advanced specimen. (B) No. 4154. (C) No. 4629. (D) No. 7394. (E) No. 6848, with an exceptionally large and straight trunk. The opaque mass dorsocaudal to the cervical sinus is the center from which the thoracic wall will spread over the heart. (F) No. 7400. (G) No. 7394. (H) No. 1620, a more advanced specimen. (I) No. 7400.

origin to the musculature of the ventrolateral body wall, and in front of them can be seen the slender mesonephric duct. Under suitable lighting the caudal cardinal vein appears as a dark band intervening between them. The segmental tributaries to the cardinal vein may give an appearance of segmentation of the overlying mammary crest (fig. 14-2A, B) (O'Rahilly and Müller, 1985). In most cases the atria are distended, and their thin walls stand out in contrast with the thick trabeculated walls of the ventricles.

In the head region the mandibular and hyoid arches are large and conspicuous (fig. 15-3), whereas the third arch in the more advanced members of the group is relatively small and partly concealed along with the depression of the cervical sinus. The hyoid arch, which in the preceding stage was already subdivided into a dorsal and a ventral segment, now tends to show a subdivision of its ventral segment. This produces a "ventralmost" segment which later will play a part in the subdivision of the sixth auricular hillock. In translucent specimens one can see much of the anatomy of the head, for example the outlines of the optic cup, the trigeminal ganglion with cells streaming into the maxillary and mandibular processes, the vestibulofacial mass extending into the dorsal segment of the hyoid arch, the otic vesicle with an elongated and well-marked endolymphatic appendage, the glossopharyngeal and vagus nerves. Winding through these various structures in a characteristic way is the primary head vein. In less-advanced members of the group the lens is indistinct. In more-advanced specimens, however, its opening stands out as a sharply outlined pore. The opening of the lens vesicle to the surface, being an especially definite characteristic, is taken as one of the criteria that determine the inclusion of a given specimen in this stage. When it is closed the embryo is moved to the next group.

The nasal plate (Bossy, 1980a) is usually flat, but it may be concave, although it has not yet acquired a distinct lip. One can usually recognize the nasal area by its thickened opaque ectoderm. If illuminated in a special way, the rim of the disc stands out in an exaggerated manner, which is the case in the photograph shown in figure 14-1D. In the same photograph the pore-like opening of the lens vesicle can be seen.

The term nasal disc (or plate) is considered useful for the peripheral feature distinct from the central components, such as the olfactory bulb etc. The term placode is avoided because of its long-standing association with supposedly "branchial sense organs" and because of its frequent usage for structures as disparate as the nasal plate and the lens disc.

Some difficulties in staging embryos, particularly stages 14 and 15, from only external criteria are mentioned in an abstract by Pearson *et al.* (1968).

CARDIOVASCULAR SYSTEM
(fig. 16-7)

The four major subdivisions of the primary cardiac tube that were seen in the previous stage are clearly defined. The atrioventricular canal is more-evenly apportioned between the ventricles (i.e., shifted relatively to the right), so that it has been claimed that the inlet of the right ventricle is probably derived from the "primitive" (left?) ventricle (Anderson, Wilkinson, and Becker, 1978). Whether the rostroventral and caudodorsal atrioventricular cushions may be beginning to be approximated is disputed, but they are not fused. The outflow tract still retains a single lumen, although functional septation has been in progress since the previous stage. Conotruncal ridges or, more probably, cushions (Pexieder, 1982) are generally described in the wall of the conus and truncus at this time, appearing at stages 12–15 (de Vries and Saunders, 1962) or 14–16 (McBride, Moore, and Hutchins, 1981). The ridges are said to be simply local remnants of disappearing cardiac jelly rather than new formations (Los, 1965). The role of the various "cushions" in the developing heart is not entirely clear; they may serve merely as a temporary adhesive. Normal cellular necrosis is a characteristic feature of the cushions (Pexieder, 1975). The sinu-atrial node is said to be identifiable (Yamauchi, 1965).

The spiral course of the aortic and pulmonary streams has been accounted for in a number of different ways: e.g., by hemodynamic factors, by differential growth, or by local absorption (Anderson, 1973; Goor and Lillehei, 1975). Pexieder (1982) has proposed that three pairs of cushions (conal, truncal, and aorticopulmonary) are simply arranged in different planes, and that their coming together inevitably leads to a spiral, without any supposed torsions and counter-torsions. Los (1978) believes that the spiral arrangement of the great

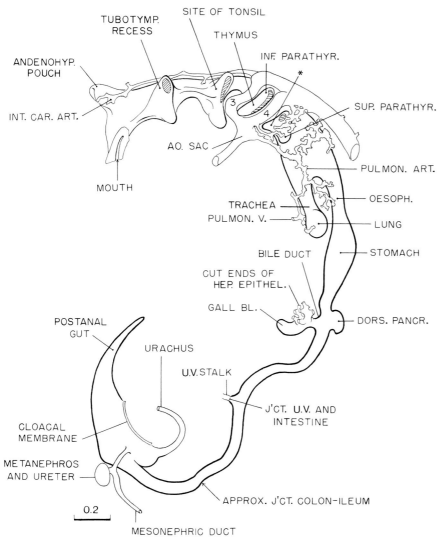

Fig. 14-4. The epithelium of the digestive system in a less advanced member of stage 14. Angiogenesis is active in the surrounding mesenchyme, which forms an ensheathing capillary network (not shown in the drawing). The large channels that serve as feeders to the capillaries of the pharyngeal and pulmonary regions are shown. The asterisk indicates the so-called "lateral thyroid." Based on a Born reconstruction of No. 1380, made by Osborne O. Heard.

vessels results from asymmetric growth of the main stem of the originally symmetric fourth and sixth pairs of arch arteries, without any twisting of the truncal septum.

The pulmonary (sixth aortic) arch is formed by a ventral sprout from the aortic sac and a dorsal sprout from the aorta (Congdon, 1922, fig. 34). At least in some instances a fifth aortic arch arises from the aortic sac or from the fourth arch and ends in the pulmonary arch (*ibid.*, fig. 22).

DIGESTIVE SYSTEM
(fig. 14-4)

The adenohypophysial (craniopharyngeal) pouch is a prominent feature of this stage. The notochord ends near its dorsal wall.

The pharyngeal pouches, which previously have been relatively simple lateral expansions of pharyngeal epithelium intervening between the aortic arches, are now more pocket-like structures. The future thymus and the "parathyrogenic zones" (Politzer and Hann, 1935) can be recognized. The thyroid pedicle (fig. 14-7D) shows further elongation but is still connected to the epithelium of the pharynx. In addition, right and left lobes and an isthmus may perhaps be presaged (Weller, 1933).

The composition of the tubotympanic recess remains unclear. Goedbloed (1960) has expressed "reservations concerning the concept that the middle ear derives from the first pharyngeal pouch" because it is claimed that the developing middle ear and pharyngeal pouch 1 do not agree topographically and belong to different periods of development: "the period in which the first pharyngeal pouch disappears is exactly the period when the new extension in the oral cavity occurs which is to become the middle ear," namely 5–10 mm (approximately stages 13–16). In another study it was concluded that, between 10 and 20 mm (approximately stages 16–20), "there is a gradual reduction in the contributions from the second arch and second pouch to the tubotympanic recess so that the tympanum and tube are formed solely from the first pouch" (Kanagasuntheram, 1967). Clearly, further work is required.

From the outset these derivatives of the lateral and ventral parts of the pharyngeal outpouchings are characterized by diverse individualities. They soon lose the uniform serial appearance that marked the pouches in their earlier and simpler form, when they were clearly secondary to the pattern of the aortic arches and to the mesenchymal masses of the pharyngeal arches. In contrast with the development of the lateral and ventral parts, the pharyngeal roof remains mostly thin and inactive. A conspicuous feature is the contact in each interaortic interval with the skin ectoderm. These contact areas, although becoming progressively smaller, are still present in stage 14. It is to be noted, however, that the telopharyngeal body is devoid of a contact area with the skin ectoderm, whereas pharyngeal pouch 3 has one. It is to be noted further that the median thyroid primordium, which is to form the main body of the thyroid gland, has no contact with skin ectoderm at any time. This structure is shown in figure 14-7D. It still retains its stalk of origin from the floor of the pharynx. It is already a bilobed structure, surrounded by a fluid-filled reticular mesenchymal

space. It comes into close relation with the aortic sac, a part of which is shown as the space at the bottom of the photograph in figure 14-7D.

A typical specimen belonging to the less advanced half of the group is illustrated in figure 14-4. When this figure is compared with figure 13-9 of the preceding stage, it is seen that the epithelial alimentary canal has become relatively more slender and the different parts are more definitely marked off from one another. The small intestine, because of its increase in length, is slightly deflected from the median plane and is deflected even more ventrally and dorsally. Thus we have the initiation of the intestinal coils. The junction of the small intestine with the colon is marked by the circumstances that the latter still lies in the median plane and is also slightly larger in diameter than the ileum.

The epithelium of the alimentary canal provides the form of the tube, which reflects the growth of its different parts. Surrounding coats appear secondarily.

The ventral pancreas (which may perhaps be distinguishable as early as stage 13) appears as an evagination from the bile duct at stages 14 (Blechschmidt, 1973) and 15. It is generally described as unpaired but, at least in some cases, may perhaps be bilobed (Odgers, 1930) or even multiple (Delmas, 1939).

RESPIRATORY SYSTEM
(figs. 14-5 and 15-6)

The hypopharyngeal eminence and arytenoid swellings appear in the floor of the pharynx, and the epithelial lamina of the larynx develops in the median plane between the arytenoid swellings (O'Rahilly and Tucker, 1973).

The trachea is recognizable. The separation point (between it and the esophagus) remains at a constant level during at least the remainder of the embryonic period proper, whereas the bifurcation point (of the trachea) descends (O'Rahilly and Müller, 1984c).

The right and left lung sacs are shown in geometric projection in figure 14-5. The eight specimens demonstrate the range of development covered from the less advanced to the more advanced members of the group. These frontal projections do not reveal the fact that the sacs, as they become larger, curve dorsally to a position lateral to the esophagus, embracing it on each side. Thus the esophagus comes to lie within the

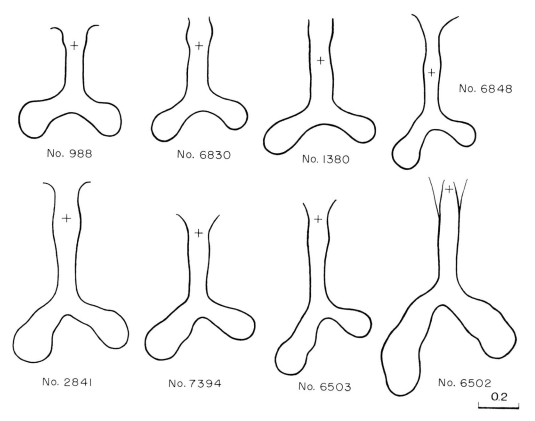

Fig. 14-5. Frontal projections of the epithelium of the trachea and primary bronchi, showing their range of development in stage 14. The level at which the laryngotracheal lumen opens into that of the digestive tube is shown by a cross.

two prongs of a fork. The right main bronchus soon shows a tendency to be longer and directed caudally, the left bronchus being shorter and more transverse.

In the preceding paragraph attention has been restricted to the epithelium, the seemingly dominant tissue of the lung. There now clusters about it a zone of condensed mesenchymal tissue, some of the cells of which are undergoing active angiogenesis. An extensive capillary network is taking the form of a basket-like envelope enclosing the mesenchymal tissue of the lung. It is fed from above, as is shown in figure 14-4, by irregular bilateral channels from the plexiform pulmonary aortic arch on each side. These channels become the pulmonary arteries. The pulmonary plexus is drained below by a short stem anastomosing with the dorsal surface of the left atrium. This anastomosis appears to be a joint product participated in by a thin fold of the atrial wall and the developing capillaries of the pulmonary mesenchyme, an example of affinity of

one endothelial outgrowth for another. It is later that subsequent adjustments transform this primary anastomosis into the paired right and left pulmonary veins. This development is facilitated by the fact that the mesenchymal zone in which it occurs is continuous between the cardiac wall and the bifurcation of the lung. The mesenchymal cells that invest the epithelial lung are derived from the overlying coelomic wall. In stage 12 the active proliferation of these coelomic cells and their detachment from the surface (fig. 12-10A) have already been noted. They can be traced as they move in toward the lung and alimentary epithelium, leaving behind them a layer of cells that will finally constitute the mesothelium. This is the condition in the present stage, as shown in figure 14-7E. The lung is thus composed of an innermost epithelial tubular system surrounded by a richly vascularized mesenchymal zone, which in turn is partially enclosed by a mesothelium (pleura) facing the coelom.

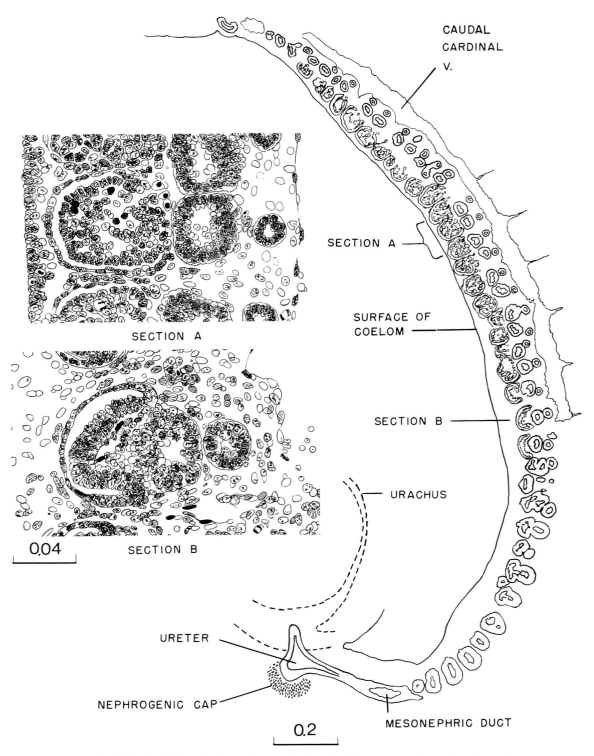

SECTION A

SECTION B

CAUDAL
CARDINAL
V.

SECTION A

SURFACE OF
COELOM

SECTION B

URACHUS

URETER

NEPHROGENIC CAP

MESONEPHRIC DUCT

0.04

0.2

Fig. 14-6. Sagittal section through the entire length of the mesonephros of No. 6500. The rostrocaudal gradient of the developing tubules is evident. Detailed drawings of section levels *A* and *B* are shown under higher magnification.

At the level shown in figure 14-7E, the mesenchymal layer of the lung is still blended with that of the esophagus. The latter can be seen in the center of the section, and the circular contours of its mesenchymal layer are marked by their deeply staining capillaries.

URINARY SYSTEM
(figs. 14-6 and 14-7)

In embryos of this stage the mesonephros is well along in its organogenesis. The steps in this process are made easier to follow by the fact that the development occurs progressively in a rostrocaudal direction. Thus in a single specimen, as shown in figure 14-6, one can retrace the gradation, from the units just starting at the caudal end as simple unattached vesicles, to the more advanced units at the rostral end, which have partially vascularized glomerular capsules, each connected by an S-shaped tubule with the mesonephric duct.

Here again is an organ in which the epithelial elements constitute its primary tissue and seem largely to determine its form. The non-epithelial mesonephric elements, though necessary complements for epithelial-mesenchymal interaction, give the appearance of being subsidiary. It has already been seen that the coelomic surface cells possess various inherent potentialities. The surface of the coelom can be mapped in definite areas in accordance with the distribution of these various kinds of surface cells. Depending on the area, there are produced such diverse tissues as cardiac muscle, the framework of the liver, and the connective tissue and muscular coats of the esophagus, stomach, and intestine. In the present case the coelomic cells give rise to epithelium. Running along each side of the median plane is a narrow strip of coelom where, by the proliferation and delamination of its surface cells, there is produced a longitudinal series of epithelial tubules that constitute the units of the mesonephros. This follows the manner in which nephric elements were formed in previous stages, and it is now about to be repeated, with certain modifications, in the development of the metanephros, which is still in the primordial state of a budding ureter with its nephrogenic capsule (fig. 14-6).

One can go a step further in regard to the inherent constitution of these coelomic epithelial tubules. Not only do they become tubules, but from the beginning they show regional differentiation. The proximal end promptly blends with and opens into the mesonephric duct, and this part of the tubule persists as a collecting duct. The distal free end at the same time begins its expansion into a highly specialized part of the tubule, namely the mesonephric corpuscle. The intervening central segment of the tubule becomes the convoluted secretory portion. Embryos in this stage are especially favorable for the study of the process of formation of the mesonephric corpuscle. As can be seen in figure 14-6, the proliferation of the tubular epithelium at the free end results in its maximum expansion. This occurs in such a way as to produce an indented flattened vesicle, known as a glomerular capsule. As seen in section, it has an arched floor-plate several cells thick and a thin, single-layered roof membrane. The two are continuous with each other but are very different in their potentialities. The roof membrane becomes attenuated as an impermeable membrane. The floor-plate continues active proliferation and many of its cells were believed by Streeter to delaminate and apparently become angioblasts, participating in the formation of the vascular glomerulus and its supporting tissues. It is now maintained, however, that the glomerular capillaries (in the metanephros) come from adjacent vessels and never develop *in situ* from epithelial cells (Potter, 1965). Further details of renal development have been provided by several authors (e.g., Potter, 1972).

The residual cells facing the capsular lumen in the mesonephros at stage 14 are reduced in the more advanced phases to a single layer, covering and conforming everywhere to the lobulations of the underlying capillary tufts.

Angiogenesis around the secretory part of the tubule is not far advanced. Angiogenic strands connect with the caudal cardinal vein, and throughout the mesonephros there are isolated clumps of angioblasts, particularly around the capsules. In figure 14-7F, G is shown a continuous row of six mesonephric tubules, covered above by coelomic mesothelium and closely adjacent to the caudal cardinal vein below. These show the typical difference in complexity of the three parts of the tubule: (1) collecting duct, (2) secretory segment, and (3) glomerular capsule. In figure 14-7H the same

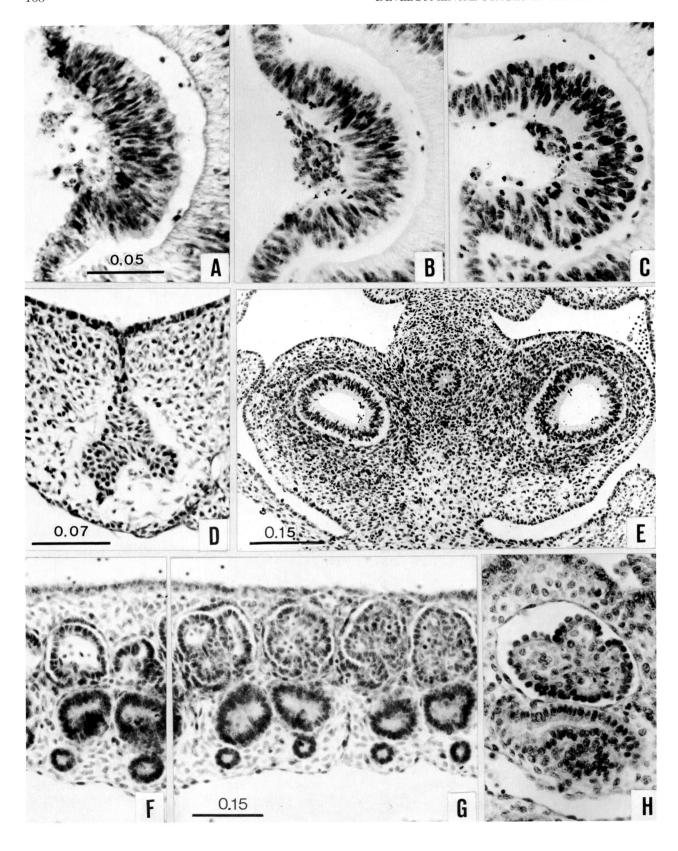

structures are shown in the same plane at a more advanced phase, at the transition into stage 15.

REPRODUCTIVE SYSTEM

The primordial germ cells migrate from the mesentery to the gonadal ridges (Witschi, 1948). Each gonadal ridge appears as a mesodermal proliferation along the medial surface of the mesonephros (Witschi, 1948; Jirásek, 1971).

NERVOUS SYSTEM

Median-plane views of three brains typical of stage 14 are shown in figure 14-8. The constancy in the detailed form of these brains is a striking illustration of the undeviating character of the process of organogenesis. All of them are definitely larger than the brains found in the preceding stage. When the representatives of the two groups are measured, it is found that the dimensions of the brain at stage 14 are about 50 percent larger than those at stage 13.

In the spinal region, the neural tube presents little variation in form from level to level, which is what one would expect from its uniformity in the mature individual. In the present stage the wall of the spinal cord is composed of three distinct zones: (1) the ventricular or ependymal zone, which contains the germinal cells from which neurons, glial cells, and ependymal cells will be derived, (2) the mantle or intermediate zone, in which characteristic clusters of precocious neurons give origin to the ventral rootlets, which thread their way ventrolaterally, and (3) the marginal zone, an expanding cell-free territory. This differentiation is more advanced in the motor or ventral half of the cord than in the dorsal half, and it is more advanced in the cervical region than in the more recently laid down caudal end. The dorsal funiculus develops in the cervical area and reaches C2.

The roots of the hypoglossal nerve have united. The cerebellar primordium is present now as a thickening of the alar plate in rhombomere 1. It consists of ventricular and intermediate layers, but does not possess a marginal layer. The sulcus limitans proceeds from the rhombencephalon throughout the mesencephalon. In the midbrain two parts can still be distinguished; the marginal layer covers three-quarters of the surface, the tectal area being the least developed. Cranial nerve 3 is present in all embryos. In the diencephalon the distinction between D1 and D2 is no longer possible. Between dorsal and ventral thalami a sulcus begins to form; it seems to be the beginning of the sulcus medius. The chiasmatic plate thickens and hence is distinct in the median plane. The preoptic sulcus (optic groove of Streeter) rostral to the optic stalk runs from the floor of one optic evagination to that of the other. The future medial striatal ridge, a part of the subthalamus, begins to form. The primordia of the corpora striata of the two sides are connected by the commissural plate. The olfactory areas also merge in this striatal field.

In the telencephalon the future hemispheres begin to be marked off by an internal crest: the velum transversum. In the median plane the telencephalon medium can be distinguished from the diencephalic roof by its thinner wall. The terminal-vomeronasal crest begins to make contact with the brain and clearly indicates the olfactory area.

Sections selected at intervals through the midbrain and forebrain are shown in figure 14-8, sections *A–E*. The levels at which they are taken are indicated by

Fig. 14-7 (facing page). A–C are all of the same enlargement. The lens in three selected embryos (No. 7394, No. 6503, No. 6502), showing the extrusion of "unwanted cells" by the lens ectoderm and their subsequent degeneration into a clump within the lens pit. (D) Thyroid primordium, showing its stalk of origin from the floor of the pharynx. The open-meshed reticulum surrounding it is characteristic. The endothelium-lined space below is the aortic sac, to which the thyroid is closely related. No. 7333, section 4-3-7. (E) Section through the pulmonary region, showing the primary bronchi surrounded by a vascularized mesenchymal zone and mesothelium (pleura). The pulmonary mesenchyme still abuts against that of the alimentary canal. No. 6502, section 21-4-1. F–H are at the same enlargement. (F,G) Six mesonephric tubules, the most caudal being on the left. They are covered above by coelomic mesothelium, and below them is the caudal cardinal vein. Differences in complexity are evident in the glomerular capsule, secretory segment, and collecting duct. No. 6500, section 1-5-7. (H) A more advanced mesonephric tubule at stage 15, for comparison. No. 7870, section 9-2-7.

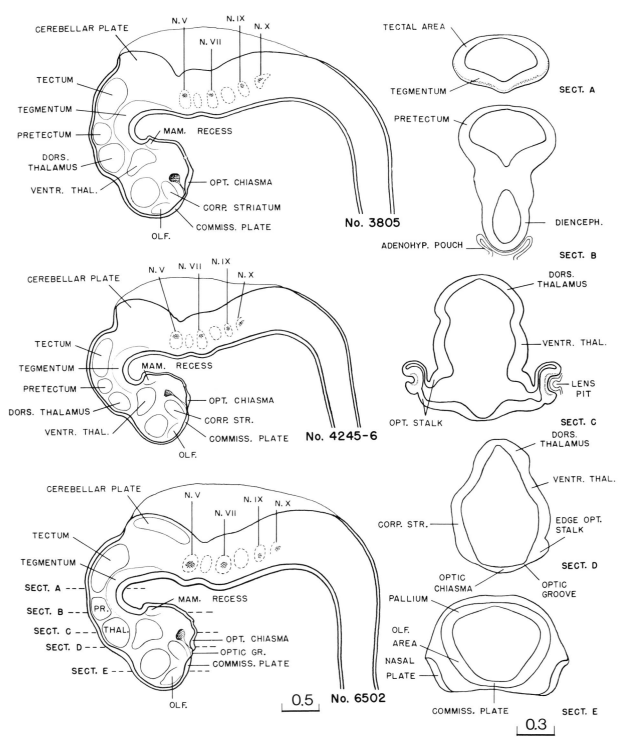

Fig. 14-8. Three brains typical of stage 14, enlarged to the same scale, showing various neural areas according to current interpretation. The pontine flexure is visible. No. 3805, No. 4245-6, and No. 6502. Based on Born reconstructions made by Osborne O. Heard. At the right are five selected sections of No. 6502, taken at the levels indicated by the interrupted lines.

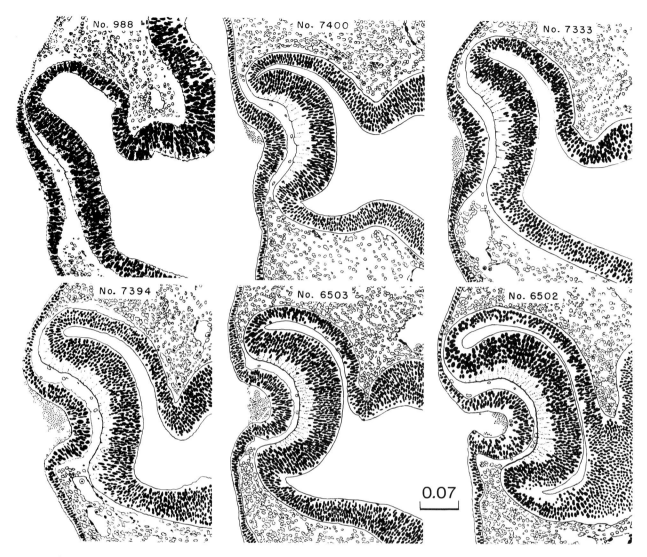

Fig. 14-9. Sections of the eye selected as typical of stage 14, arranged in order of the indentation of the lens disc. Discarded material within the lens pit is shown also in figure 14-7A–C. All drawings are enlarged to the same scale.

dotted lines on the drawing of the third brain. In these sections it can be seen how the various areas at this time are marked off from one another by ridges or grooves. The thickness of the wall may be misleading if the section is partially tangential. Thus one can identify functional areas by the contours of the wall long before the component cells have acquired individualities in form. Section C is a particularly good example of well-defined territories, such as can be seen in carefully preserved specimens.

The three brains of embryos belonging to this stage,

illustrated in figure 14-8, show a convincing uniformity in the outlines of their respective functional areas. Each area has its own individual site, size, and form.

To summarize the main subdivisions of the brain, it has been seen that (1) the prosencephalon, mesencephalon, and rhombencephalon can be distinguished as regions in the completely open neural folds at stage 9, (2) the diencephalon and the telencephalon medium can be detected in stage 10, and (3) the future hemispheres and the cerebellar plates appear by stage 14.

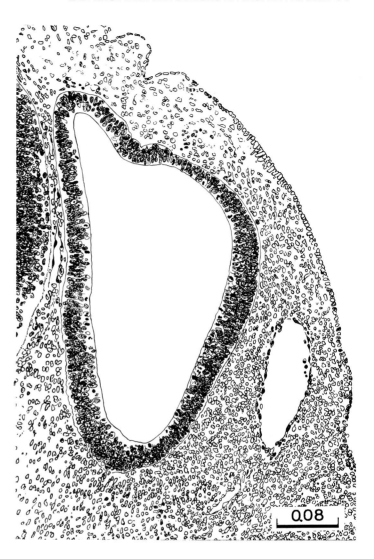

Fig. 14-10. The otocyst at stage 14. The endo-lymphatic appendage is tapered and well defined. Active proliferation in various areas of the vesicular wall presage special parts of the membranous lab-yrinth. The ventral part of the otic vesicle is the primordium of the cochlear duct. No. 6503, section 6-4-7.

The pons of the postnatal brain, in the sense of the apparent bridge shown by Eustachius and Varolius in the 16th century, appears early in the fetal period but does not possess a counterpart during the embryonic period proper. The pontine region, however, can be distinguished very early by the attachment of the appropriate cranial nerves (7/8 at stage 10, 5 at stage 11, and 6 at stage 15) and in relation to the summit of the pontine flexure (by about stage 16). The pontine flexure appears gradually during stages 14–16 but its initial appearance is not readily visible in lateral views.

The spinal nerves are now attached to the muscular primordia, and rami communicantes are present (Bossy, 1980c).

The innervation of the upper limb buds begins at stage 14, that of the lower limb buds at stage 15. The cutaneous innervation follows the external form but is one or two stages behind (Bossy, 1982). Diagrams purporting to show the dermatomes during the embryonic period are, at least in the present stage of knowledge, figments of the imagination.

Eye
(fig. 14-9)

In stage 14 the lens disc shows various degrees of indentation, and in the more advanced members of the group it is cup-shaped, communicating with the surface by a narrowing pore. There may be a slight variation between the right and left vesicles, but as long as one of them is definitely open to the surface of the embryo, the specimen is included in this stage. The final closure and pinching off occur subsequently.

Sections of the eye, typical of stage 14 and arranged in order of the indentation of the lens ectoderm, are shown in figure 14-9. It will be seen that the lens closely follows the retina in the rate of invagination, and as it does this it becomes partly enclosed by the latter. A significant and constant accompaniment of lens development is the accumulation of a clump of disintegrating cell remnants in the lumen of the lens pit. Photographs of this material are shown in figure 14-7A–C. From an examination of these and the serial sections themselves one concludes that they are nuclear remnants extruded by the lens ectoderm. The latter is in a state of active cell division, and many of the daughter nuclei can be seen migrating or perhaps being crowded to the surface. Different stages in the emergence of these "unwanted nuclei" and their aggregation in free clumps in the lens depression can be recognized.

A uveocapillary lamina becomes defined. As the retinal disc is invaginated to form the optic cup, the retinal ("choroid") fissure is delineated. The inverted layer of the optic cup comprises a terminal bar net (the future external limiting membrane), proliferative zone (the mitotic phase), primitive zone (the intermitotic phase), marginal zone, and an internal limiting membrane (O'Rahilly, 1966). The developing cerebral stratum of the retina is closely comparable to the developing cerebral wall (*ibid.*, fig. 8).

Ear

Aside from becoming about one-fourth larger and showing an increased delineation and tapering of its endolymphatic appendage, there are no striking characteristics in the otic vesicle at this stage that are not already present in the more advanced members of the preceding group. If, however, three-dimensional reconstructions are made of them, it is seen that the oval vesicle of stage 13 has become elongated by the ventral growth of the primordium of the cochlear duct. One can also recognize the beginning differential thickening of the walls of the vesicle, the thicker areas marking the location of what are to be the definitive parts of the labyrinth. A section typical of this stage is shown in figure 14-10. It can be compared directly with those illustrated in figure 13-12.

Proliferation of mesodermal cells indicates the beginning of the condensation that precedes the cartilaginous otic capsule, which will enclose the otic vesicle.

Specimens of Stage 14 Already Described

H. Braus, 6-mm embryo, Heidelberg. Enlarged views of this well-preserved curettage specimen are included in the Hochstetter (1907) portfolio of pictures of the outer form of a series of human embryos. The nasal plate is more advanced than in others of this stage, but the limb buds are like those of the older members of the group.

E. Gasser, 6.5-mm. Leyding embryo, Marburg Anatomisches Institut. Description of this advanced embryo is in the Keibel and Elze *Normentafeln* (1908).

J. A. Hammar, 5-mm Vestberg embryo, Anatomisches Institut, Uppsala. Embryo described by Hammar in the Keibel and Elze *Normentafeln*. Typical sections and models of the pharyngeal region and gut are illustrated. This well-preserved embryo has been studied by several investigators, including Hammar on the development of the foregut, salivary glands, and tongue, and Broman on the development of the diaphragm and omental bursa.

His, embryo R, 5.5 mm. Illustrated by His (1885). It was concluded by His that this embryo approximated the Fol embryo (stage 13). The lens pit indicates stage 14. This assignment is supported by other features: e.g., the ductus venosus.

His, embryo B, 7 mm, and embryo A, 7.5 mm. These two embryos are described jointly, in great detail, by His (1880). Embryo A is evidently a little more advanced than embryo B and perhaps should be placed in stage 15.

Keibel, 6.5-mm embryo "forensis." Embryo described in the Keibel and Elze *Normentafeln*. This embryo was used by Keibel in a series of studies on the development of the urogenital system.

Keibel, 6.8-mm embryo, No. 501. Embryo included in the Keibel and Elze *Normentafeln*. It is described in monographic form by Piper (1900).

Strahl, 6.75-mm embryo (Walther), Giessen. Described in the Keibel and Elze *Normentafeln*. The external form is pictured by Hirschland (1898).

6.5-mm embryo, University of Minnesota. Drawings of external views of this and of a 2.9-mm (stage 11) embryo were published by Wells and Kaiser (1959).

Free Hospital for Women, Brookline, Massachusetts, No. 33, 6 mm, No. 29, 7 mm, and No. 31, 7 mm. The histochemistry of these embryos of stage 14 was studied by McKay *et al.* (1956).

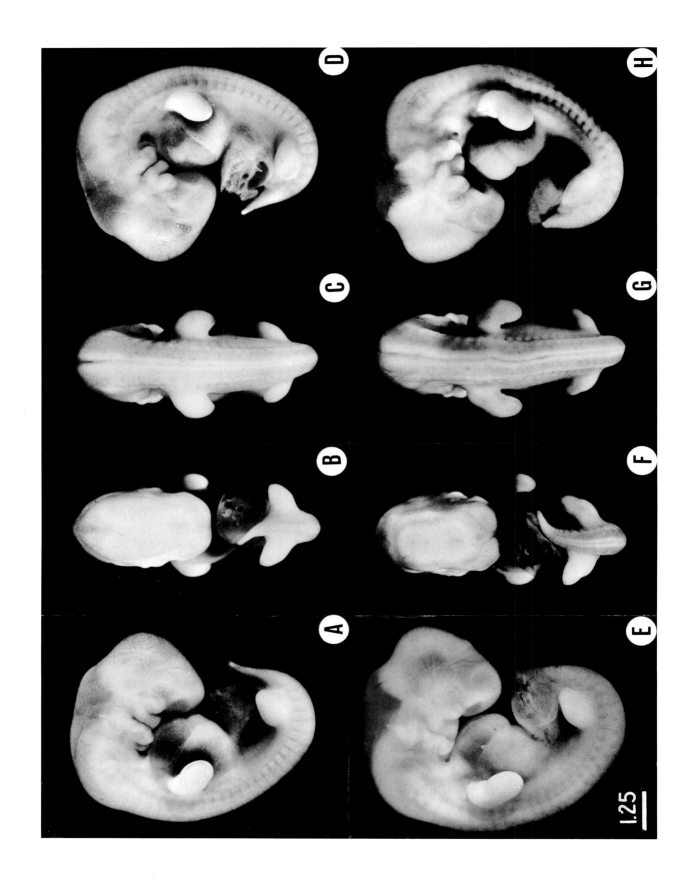

1.25

STAGE 15

Approximately 7–9 mm

Approximately 33 postovulatory days

SUMMARY

External: lens vesicles are closed; nasal pits are appearing; hand plates are forming.

Internal: foramen secundum begins to develop in the heart; a definite intestinal loop and caecum are present; lobar buds appear in the bronchial tree; the pelvis of the ureter develops, and the primary urogenital sinus forms; the future cerebral hemispheres are better delineated, the future paleostriatum and neostriatum become distinguishable, and the primordium of the epiphysis cerebri becomes recognizable; retinal pigment appears.

SIZE AND AGE

Approximately 80 percent of the embryos after fixation range from 6.5 to 8.5 mm. This range may be taken as the expected length at this stage, and many of these embryos are from 7 to 8 mm. A few, however, are smaller (6 mm) or larger (11 mm).

The size of the chorion is even more variable. Its greatest diameter is generally 30–40 mm.

The age of the embryos of stage 15 is believed to be approximately 33 postovulatory days (Olivier and Pineau, 1962) but may extend to 38 days (Jirásek, 1971). One specimen with known coital history was 36½ days in age (Windle, 1970).

EXTERNAL FORM
(figs. 15-1 to 15-3, and 16-4)

Up to this time the central nervous system appears to have played the principal role in determining the contours of the head and trunk of the embryo. Other details in its form are provided by the heart, the limb buds, and the condensed masses that are to form the mandibular and hyoid regions (the pharyngeal arches). As in stage 14, the embryo resulting from these influences is bilaterally flattened, having a curved or partially spiral axis. In the embryos of stage 15, the relative width of the trunk region (fig. 15-1) has become greater because of growth of the spinal ganglia, the muscular plates, and the mesenchymal tissues associated with them, all of which add to the bulk of the trunk. Thus when viewed from the back, embryos of this stage appear wider from side to side than those of stage 14. This increase in relative width of the trunk becomes still greater in the succeeding groups. The result is that

Fig. 15-1 (facing page). Four views of each of two embryos illustrate the respective characteristics of less-advanced and more-advanced members of stage 15. In the first specimen the hand plate is marked off from the rest of the limb, and the distinction is more pronounced in the second embryo. When filled with blood the marginal vein can be seen. The lower limb bud is larger and rounded opposite the lumbar levels, and more tapering opposite the sacral levels. The tip of the latter will form the foot (E,F). The muscular plates and the ganglia can be seen distinctly from the occipital region to the caudal end of the body. The head region shows the most-advanced characters. The nasal plate, a shallow depression, is visible in profile view. A subdivision of the maxillary growth center forms the lateral border of the nasomaxillary groove. In all the profile views shown here, the trigeminal nerve and its divisions can be discerned. On the mandibular arch, one can distinguish the auricular hillocks that are to form the crus and tragus of the external ear. The hyoid arch with its three hillocks is large and partly crowds over onto the third pharyngeal arch. The latter can be seen in H with a depression caudal to it, known as the cervical sinus. The swelling closing around this is the primordium of cervical muscles and associated tissues that are to spread downward over the heart, making the thoracic wall. At this time most of the brain is very thinly covered. In E and H the form of the otic vesicle can be seen. Most of the photographs in this study were taken by Reather. A–D, No. 3441. E–H, No. 3512. All photographs are enlarged to the same scale.

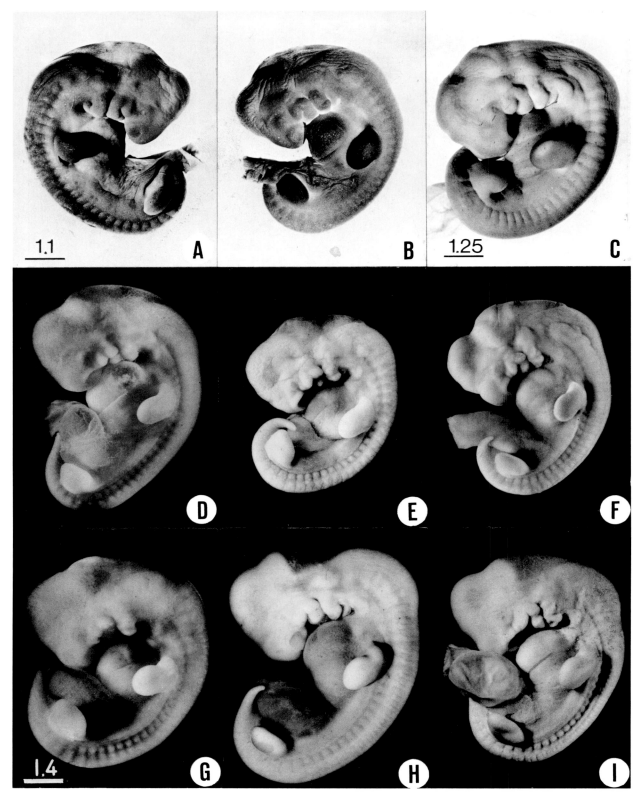

Fig. 15-2. All the embryos shown here have the essential morphological characteristics of stage 15. The variations are caused by differences in fixation, shrinkage, and original condition of the specimens. The embryos shown in the upper row (A–C) were stained in alum cochineal to portray the surface markings better. The form of the limb buds is one of the most constant characteristics, but it may be misleading because of illumination. (A) No. 3216. (B) No. 3216. (C) No. 810. (D) No. 6595. (E) No. 3953. (F) No. 5892. (G) No. 7199. (H) No. 3385. (I) No. 6506. C–F, H, and I are at the same enlargement, and so are A and B.

the greatest transverse diameter, which originally is in the dorsoventral axis, eventually coincides with the side-to-side width of the embryo. In stages 15–18 this increase in relative width of the trunk is rapid enough to serve as one of the criteria for determining the developmental status attained by a given embryo. Allowance must be made, however, for the fact that the occipitocervical region is more advanced and is consequently wider than the lumbosacral because of the rostrocaudal gradient in growth. New factors greatly complicate the picture in more-advanced stages, where special modifications occur in the relative diameters of the trunk in its different regions and where its width varies correspondingly.

Five characteristics are present in stage 15. (1) The lens vesicles have closed, and on each side the pores by which the vesicles had communicated with the surface have disappeared. (2) The nasal discs, because of the relatively greater growth of the surrounding tissues, begin to recede from the surface, acquiring the form of large oval depressions (i.e., the nasal pits). In the less advanced members a low ridge marks the frontal and lateral borders of the depression. In the more advanced members this ridge has become a slightly overhanging lip. It is this rapidly growing ridge that will subsequently form the nostril on its side of the head. (3) Before this period the hyoid arch has already been differentiated into a dorsal and a ventral segment, but now its ventral segment acquires a subsegment, or ventralmost segment, which is the primordium of the antitragus. (4) The active transformations occurring in the upper limb buds contribute to the precision with which embryos can be identified as belonging, or not belonging, in stage 15. In stage 14 one could speak of an elongating upper limb bud. In stage 15, as shown in figures 15-1 and 15-2, one can recognize the developmental steps by which the upper limb bud becomes regionally subdivided into a distal hand plate and a proximal forearm, arm, and shoulder region. The less precocious lower limb bud exhibits a beginning differentiation into a rounded rostral half and a more tapering caudal half (fig. 16-4). It is the tip of the latter that will form the foot. (5) As in less-advanced embryos, in all the members of this group the muscular plates, somites, and underlying spinal ganglia produce characteristic elevations which can be seen sufficiently well for fairly accurate counting, through-

out the length of the cord, from the occipital region to the coccygeal levels. In transparent specimens they appear as white opaque condensations. In subsequent stages, the ganglia and somites will become covered over with mesenchymal tissues so that they can no longer be seen from the surface. This occurs first in the occipitospinal region, whence it spreads caudalward.

The developing facial region at three successive stages is shown in figure 15-3. The mandibular processes are more prominent than the maxillary. In stage 13 the nasal discs consist merely of areas of thickened surface ectoderm. In stage 14 the nasal disc has undergone active cellular proliferation, with the result that it is larger and thicker. It has also acquired a shallow central depression and its margins are elevated. In stage 15 a nasal pit is produced, and a dorsolateral lip known as the lateral nasal process develops. The two nasal pits are relatively wide apart at the outset.

The lateral and caudal portions of the mandibular arch contribute to the formation of the external ear, shown by stippling in the figure.

CARDIOVASCULAR SYSTEM
(figs. 15-4, 15-5, and 16-7)

The vascular system is highly adaptable. Streeter was impressed by the circumstance that the venous drainage of the enlarging brain undergoes a continuous series of modifications, and that many of the constituent channels of a blood pattern have ephemeral importance. On the other hand, some of them persist as adult vessels with only minor modifications. During this same time, however, the heart itself undergoes marked alterations, changing from a relatively simple bulbous pump to a two-current pump with valves. These changes are sufficiently marked to be detected between successive stages in ordinary serial sections. Thus the structure of the heart can be included with advantage in listing the syndromic features that characterize developmental stages.

In earlier stages (compare figs. 11-7, 12-6, 12-7, 13-3, and 13-4) the origin of the venous end of the heart (i.e., the sinus venosus and atria) has been traced from specialized parts of the vitelline plexus which form a vascular saddle astride the neck of the umbilical vesicle. From the very outset the arterial part of the heart, the part from which the ventricles are derived, is clearly demarcated from the venous part coming from the vitelline plexus. This is shown in figure 12-7. The arterial part of the heart is further illustrated in figure 15-4. Comparison of the four levels shown in the latter figure reveals that throughout that period one can speak of an arterial part that starts abruptly at the atrioventricular junction and curves rostrally to terminate in the aortic sac. The cardiac jelly is found mostly in the arterial part and fills the myo-endocardial interval. This layer appears to act as a closure cushion that facilitates the emptying of the tube and at the same time checks regurgitation from the aortic sac, biding the time when specialized cardiac valves will become established. In arriving at more-advanced stages the cardiac jelly acquires more cells, and one can then speak of it as a gelatinous reticulum or cardiac mesenchyme. In more-condensed form this may become converted into the

semilunar valves, and it finally disappears in the formation of the atrioventricular valves and the membranous part of the interventricular septum.

At stage 15 the distribution of the thick layer of cardiac mesenchyme can be seen in typical sections selected from a sagittal series shown in figure 15-4. It still exists as a continuous sleeve around the arterial part of the tube, beginning at the atrioventricular canal and stopping before reaching the aortic sac. In figure 15-5, this part of the tube is shown at four levels of development. These drawings were made from three-dimensional reconstructions of the endocardial surfaces and therefore correspond to casts of the cavities of the heart. The form of the atria is largely influenced by the state of their contraction and consequent distention by the contained blood. The variation in the arterial part is less marked, and, with the gelatinous reticulum removed, its form is fairly constant for each

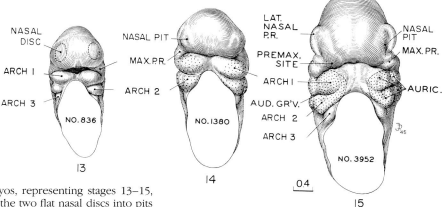

Fig. 15-3. These three embryos, representing stages 13–15, illustrate the transformation of the two flat nasal discs into pits from which the nasal passages will be derived. (Cf. figs. 16-5, 17-3, and 18-3.) Together, the three form a series illustrating the morphogenesis of the face. The prominent lateral border of the nasal pit in stage 15 (No. 3952) is the primordium of the nasal wing and has usually been designated as the lateral nasal process. The medial border of the pit is less prominent, but out of deference to its lateral associate is commonly spoken of as the medial nasal process. It is to be noted, however, that if the premaxillary center is not included with it, it plays but the small role of becoming the medial rim of the nostril. The mandibular arches are uniting to form a lower jaw. The upper jaw is less precocious and is represented only by the widely separate right and left maxillary centers. One can see, however, where the premaxillary centers will form. The nerve trunks of the mandibular division of the trigeminal nerve appear to the casual glance more advanced than those of the maxillary division, and thus are associated with the precocity of the lower jaw. Drawings made by James F. Didusch from reconstructions made by Osborne O. Heard. All drawings are enlarged to the same scale.

developmental level. In passing from stage 13 to stage 15 it becomes relatively more voluminous, and its distended parts mark what are becoming the aortic and pulmonary channels.

A major feature of the heart at stage 15 is that the flow of blood through the atrioventricular canal is already divided into left and right streams (de Vries and Saunders, 1962), and continues as separate streams through the outflow tract and aortic sac (McBride, Moore, and Hutchins, 1981).

The aorticopulmonary septum, a controversial feature, is regarded by Los (1978) as "an artifact of two-dimensional histology" and merely a section through the condensed mesenchyme that forms the dorsal wall of the aortic sac.

Foramen secundum appears in septum primum from stage 15 to stage 17, and the semilunar cusps appear at the same time (McBride, Moore, and Hutchins, 1981). The level of the semilunar valves (at the dorsal bend of the outflow tract, according to de Vries and Saunders, 1962) has been disputed by some workers. The semilunar valves are said to be derived from the truncal ridges (Los, 1978) or cushions (Pexieder, 1982).

The trabeculated parts of the ventricles show endocardial diverticula along the peripheral edge of the cardiac tube. These diverticula interlock with corresponding slender trabeculae from the overlying myocardium, as was illustrated in figures 13-6 and 13-7B, D. Thus in these two areas, instead of having a thick covering of gelatinous reticulum, the cardiac tube extends peripherally in the form of two trabeculated side-pouches which are the primordia of the right and left ventricles. These side pouches can be recognized as early as stage 11 while the cardiac tube is a simple

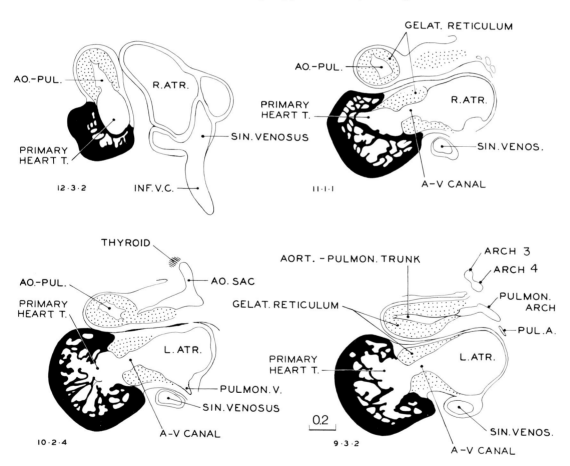

Fig. 15-4. Selected sagittal sections through heart of No. 6504. This figure illustrates that the heart is composed of three tissue types: the venous type of the atria, the gelatino-reticular type of the primary cardiac tube, and the highly specialized muscular ventricles, opening out of the primary tube.

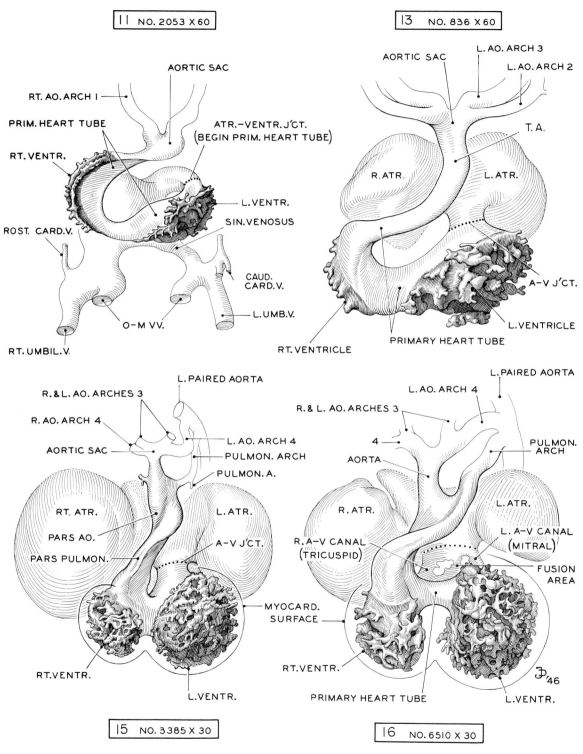

11 NO. 2053 X 60

AORTIC SAC

RT. AO. ARCH I

PRIM. HEART TUBE

RT. VENTR.

ATR.–VENTR. J'CT.
(BEGIN PRIM. HEART TUBE)

ROST. CARD.V.

L. VENTR.

SIN. VENOSUS

CAUD.
CARD. V.

O–M VV.

L. UMB. V.

RT. UMBIL. V.

13 NO. 836 X 60

AORTIC SAC

L. AO. ARCH 3

L. AO. ARCH 2

T. A.

R. ATR.

L. ATR.

A–V J'CT.

L. VENTRICLE

RT. VENTRICLE

PRIMARY HEART TUBE

15 NO. 3385 X 30

L. PAIRED AORTA

R. & L. AO. ARCHES 3

R. AO. ARCH 4

AORTIC SAC

L. AO. ARCH 4

PULMON. ARCH

PULMON. A.

RT. ATR.

L. ATR.

PARS AO.

A–V J'CT.

PARS PULMON.

MYOCARD.
SURFACE

RT. VENTR.

L. VENTR.

16 NO. 6510 X 30

L. PAIRED AORTA

L. AO. ARCH 4

R. & L. AO. ARCHES 3

4

AORTA

PULMON.
ARCH

R. ATR.

L. ATR.

R. A–V CANAL
(TRICUSPID)

L. A–V CANAL
(MITRAL)

FUSION
AREA

MYOCARD.
SURFACE

RT. VENTR.

PRIMARY HEART TUBE

L. VENTR.

Fig. 15-5. Reconstructions illustrating the primary cardiac tube, as distinct from the atrial parts. Only the endocardium is shown. The latter opens out as two trabeculated sacs in two areas, the right and left ventricles. Here the cardiac mesenchyme (gelatinous reticulum) is replaced by processes from the myocardium which interdigitate with the reticulated endocardium. As the ventricular sacs form, the tube becomes distended and gradually divided into two channels in a manner indicating separate blood currents, in accommodation to the functioning of the right and left ventricles. Drawings made by James F. Didusch and reconstructions made by Osborne O. Heard.

channel. Contractions of the right ventricular sac would result in a current directed along the pulmonary border of the cardiac tube, whereas the left ventricular sac would favor a cross current toward the aortic border of the tube. It therefore seems possible that these two ventricular sacs may be factors in producing respectively the pulmonary and aortic currents.

Other features of the heart at stage 15 are that the left ventricle is more voluminous and thicker-walled than the right (de Vries and Saunders, 1962). The lumen of the outflow tract is H-shaped. The atrioventricular cushions are apposed. The atrioventricular bundle has been detected (Mall, 1912).

DIGESTIVE SYSTEM
(figs. 15-7 and 15-8)

The thyroid primordium may be detached from the pharyngeal epithelium in some instances. The gland rests near the rostral border of the aortic sac.

The esophagus is longer and is straddled in front by the primary bronchi (fig. 15-8). From one stage to the next the intestine appears to become more slender. At least, the epithelial tube becomes steadily longer relative to its diameter.

The elongation of the ileum has produced a definite intestinal loop, which is more marked than the slight

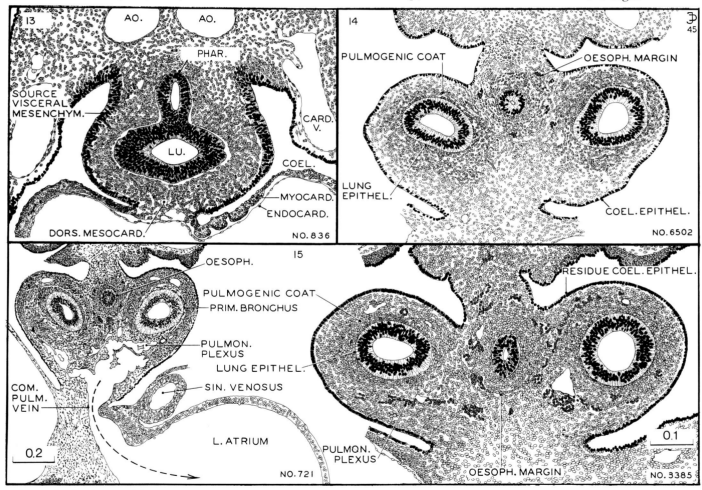

Fig. 15-6. The degree of differentiation of the mesenchymal tissues of the pulmonary and esophageal regions characteristic of stages 13–15. In the least advanced (stage 13) one can still see migrant cells from the proliferating coelomic epithelium. In stage 14 the coelomic epithelium has virtually ceased its proliferative activity and the mesenchyme is arranging itself in zones. Angioblasts are forming a net that outlines the esophagus; a photograph of this section is shown in fig. 14-7E. In stage 15 angiogenesis is taking place around the primary bronchi. Large meshes of the pulmonary plexus communicate with the common pulmonary vein, and through it the blood reaches the floor of the left atrium. This is shown in embryo No. 721 of stage 15. The other three sections are drawn to the same scale. All drawings made by James F. Didusch.

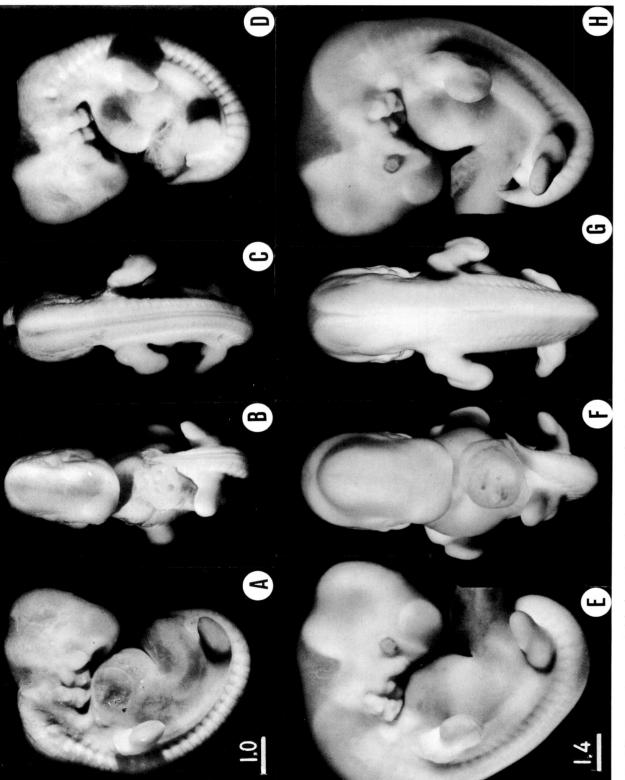

Fig. 16-2. Two embryos: one of the least advanced and one of the most advanced members of stage 16. The differences are exaggerated by the fact that the first specimen was fixed in formalin and then became shrunken. The examples illustrate the uncertainty of depending entirely on external form for alignment of embryos in their developmental order. Both specimens qualify for this stage on the basis of their internal structure. A and C show shrinkage and sinking in of the roof of the fourth ventricle. The distinctness of the ganglionic and somitic masses is also an effect of the shrinkage. The auricular hillocks and the limb buds are found to provide the most reliable of the surface characteristics for this period of development. (A–D) No. 6054. (E–H) No. 8112.

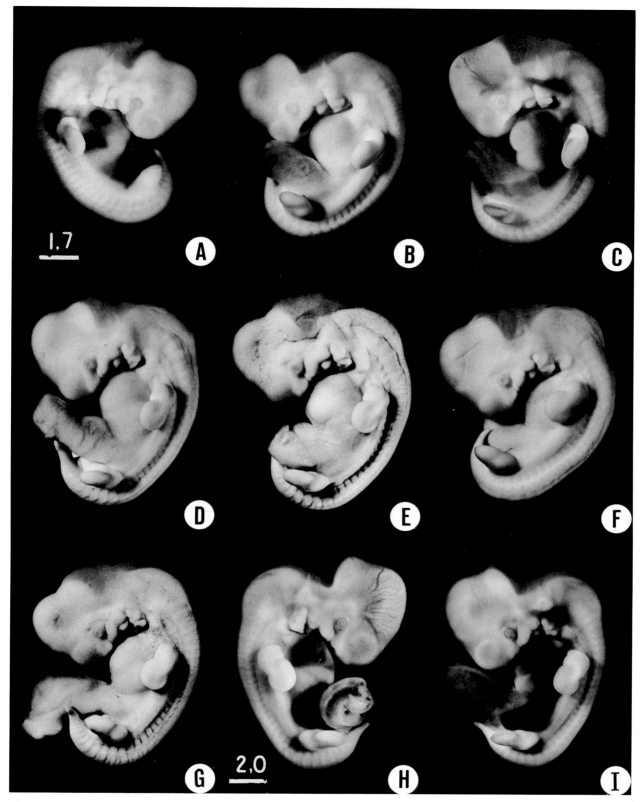

Fig. 16-3. These embryos have been sectioned serially and in their microscopic structure qualify as members of stage 16. The differences between them are for the most part accounted for by the factors of fixation, shrinkage, manner of illumination, and original condition of the specimen. The otic vesicle, where it can be seen, the auricular hillocks, the lateral nasal wing, the disappearing third pharyngeal arch, the distinct hand plate, and the rounded foot plate with its early marginal vein are characteristics common to all these specimens. (A) No. 6750. (B) No. 7115. (C) No. 7804. (D) No. 6517. (E) No. 6511. (F) No. 6510. (G) No. 6514. (H) No. 8179. (I) No. 7629. A–G are at the same magnification, H and I are slightly less.

active proliferation and supply the visceral mesenchyme that gives origin to the vascularized muscular and connective-tissue coats of the viscera, whereas the residual surface cells become permanent serous membranes and serve as the pericardium, pleura, and peritoneum. These mesenchymal components, of primitive-streak ancestry, can be followed without much difficulty.

Especially in the head region, other mesenchymal cells are known (chiefly from experiments on the chick) to be derived from the neural crest. A third source, the prechordal plate, furnishes cells for the muscles

of the orbit (Gilbert, 1957) and probably for the meninges (O'Rahilly and Müller, 1986b).

Another characteristic of head mesenchyme is the prevalence of greater thickness of the skin ectoderm over its more condensed areas, suggesting increased functional activity. This is notable in the ventral parts of the head, particularly the mandibular and hyoid regions. The thick areas are part of the ectodermal ring (O'Rahilly and Müller, 1985). Such areas stand out in contrast with the loose reticular mesenchyme found over the dorsal parts of the head, where the skin ectoderm is thin, apparently merely adapting itself to the

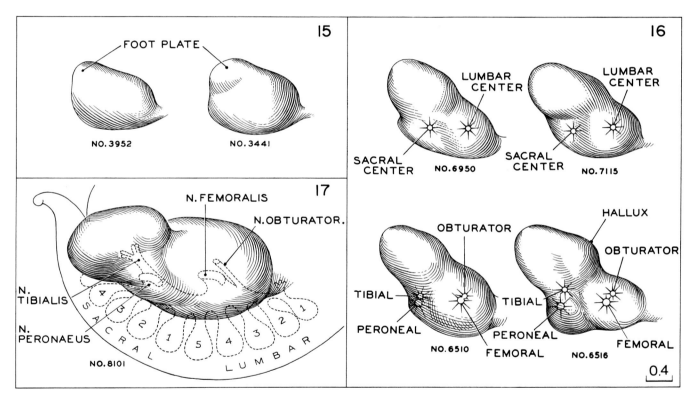

Fig. 16-4. Differentiation of the lower limb bud at stages 15–17. At stage 17 the primary divisions of the limb are clearly indicated by the nerve trunks, which branch in a characteristic pattern from the lumbosacral plexus. The femoral and obturator trunks lead to the thigh and, together with the condensed center surrounding them, are responsible for the bulging mass on the proximal part of the limb bud. Coincidently with the breaking apart of this mass into subcenters (muscles), the femoral and obturator trunks split into their respective branches. The trunks from the sacral plexus form the central core of the condensed mass of the caudal half of the limb bud; one trunk (N. tibialis) reaches distally to the plantar region of the foot plate. Thus the tibial and peroneal trunks delimit the primary parts of the limbs below the knee. This lumbosacral distribution might be expected from the fact that when the lower limb bud is first discernible at stage 13, its caudal half lies opposite the sacral nerve-ganglion masses, whereas its cranial half similarly lies opposite the lumbar ones. In stage 16, one can still identify the thigh and the leg by their neural relationships. The foot plate is already determined, and among the more advanced members of the group one can recognize the region of the hallux. Stage 15 marks the emergence of the foot plate. The stage is represented only by more-advanced members of the group. Among the less advanced members one finds less-discrete elevations of the limb bud.

expanding size of the underlying brain. Thick skin ectoderm (the apical ectodermal ridge) and marked proliferation of the mesenchyme with which it is in contact are likewise characteristic of the limb buds, and are an expression of interaction between the two tissues. The limb buds and the group of mesenchymal ridges that form at the sides of the mouth and pharynx around the termination of the large cranial nerves are the product of the same kind of developmental relation between the skin ectoderm and the underlying blastema, together with whatever the nerves may contribute.

In stage 16, between the thin skin ectoderm and the brain, there is found a sparse amount of loose embryonic connective tissue (the primary meninx) through which passes the network of capillaries and blood vessels supplying the brain wall and cranial nerves. Standing out in contrast are some fields where the mesenchymal cells by active proliferation have produced condensed areas, or detached foci of growth.

They are found in the region of the eye, and surrounding the otic vesicle and the nasal plate. To some extent these condensations influence the surface form of the embryo, as seen in the lateral nasal process or wing.

In the more ventral parts of the head, mesenchymal condensation exhibits relative precocity. One can recognize a rather dense maxillary field that bulges on the surface as a prominent ridge (fig. 16-5, No. 1121). Under the surface this field blends with the adjacent condensations surrounding the nasal pit and eye of the same side. The right and left maxillary fields are, however, still widely separated. Between them is the broad region that is to become the roof of the mouth. The only surface markings of this region are two rounded, low elevations produced by incipient bilateral (premaxillary) condensations constituting the primordia of the primary palate. Apart from these modest representatives, there is lacking any future upper jaw. In many respects the ventral part of the cranium and the floor of the mouth are more advanced than its

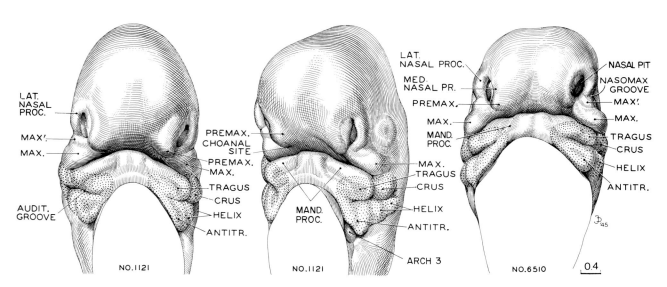

Fig. 16-5. Representative views of the nasal pits and oral region at stage 16. The two views of No. 1121 show a less advanced member of the group, whereas No. 6510 belongs among the more advanced ones. The right and left nasal pits show no evidence yet of uniting to form a nose. The interval between them consists of undifferentiated tissue extending from the roof of the stomodeum "forward" and "upward" over the frontal region of the head. This is sometimes spoken of as the "frontal process," but if that term is to be applied at stage 16 one must be satisfied with an idea rather than with a recognizable structure. The growth centers that are to form the upper jaw are

widely separated, like the nasal pits, and are present only as bilaterally placed masses. These include the premaxillary (globular process of His) and maxillary centers, together with a characteristic subdivision of the latter (marked *MAX'.*). Though one cannot yet speak of an upper jaw, the future lower jaw is definitely marked off and hence has the distinction of being the first part of the facial equipment to become thus established. The auricular hillocks on the mandibular and hyoid arches are given labels with the parts of the external ear that they are to form. Drawings made by James F. Didusch. Reconstructions made by Osborne O. Heard. The drawings are all at the same scale.

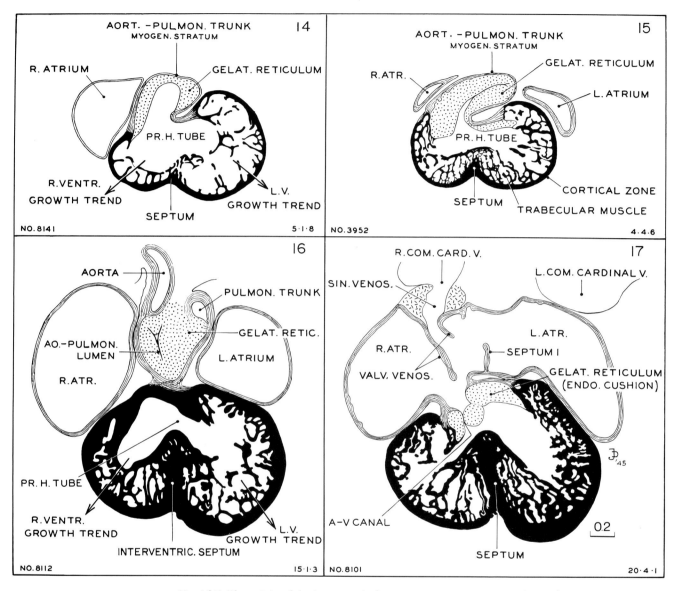

Fig. 16-7. The origin of the interventricular septum, as seen at stages 14–17. The sections of the first three stages are taken from embryos cut coronally and the fourth from one sectioned transversely. This makes them easily comparable. It will be seen that the two ventricles start as separate reticulated pouches, but as they expand their myocardial shells coalesce in the formation of a party wall. The crest of the latter is its oldest part.

caused by displacement of the conus to the left, by reduction of the conoventricular flange, or by conal absorption.

The aortic arches, in ventral view, appear to be more or less symmetrical at stages 11 and 12 but have begun to be asymmetrical at stage 16 and are definitely so from stage 17 onward (Congdon, 1922, figs. 1–16).

DIGESTIVE SYSTEM

The outlines of the epithelial canal for stages 15–17 (figs. 15-8, 16-8, and 17-8) were made for direct comparison of such features as relative length, diameters, flexures, and general form.

A striking feature of the alimentary epithelium is the

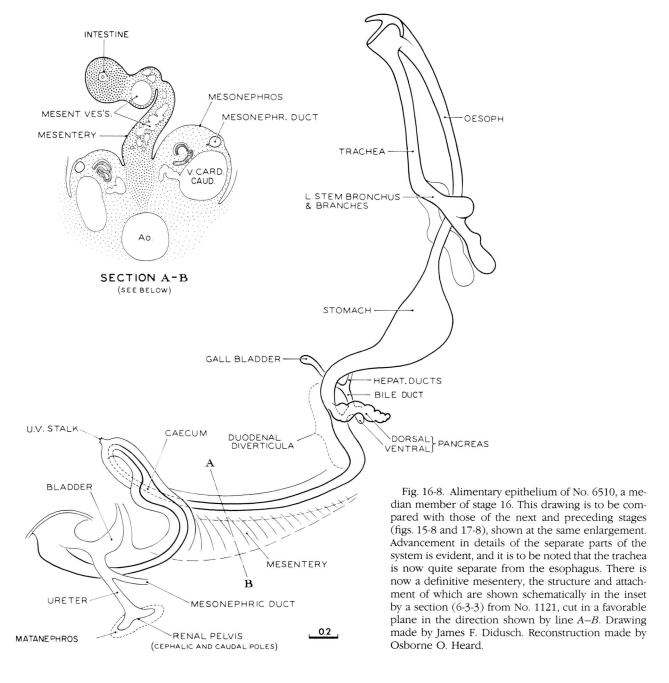

Fig. 16-8. Alimentary epithelium of No. 6510, a median member of stage 16. This drawing is to be compared with those of the next and preceding stages (figs. 15-8 and 17-8), shown at the same enlargement. Advancement in details of the separate parts of the system is evident, and it is to be noted that the trachea is now quite separate from the esophagus. There is now a definitive mesentery, the structure and attachment of which are shown schematically in the inset by a section (6-3-3) from No. 1121, cut in a favorable plane in the direction shown by line A–B. Drawing made by James F. Didusch. Reconstruction made by Osborne O. Heard.

seeming leadership it exhibits in the delineation of the different parts of the system, and this applies also to such offspring as the pulmonary epithelium, biliary passages, and pancreas. These regions, which could be identified earlier, now stand out in advanced detail (fig. 16-8). It is to be noted particularly that one can now speak of a definitive mesentery, beginning near the caudal end of the duodenum and extending caudally to include the rostral half of the colon. It provides the framework for the primary intestinal loop. The section A–B in this figure shows schematically the structure of this mesentery and its terminus in the primordium of the gut wall. The mesenteric vessels are conspicuous. Here as elsewhere, distinct gut epi-

and begins to acquire a slight lumbar flexure, the caus-ative factors for which are to be found in the trans-formations of the inner structures. The caudal termination of the trunk, instead of tapering smoothly as heretofore, now begins to have an abrupt recessive character that will result in the caudal filament of later stages.

A distinct nasofrontal groove is constant in profiles of all specimens of the group. The nasal pit opens ventrally and cannot be seen in full-profile views. To examine the nostril it is necessary to have decapitated specimens or models.

The auricular hillocks exhibit their characteristic form at stage 17. Shown in figures 16-5 and 17-3, they consist of six circumscribed superficial condensations, three (Nos. 1–3) on the mandibular arch and three (Nos. 4–6) on the hyoid arch. The latter are more prominent and are destined to form the auricle of the ear. The three on the caudal surface of the mandibular bar are less sharply outlined. The ventralmost of them be-comes the tragus, and the dorsal two join in the for-mation of the crus helicis. Between these two rows of hillocks the hyomandibular groove increases in width and depth, thereby initiating the formation of the con-cha and the external acoustic meatus. It is common for the hillocks to coalesce at this time and take the form of a key-plate. The opening for the key is en-croached upon by hillocks 2 and 5, and the key slot is thus separated into dorsal and ventral parts, like the numeral 8.

The transformation of this region into the external ear has been described by Streeter (1922), Hochstetter (1948), and Blechschmidt (1965). According to Stree-ter, only minimal and superficial parts of the mandi-bular and hyoid arches participate in the building of the external ear. The importance of the auricular hil-locks has long been in dispute. In spite of their ap-parent independence of other structures, the development of the external ear keeps in step with that of other organs, and one can fairly well determine, from the status of the external ear, the stage to which a given embryo belongs.

The upper limb bud at stage 17 is distinguished from that of the previous stage by the acquisition of finger rays. They are only slightly indicated in the less ad-vanced members of the group, but are clearly demar-cated in all others. The hand plate of the most advanced

members begins to have a crenated rim caused by the projecting tips of the individual digits. This crenation becomes a prominent characteristic at the next stage.

An outline of the lower limb bud at stage 17 is shown in figure 16-4. Apart from having increased in length and general mass, it now has a rounded digital plate, set off from the tarsal region and leg. One can also begin to see, at the junction of the limb bud and trunk, evidence of slower-developing tissue that will even-tually become the muscles and bones of the pelvic girdle.

Turning to the somites, it is found that these do not influence the surface markings except in the lumbar and sacral regions, where they stand out as definite elevations. In less-advanced members of the group they can be seen as far rostrally as mid-thoracic levels. Throughout the cervical and upper thoracic regions, the increase in superficial embryonic connective tissue obscures the spinal ganglia. When embryos are unu-sually translucent the ganglia can be seen even here.

Face

By stage 17 the face has emerged as a consequence of the enlargement and fusion of several growth cen-ters which are generally spoken of as facial processes. As they merge, these produce structures recognizable as the definitive nose and upper jaw. The important steps in this transformation are illustrated in figure 17-3. Ever since the pioneer descriptions of His, they have been designated as facial processes. To call them that, however, has the disadvantage of oversimplification. In reality they are not prolongations having free ends that meet in the nasal region; nor is the ectoderm absorbed over their abutting surfaces. In transverse series of embryos the facial region is likely to be cut coronally (i.e., tangentially), which gives an exagger-ated idea of their length. The alternate sections of the series used by His are now in the Carnegie Collection, catalogued as No. 7317. It is more precise to speak of these structures as swellings or ridges that correspond to centers of growth in the underlying common mes-enchyme. The furrows that lie between them on the surface are smoothed out as the proliferation and fu-sion of the growth centers fill in beneath: i.e., merging occurs rather than fusion (Patten, 1961). Under these

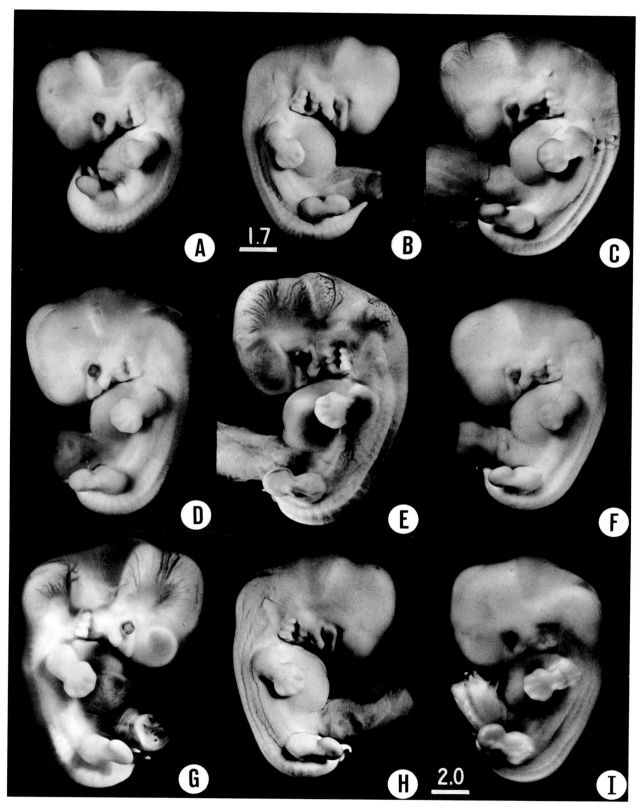

Fig. 17-2. These photographs show the variation in form encountered in stage 17, a two-day period of development. In spite of variations in fixation, shrinkage, and original condition of the embryos, their external characteristics apply fairly well to this whole group: i.e., the presence of the lateral nasal wing, the prominence of the three-hillock plate behind the hyomandibular groove, the disappearance of the third pharyngeal arch, the presence of finger rays of the hand plate, and the absence of toe rays except for the prominence of the great toe. (A) No. 6742. (B) No. 6519. (C) No. 8118. (D) No. 6631. (E) No. 1267A. (F) No. 6521. (G) No. 6258. (H) No. 6520. (I) No. 5893. All are at the same magnification except B, which is slightly greater in magnification.

circumstances no ectoderm requires absorption; it is simply flattened out in adaptation to the changed surface. This is in confirmation of the observations of Peter (1913), who found that the grooves separating the facial processes do not disappear as a result of the fusion of their edges. Instead they become more shallow and eventually smooth, as the increase in mass produces a new surface level. This point is to be kept in mind in analysis of the factors involved in the deformities that accompany harelip.

In the formation of the face certain aspects require emphasis. First, the component growth centers are bilateral, and the right and left groups are originally widely separated from each other. Secondly, these growth centers on each side include (1) a ventromedial extension of the maxillary arch (maxillary process), (2) the ridge, or lip, forming the dorsolateral boundary of the nasal pit, destined to become the nasal wing on that side (lateral nasal process), (3) the rounded medial rim of the nasal pit (medial nasal process), which subsequently in cooperation with its mate and the intervening tissue unites in the formation of the septal elements of the nose, together forming a single median structure, the composite nasal septum, and (4) the growth center at the ventral end of the medial nasal rim, but discrete from it, destined to form the premaxilla (premaxillary center). The last is the globular process of His and is commonly included as part of the medial nasal process. It could equally well be termed the intermaxillary or incisive center. The term frontal process has been applied to the median field lying between and dorsal to the nasal pits. In stage 17 the frontal field is marked by the absence of any condensation, and it is premature to speak of a "process."

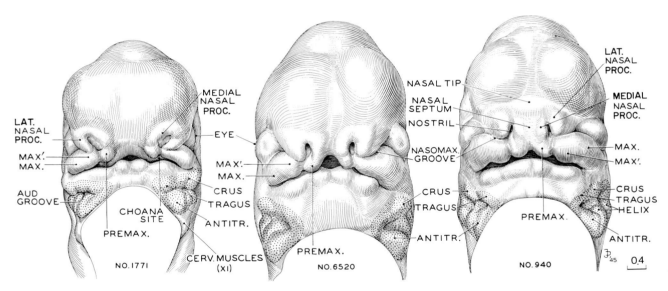

Fig. 17-3. This is the period of the emergence of the nose and future upper jaw. Less-advanced, intermediate, and more-advanced representatives of stage 17 are illustrated. Similar views of the preceding stage are shown in figure 16-5, and the following stage is shown in figure 18-3. All are at the same magnification and hence can be compared directly. One can see the facial parts coming into existence as a consequence of the proliferation of the underlying mesenchymal growth centers. These undergo a coalescence of ridge-like masses, each mass differentiating into the various structures of its own region. Both the overlying epithelium and the precocious trigeminal and facial nerve strands appear to participate with the mesenchyme in the regulation of the form of the developing facial components. The field marked by the presence of the auricular hillocks is stippled, and the hillocks are indicated in accordance with the parts of the external ear derived from them.

AUD. GROOVE, hyomandibular groove. (As it becomes wider and deeper because of the elevation of the surrounding structures, the hyomandibular groove is transformed into the concha and external acoustic meatus.) CERV. MUSCLES, cervical muscle center at tip of accessory nerve. MAX., maxillary growth center. MAX'., supplementary maxillary growth center. MEDIAL NASAL PROC., medial nasal process. NASOMAX. GROOVE, nasomaxillary groove. NASAL SEPTUM, ventral border of septum as it projects between the two nostrils. NASAL TIP, tip of nose, as found in more-advanced members of this stage. (The nose at first is like a raised awning, and it will subsequently come down as its roof forms.) LAT. NASAL PROC., lateral nasal process. PREMAX., premaxillary or incisive center (globular process of His). Drawings made by James F. Didusch. Models made by Osborne O. Heard.

The latter will come considerably later as a part of the building of the elongated dorsum of the nose. Thirdly, the above-mentioned growth centers blend with each other and, in some cases, meet across the median plane. As they do so, they exhibit in each instance the ability to form the various structures and strata required in their particular region, such as lip, alveolar and palatine processes, and finally teeth.

According to Politzer (1936), two more or less parallel furrows are found cranial to the maxillary process. He maintained that the cranial is the nasolacrimal groove whereas, contrary to the usual description, the caudal, in his view, is merely the limiting furrow of the maxillary process (*Grenzfurche des Oberkieferfortsatzes*), or what is generally termed the nasomaxillary groove.

The establishment of the face can be traced in figures 16-5, 17-3, and 18-3. Scanning electron micrographs have been published by Hinrichsen (1985).

Nasal Passages

The transformations of the right and left nasal pits lead to the establishment of bilateral respiratory passages that by-pass the mouth. Already at stage 16 the epithelium of the nasal pit shows evidence of regional specialization. Because of this and the accompanying proliferation of the underlying mesenchyme, one can now recognize the outlines of the wings of the future nose and the median rim of each nostril.

From the edges of the nostril, and sharply demarcated from the abutting skin ectoderm, the nasal epithelium extends deeply into the preoptic region as a flattened pocket, constituting the nasal sac. Along the ventral fold of the latter, the epithelium exhibits a characteristic growth activity. It proliferates in the form of a plate-like fin or keel which maintains an epithelial continuity between the nasal sac and the roof of the

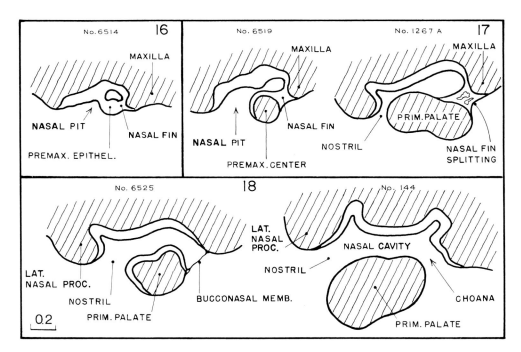

Fig. 17-4. Simplified outlines of selected sagittal sections showing the steps in the formation of the respiratory by-pass in stages 16–18. Judging from its prominence and precocity, the epithelium of the nasal pit appears to be an important determining factor. This same epithelium is a mosaic of at least four specialized areas. One forms the zone of olfactory cells; another becomes the vomeronasal organ; another participates in the formation of the system of nasal conchae; and another is the plate-like nasal fin, which by a characteristic splitting phenomenon produces the choana. The underlying mesenchyme is an important partner in these changes. It is from the maxillary and premaxillary centers that the primary palate spreads forward and across, thereby separating the nasal passage from the mouth. The nasal ectoderm is much thicker than the contiguous skin ectoderm, but allowance is to be made for exaggeration in some places because of the tangential section, notably in the first two phases. In each case the outlines represent camera lucida drawings of single sections, with the exception of the last, which is a composite of two sections.

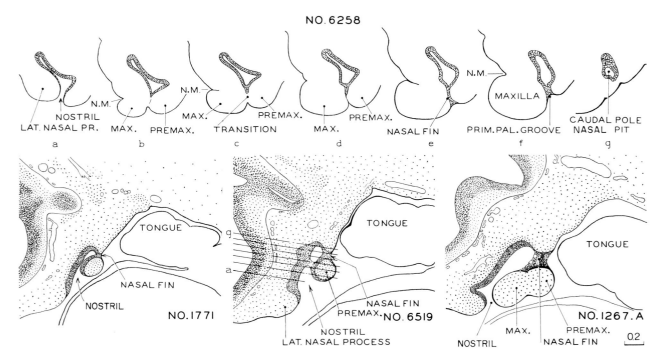

Fig. 17-5. Upper row, camera lucida drawings of transverse sections (in most instances, every fifth section) through right nasal pit of No. 6258. This embryo corresponds closely to No. 6519, a sagittal section of which is shown in the lower row. To facilitate comparison of the two, the approximate section levels of the tracings of No. 6258 are superimposed upon the latter. The sagittal drawings in the lower row show less-advanced, intermediate, and more-advanced representatives of this stage, a period of rapid transformation in the nasal region. It is to be noted that the primary characters of this respiratory by-pass are acquired in miniature and before the attainment of its topographical relation to the tongue.

LAT. NASAL PR., lateral nasal process; *MAX.*, maxillary growth center; *N.M.*, nasomaxillary groove; *PREMAX.*, premaxillary growth center.

mouth. The location of the nasal fin is indicated on the surface by a groove, at first shallow, later becoming deeper and marking the boundary between the premaxillary and maxillary growth centers. This is the primitive palatine groove of Peter (1913).

Except for that maintained by the nasal fin, the continuity between the nasal sac and the roof of the mouth becomes interrupted by the active proliferation of the mesenchyme of the premaxillary and maxillary growth centers, which blends across from one center to the other, in front of the nasal fin. There is thereby established the primordium of the palate. The right and left primary palates are derived from the premaxillary centers and unite in the median plane. That part (secondary palate) derived from the maxillary centers takes the form of lateral elevations on the two sides.

The developmental function of the nasal fin begins to express itself already in stage 16, at which time there

is scarcely more than a nasal pit. In stage 17 the primary palate makes its appearance, and the nasal fin becomes transformed from an epithelial plate to an epithelium-lined passage in consequence of the coalescence of its cleavage spaces and through adaptation of its rapidly proliferating cells. As long as the end of this passage is obstructed by incomplete cleavage of the epithelium, it constitutes a cul-de-sac, the *hinteren Blindsack* of Peter. In stage 18, among the less advanced members of the group, an epithelial membrane-like remnant (the bucconasal membrane of Hochstetter) still stretches across the opening. In more-advanced members, the last strand has been retracted and a free respiratory passage exists from the nostril through the choana to the nasopharynx. The steps in the laying down of the primary nasal passage can be seen in simplified form in sagittal sections, as is illustrated in figure 17-4. Sections taken from four embryos belonging to stage 17

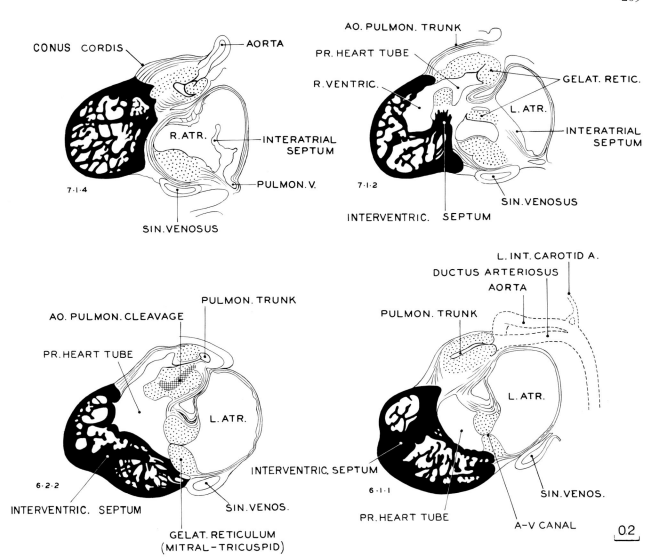

Fig. 17-6. Four selected sagittal sections through the heart of No. 1771, a less advanced member of stage 17. The aortic and pulmonary trunks are undergoing cleavage, a process that (according to Streeter), starts distally and extends proximally into the heart. At this time the trunks have been separated to a point proximal to the semilunar valves, which are now present in rough form.

are shown in greater detail in figure 17-5. These illustrate the nasal fin during its maximum prominence, as seen in both transverse and sagittal sections.

CARDIOVASCULAR SYSTEM

Heart

The cleavage of the primary cardiac tube continues during stage 17, advancing the separation of the pulmonary and aortic channels. In addition, the right and left atrioventricular canals become completely separate. As shown in figure 17-6, the primary cardiac tube and its surrounding mesenchyme (gelatinous reticulum) still form a considerable part of the field and stand out in contrast with the trabeculated muscular sacs that are forming the right and left ventricles. As has been pointed out, the right and left ventricular pouches, as they increase in size and pulsating force, tend to give rise to two diverse currents corresponding to their separate directional axes. Apparently this finds

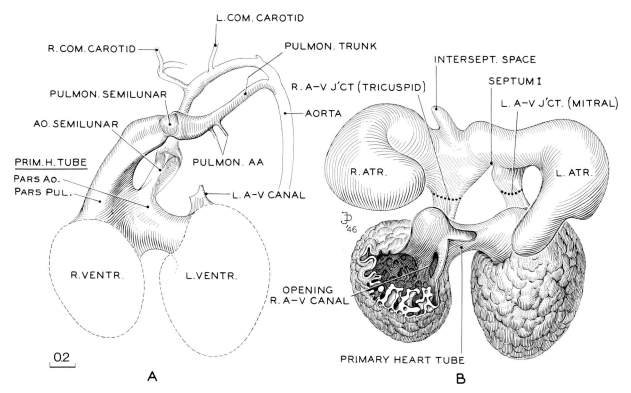

Fig. 17-7. Reconstruction of the endocardium of the heart and its arterial trunks in No. 6520, a member of the median third of stage 17. It is shown in two parts, A and B. In A, only the derivatives of the primary cardiac tube are shown. In B, enough of the primary tube is removed to expose the venous part of the heart. The latter, being in a contracted state, reveals in an unobstructed view the right and left atrioventricular canals, now clearly separated, each leading forward into its respective ventricle. It will be noted that the primary cardiac tube is connected with the venous part of the heart only at the two atrioventricular junctions. When the latter are severed, the arterial portion can be freely separated from the venous part. In A, the cleavage has not yet crossed the crest of the septum, and both arterial trunks lead off from both ventricles. From the distention of the endocardium of the primary cardiac tube, however, one can see that the left ventricle favors the aorta, and the right ventricle the pulmonary trunk. Drawings made by James F. Didusch. Reconstruction made by Osborne O. Heard.

its expression in the expansion of the endocardial lumen into two main channels (aortic and pulmonary), as seen in embryos Nos. 3385 and 6510 in figure 15-5. According to Streeter, the endocardium between them is consequently subject to less distention, resulting in its final absorption. Thereupon the supporting mesenchyme fills in along that spiral path of less stress. Under such circumstances the adaptation of endothelium to the existence of two blood currents must rank high as a factor in the cleavage of the aortic and pulmonary trunks, whereas conotruncal ridges are merely the remains of the cardiac mesenchyme, a filling-in behind the reshaping of the endothelium. An increase in the supporting reticular cells is found, and

such a condensation is seen particularly in the plane where the aortic and pulmonary channels are undergoing cleavage. An area of that kind is illustrated in section 6-2-2 in figure 17-6, and it signifies that one is close to an endothelial surface.

A complicated organ like the heart can be studied with advantage in three-dimensional reconstructions (fig. 17-7). In the embryo selected, the atria were contracted, thus favoring the viewing of the two atrioventricular canals. The reconstruction is shown at two levels, one (A) in front of and to be superimposed upon the other (B). The front model (A) shows the pulmonary and aortic trunks leaving the heart, and the part they take in the formation of the left dorsal aorta.

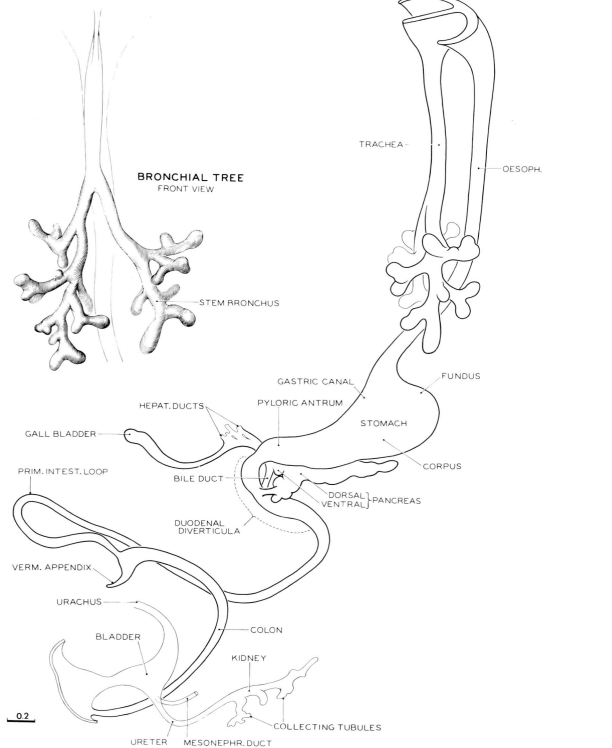

BRONCHIAL TREE
FRONT VIEW

STEM BRONCHUS

TRACHEA

OESOPH.

GASTRIC CANAL

FUNDUS

HEPAT. DUCTS

PYLORIC ANTRUM

GALL BLADDER

STOMACH

PRIM. INTEST. LOOP

CORPUS

BILE DUCT

DORSAL
VENTRAL PANCREAS

DUODENAL
DIVERTICULA

VERM. APPENDIX

URACHUS

COLON

BLADDER

KIDNEY

COLLECTING TUBULES

URETER   MESONEPHR. DUCT

0.2

Fig. 17-8. Reconstruction of the epithelial core of the alimentary canal typical of the median members of stage 17 (No. 6520). It will be noted that the epithelium has acquired a pattern in which one can recognize many details approximating the regional forms of the mature canal; the elements of this epithelial pattern are already present at stage 16 (fig. 16-8). Antedating stage 16 is a level with yet simpler expression of the same parts, and so on, back to the primordial system. Thus starting from the primary form this precocious epithelium of the gut progresses in its development step by step, always in the direction of its inherent plan and at no place deviating from it. Considering the relative backwardness of the other coats of the gut during this period, one must attribute a high degree of intrinsic potency to the different regions of the epithelium.

In stage 17 the vermiform appendix becomes marked off from the caecum. In the kidney the pelvis has become branched. The intestinal loop herniates into the umbilical cord without rotation or coils. Drawing made by James F. Didusch. Reconstruction made by Osborne O. Heard.

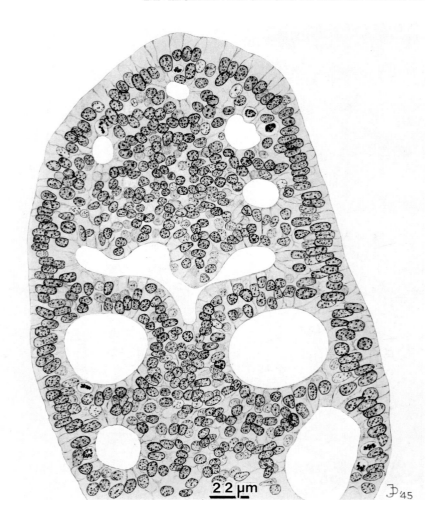

Fig. 17-9. Section through duodenal epithelium of No. 6520. (Cf. fig. 17-8.) In its proliferative activity it forms diverticula opening from the central lumen and also isolated follicles. Because of the exuberant growth of its epithelium there are produced the two fusiform enlargements of the duodenum, above and below the combined pancreatic and bile ducts. Drawing made by James F. Didusch. Section 48-3-3.

It also shows the progress of cleavage of the endocardial aortic and pulmonary channels. At the semilunar valves (which appeared already at stage 16) the endocardium preserves the continuity of the lumen, whereas the condensing mesenchyme fills in behind it, forming three characteristic rounded occluding masses. The narrow lumen through the valve appears on section as a three-limbed cleft. This, therefore, is a weak spot, and when one attempts to make a cast of the lumen of these trunks, a break at the semilunar sites is likely to result. Proximal to the valves the primary cardiac tube is still relatively voluminous, and the larger parts correspond more or less to channels suited to the two main blood currents. In the formation of the semilunar valves, if mechanical factors enter in, they certainly must be much more complicated than those suggested to account for the separation of two

main blood channels. But even in these valves one would hesitate to rule out the possibility of some mechanical influence at these sites, associated, for instance, with the back-thrust of the systemic blood columns which would, already at this time, follow each heartbeat.

The posterior model (B) shown in figure 17-7 is visualized as dissected free from the more anteriorly situated part (A). The cut edge of the primary cardiac tube (B) is arranged so as to leave uncovered the entrance of the right atrioventricular canal. From examination of both views (A and B) one finds that the separation of the aortic and pulmonary channels is complete to the region proximal to the semilunar valves. From there proximally, the primary cardiac tube still consists of a single voluminous cavity, common to right and left sides. Into it the incoming blood enters sep-

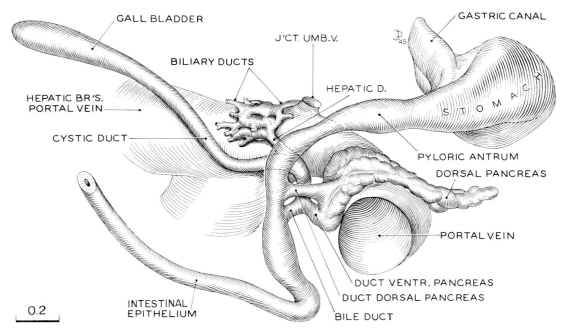

Fig. 17-10. Reconstruction of the epithelial core of the two pancreatic ducts, showing also the biliary ducts and their relation to the alimentary epithelium, typical of stage 17 (No. 1267A). It can be seen that the dorsal pancreas, although fused with the ventral pancreas, still retains its original duct. Drawing made by James F. Didusch. Reconstruction made by Osborne O. Heard.

arately from the right and left atria. These canals mark the sites of the mitral and tricuspid valves, which are still in the form of condensing mesenchyme.

By stage 17 foramen primum is obliterated and foramen secundum is wide. The membranous part of the interventricular septum is formed from cushion material that does not close the primary interventricular foramen (McBride, Moore, and Hutchins, 1981). Interventricular foramen 2 is finally bounded by the conal septum (especially by the right conal ridge) and the fused atrioventricular cushions (Wenink, 1971). The outflow tract is said to have been undergoing a counterclockwise rotation. It should be stressed, however, that "the formation of the septal system of the truncus and conus is more complex than is usually recognized" (Kramer, 1942).

DIGESTIVE SYSTEM

Six zones (four maxillary and two mandibular) of odontogenic epithelium have been identified (Nery, Kraus, and Croup, 1970).

In figure 17-8 is shown in outline the epithelial al-

imentary canal that is characteristic of stage 17. Over and above its relative increase in length, various regional morphological details are making their appearance. In addition to a caecum, one can now distinguish the vermiform appendix. The primary intestinal loop projects further into the umbilical cord as the normal umbilical hernia, which persists until approximately 40 mm. The elongating colon seems to be providing the thrust that will aid in bringing the caecum to the right side of the body.

The duodenal region is an especially active center of epithelial proliferation, resulting in two fusiform enlargements, one proximal to the entrance of the bile and pancreatic ducts and the other distally. In the region of these enlargements the epithelium in its accentuated growth acquires a follicular arrangement in which the epithelium is oriented around small discrete cavities (Johnson, 1910). In some cases these constitute isolated follicles and in others they consist of diverticula, communicating with the partially obliterated original lumen of the gut (fig. 17-9) (Boyden, Cope, and Bill, 1967). Traces of this exuberant type of epithelial

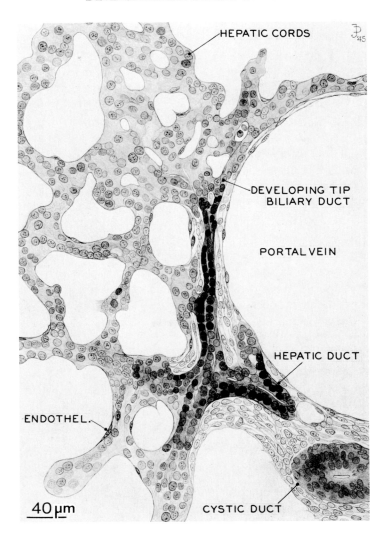

Fig. 17-11. Histological appearance of the abrupt transition from the biliary ducts to the hepatic epithelium. It supports the assumption that at the tips of the ducts some of the hepatic epithelium becomes redifferentiated into the compact, deeply staining, duct-forming cells. This process of redifferentiation progresses outward through the embryonic connective-tissue coat of the portal vein and its branches. The growth of new connective tissue and the ductal formation keep in close step. Drawing made by James F. Didusch. No. 1267A, section 5-1-1.

proliferation with its characteristic follicular tendency are found also in other parts of the canal, notably in the esophagus.

The relations of the ventral and dorsal pancreas and of the biliary ducts to the intestine are shown in figure 17-10. One can see that the ventral pancreas, which had sprouted from the bile duct, has now fused with the dorsal pancreas. Each pancreas, however, still retains its original duct, that of the ventral pancreas emptying into the bile duct and that of the dorsal pancreas, further rostrally, directly into the duodenum. Finally, following anastomosis of the ductal systems of the two parts, the more favored passage for the pancreatic secretions from the whole gland leads through the ventral pancreatic duct beside the bile duct, and the dorsal pancreatic duct may disappear in the process.

Liver

The liver has already taken form as the joint product of angioblastic tissue arising from the coelomic surface cells (fig. 11-6) and of epithelial columns coming from the opposite direction, sprouting from the hepatic evagination of the gut epithelium (fig. 12-5). The two tissues in this combination undergo continued rapid proliferation, and there is soon produced the typical, large trabeculated epitheliovascular organ known as the liver. The liver shows signs of functional activity important to the embryo from the beginning of blood circulation and thereafter. If its first functional assignment were to be its sole function, there appears no reason that it should not become detached from the gut wall and carry on by itself. It does not, however, become detached. There remains an epithelial stem that preserves the continuity between the hepatic epithelium and that of the gut. This stem is partially plexiform, and by stage 17 it is readily recognized as the hepatic duct.

The nature of the abrupt terminal endings of the hepatic duct is illustrated in fig. 17-11. It does not yet penetrate far into the hepatic substance and is found only at the hilum in the connective tissue of the wall of the entering portal vein. At its elongating tips, it is directly continuous with the hepatic epithelium, and its further peripheral growth is accomplished at the expense of the latter, which cell by cell at these tips is transformed into smaller, darkly staining ductal cells. This differentiation keeps step with the formation of the connective tissue coat of the portal vein, along the branches of which the biliary ductal system spreads. Near the hepatic duct, but essentially separate in origin, is the gall bladder and its duct. The hepatic duct and the plexiform terminations of its biliary tributaries, in the reticulum along the wall of the portal vein, have been reconstructed in three dimensions and are shown in figure 17-10. Information on the development of the intrahepatic biliary ducts is available (Koga, 1971).

RESPIRATORY SYSTEM

The separation of the lungs from the digestive system is essentially complete by stage 17, and the pseudoglandular phase of pulmonary development is under way. The form of the epithelial bronchial tree is illustrated in figures 17-8 and 17-14. One can more definitely recognize the groupings that will make up the three lobes on the right side and two on the left. Segmental buds represent the bronchopulmonary segments. In addition to the growth and branching of the epithelial tube, the surrounding visceral mesenchyme, which, in part at least, was derived from the coelomic epithelium, is advancing in its differentiation, and one can now recognize condensations that are to become tracheal cartilages. The vagus nerves have increased progressively in size. Figure 15-7c shows that the esophagus, lying behind the trachea, is acquiring a submucous coat enclosing the epithelium, which coat is practically absent from the trachea. It is also to be noted that the right and left pulmonary arteries have become more prominent.

URINARY SYSTEM
(fig. 17-14)

The mesonephros shows epithelial plaques in the visceral layer of the glomerular capsule and hence can produce urine (Silverman, 1969). The pelvis of the ureter usually shows three main divisions, and calices appear. The urogenital sinus presents a pelvic part (vesico-urethral canal) and a phallic part (definitive urogenital sinus).

REPRODUCTIVE SYSTEM

The structure of the gonad is shown in figure 18-9. The paramesonephric ducts, which may appear at the previous stage, arise as invaginations of the coelomic epithelium. The genital eminence forms the phallus at stage 17 or stage 18. The nipples appear as buds on the mammary crest (Bossy, 1980b).

SKELETAL SYSTEM

Some of the vertebral centra, which appear at stage 15, begin chondrification at stage 17 (Sensenig, 1949). The neural arch begins as right and left neural processes at stage 15. The skeleton of the upper and lower limbs becomes visible as mesenchyme at stages 15 and 16, respectively, and chondrification commences at stages 16–17 (e.g., in the humerus and radius) and 17–18 (e.g., in the femur) (O'Rahilly and Gardner, 1975). A general view of the mesenchymal skeleton at stage 17 shows also the beginning chondrocranium (Blechschmidt, 1963, plate 24).

NERVOUS SYSTEM
(fig. 17-12)

The rhombomeres are still visible, but the rhombic grooves are limited to the side and absorbed in the surrounding surface, so that they are no longer visible in a median view. Migration of cells from the medioventral cell column to the definitive sites of the special visceral motor nuclei is still proceeding. The first nucleus to settle down is that of the trigeminal nerve. Vestibulocerebellar and trigeminocerebellar fibers run toward the cerebellum, which grows in thickness. The

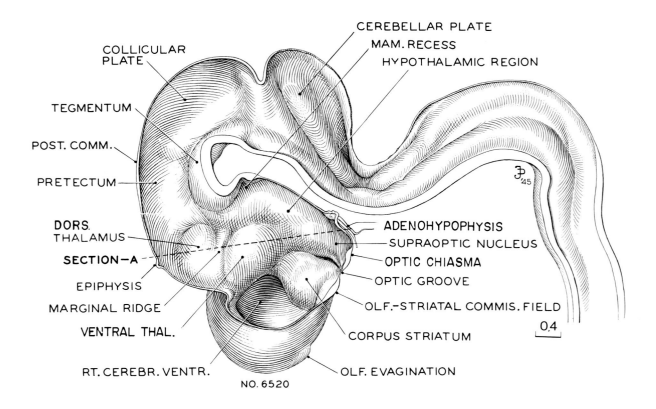

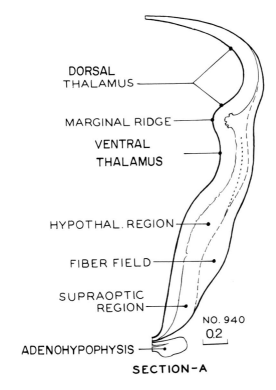

Fig. 17-12. Reconstruction of right half of brain of an embryo (No. 6520) belonging in the middle third of stage 17. The marginal ridge, projecting into the lumen and separating the dorsal thalamus from the ventral thalamic region lying rostral to it, is now plainly seen. The contours of the wall are seen in section A. This drawing was made from No. 940 of the same stage, and it corresponds to a transverse section along the dotted line shown in the sketch of the reconstruction, passing caudal to the epiphysis, with its lower end transecting the hypophysis. It will be noted that above the marginal ridge the wall is behind in development, and ventral to it the wall is precocious. The ventral thalamic region has a nuclear area comparable to a mantle zone. In the hypothalamic region there is a large fiber field which appears to unite later with the peduncular system. The neuro-hypophysis forms a deep ventral pocket with characteristic foldings of its caudal wall. The adenohypophysis is flattened dorsoventrally, but spreads widely, enclosing the infundibulum on each side with its two wings: it is therefore larger than is shown in a median section. Finally, it is to be noted that the olfactory evagination is just making its appearance. Drawings made by James F. Didusch. Reconstruction made by Osborne O. Heard.

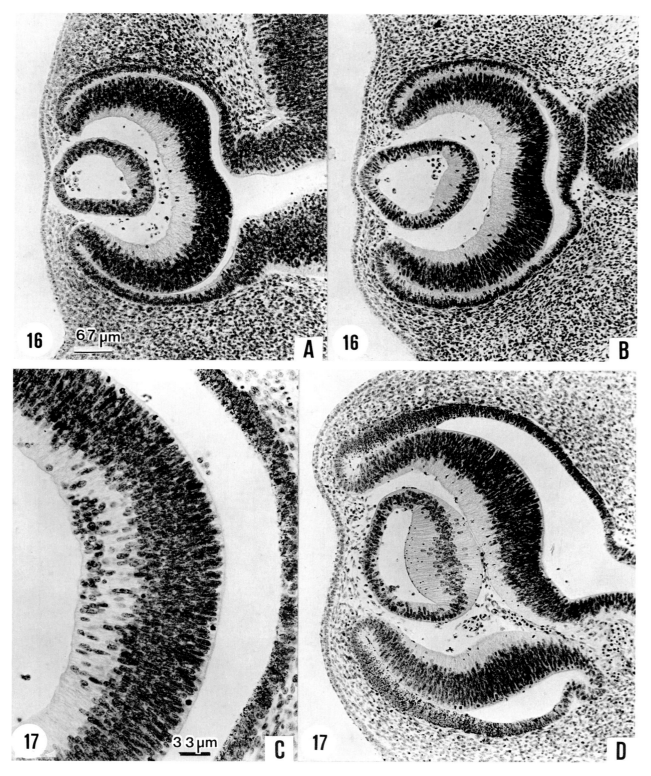

Fig. 17-13. These photomicrographs show the characteristics of the eye, as seen under the microscope, in stages 16 and 17. In stage 16 the lens vesicle has a large lumen. One can see rather sharply demarcated the section of its wall that is to become the lens disc, distinct from the epithelium that is to remain as the thin epithelial layer over the front of the lens in the mature eye. In stage 17 the lens disc, in the histogenesis of lens fibers, becomes much thicker and encroaches upon the lens cavity, reducing it to a crescentic shape. Another decisive advance is the formation of the internal neuroblastic layer of the retina by migration from the primary zone (O'Rahilly, 1966), as seen in C. The starting point of this migration occurs at about the location of the future macula. In the next stage the spread is much wider. (A) No. 6509, 12-1-3. (B) No. 6507, 7-2-3. (C) No. 6520, 22-2-3. (D) No. 6521, 24-3-4. A, B, and D are at the same magnification.

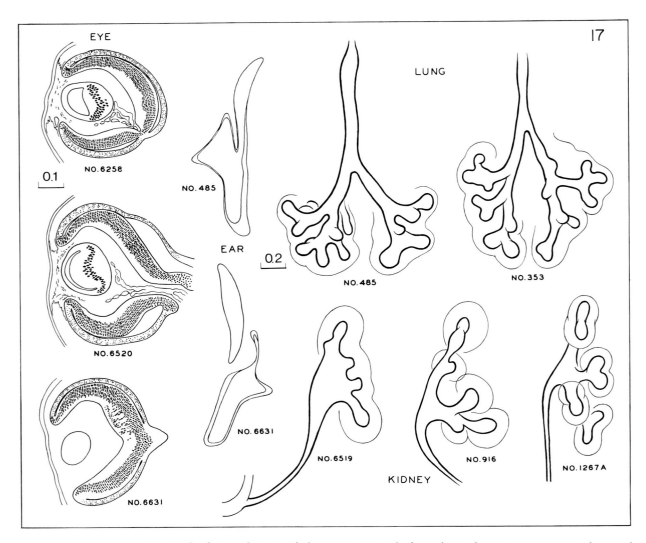

Fig. 17-14. Cluster of structural characters required of members of stage 17. Formation of internal neuroblastic layer of retina (fig. 17-13C) by migration. At this time the migration is limited to a restricted field, approximately at the site of the macula. The cavity of the lens vesicle, as seen in section, shows various phases in becoming a crescentic cleft. In the inner ear the walls of the labyrinth, save at its thick rims that are to be the ducts, are beginning to sink inward, preparatory to absorption of their thin parts. In the lungs, segmental buds are appearing in the bronchi. In the kidney, the pelvis begins to exhibit well-marked calices.

geniculate ganglion is now separated from that of the vestibulocochlear nerve. The cerebellar plate (*innerer Kleinhirnwulst* of Hochstetter) is present as a clear thickening. The mesencephalon now possesses an intermediate layer throughout most of its extent. The posterior commissure between the midbrain and the diencephalon is prominent. The ventral thalamus, lying rostral to the marginal ridge, is well in advance of the dorsal thalamus. The former possesses an intermediate layer, whereas the latter begins its development only now. The neurohypophysis is a distinct evagination in all embryos; the adenohypophysis is still open toward the pharyngeal cavity. The epiphysis cerebri, a thickening in the roof of the diencephalon, develops an intermediate layer. The corpus striatum bulges into the ventricular cavity, and, together with the ventral thalamus, delimits the interventricular foramen. The area overlying the corpus striatum is slightly flattened and represents the future insula. One-third of the length of the cerebral vesicles reaches more rostrally than the lamina terminalis. The olfactory tubercle is characterized by cellular islands; both the olfactory tubercle and the future olfactory bulb are marked by a slight elevation at the surface of the brain. The olfactory fibers form a compact bundle that runs from caudal to rostral, where the fibers enter the brain wall. A medial strand, containing the future vomeronasal and terminal nerves, can be distinguished from a lateral one (Bossy, 1980a). All parasympathetic ganglia of the cranial nerves, except the otic, are present (Woźniak and O'Rahilly, 1980). The dural limiting layer begins to form in basal areas of the brain, and pori durales for some of the cranial nerves are present (O'Rahilly and Müller, 1986b).

Eye

Retinal pigment is clearly visible even under low power (figs. 17-13C,D and 18-12B). The retinal fissure is largely closed. Further changes are occurring in retinal differentiation (O'Rahilly, 1983b), particularly in the future macular region. The cavity of the lens vesicle changes gradually from D-shaped to crescentic (fig. 17-13D).

Ear

The membranous labyrinth is shown in figure 17-14. The endolymphatic appendage is a relatively large, thin-walled, fusiform sac. The future cochlear duct is elongating at the tip of the labyrinth. The walls of the vestibular part are becoming thinner and approximated, making imminent the absorption of the contacting surfaces and the resulting formation of the semicircular ducts. Only those specimens in which absorption has not yet occurred are admitted to this stage, and consequently in none of them is a semicircular duct yet present. The auditory ossicles are defined in mesenchyme.

Specimen of Stage 17 Already Described

12-mm embryo. The peripheral nervous system was described by Volcher (1959) in an embryo of stage 17.

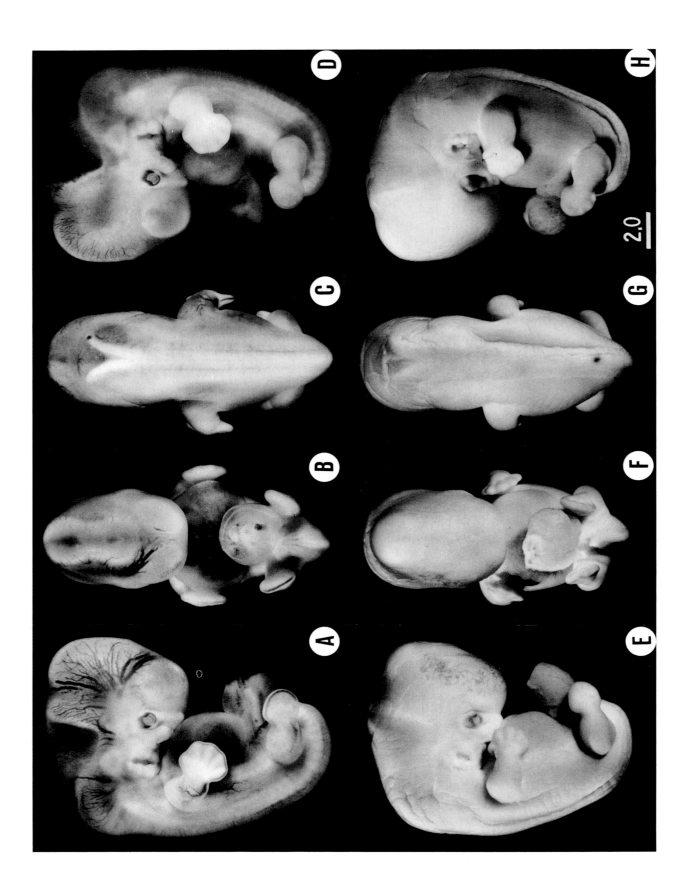

2.0

STAGE 18

Approximately 13–17 mm

Approximately 44 postovulatory days

SUMMARY

External: the body is more of a unified cuboidal mass, and both cervical and lumbar flexures are indicated; the limbs are longer, the digital plate of the hand is definitely notched, the elbow region is usually discernible, and toe rays can be identified in some specimens; eyelid folds are present in the more advanced embryos; a distinct tip of the nose can be seen in profile; auricular hillocks are being transformed into specific parts of the external ear.

Internal: in the heart, septum secundum and the associated foramen ovale are appearing; the membranous part of the interventricular septum is beginning to take form; the vomeronasal organ is represented by a groove; choanae develop; some subsegmental buds develop in the bronchial tree; collecting tubules develop from the calices; testicular cords may begin to appear in the male gonad; the paramesonephric duct grows rapidly down through the mesonephros; 1–3 semicircular ducts are present in the internal ear.

SIZE AND AGE

Less-advanced embryos of stage 18 may be expected to have a greatest length of about 14.5 mm, whereas more-advanced examples would in most instances be about 16 mm. Nearly two-thirds of all embryos at this stage range from 14 to 16 mm.

Although the data are not extensive (only eight specimens), the greatest diameter of the chorion usually ranges from 40 to 51 mm, and all three principal diameters are approximately equal.

The age is believed to be approximately 44 postovulatory days.

EXTERNAL FORM
(figs. 18-1 to 18-3)

From external form alone it is not always possible to distinguish between less-advanced specimens of stage 18 and more-advanced ones of stage 17. In drawing an arbitrary borderline between the two groups, as has been done in this study, one must rely on selected structural characters of the internal organs that are revealed in sections. Indeed, in several instances, it has been found necessary to change the placement of certain embryos from a provisional one based on their external form to one in an adjacent group, based on the study of the same embryos after they had been cut in serial sections.

To gauge accurately the level of development of an embryo, its internal structure must be taken into account. There are many things, however, to be learned

Fig. 18-1 (facing page). (A–D) Four views of a less advanced member (No. 8097) of stage 18. One can see the vascular patterns and details of inner structure. The inner ear, and also the trigeminal nerve and details of the eye, can be seen in the profile views. A number of details in the form of the brain, notably the cerebral hemispheres, are discernible (cf. O'Rahilly, Müller, and Bossy, 1982).

(E–H) Four views of a more advanced member (No. 7707) of stage 18. Because of the particular fixation, the tissues are opaque, making the specimen suitable for the study of surface features. The embryo has become wider from side to side, and it is now more or less cuboidal (F, G). The finger rays have become more distinct, and the rim of the hand plate is moderately crenated; one can recognize the bend of the elbow. Toe rays are visible (H). Small condensed masses are creeping forward over the retina, and the upper eyelid is beginning. The three-hillock plate, to the rear of the hyomandibular groove, exhibits different stages in its resolution into definitive parts of the external ear.

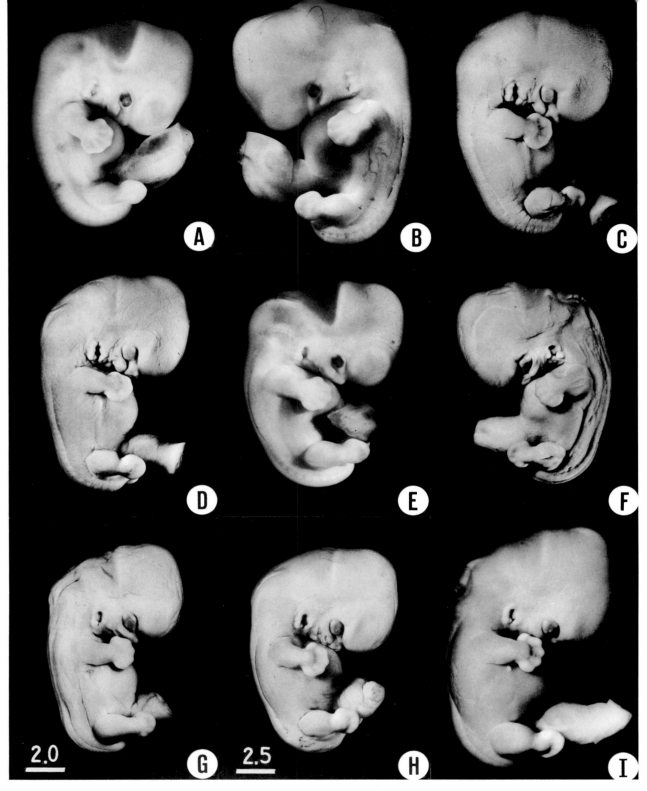

Fig. 18-2. Photographs illustrating the variations in form encountered in stage 18. It should be appreciated that certain appearances are the result of fixation, shrinkage, and the original condition of the embryo. All these specimens have been sectioned, and in their microscopic structure all qualify as members of this stage, in which semicircular ducts are acquired by the inner ear, in which the paramesonephric duct descends along the margin of the mesonephros, and in which the gonads show initial sexual differentiation. In general the embryos in the upper part of the plate are less advanced and those toward the lower part are more advanced. The embryo shown in I is near the borderline. It was fixed in a corrosive acetic mixture, which accentuates its surface features. The right nipple is visible immediately below the forearm. (A) No. 1909. (B) No. 5935A. (C) No. 6525. (D) No. 6528. (E) No. 5542B. (F) No. 6533. (G) No. 6522. (H) No. 6529. (I) No. 4430. B, C, D, F, G, and I are at the same magnification, whereas A, E, and H are slightly less magnified.

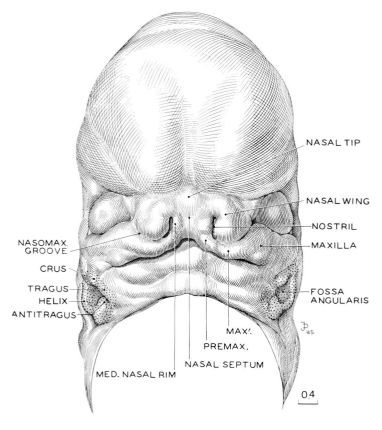

NASAL TIP

NASAL WING

NOSTRIL

MAXILLA

NASOMAX.
GROOVE

CRUS

TRAGUS
HELIX
ANTITRAGUS

FOSSA
ANGULARIS

MAX'.

PREMAX.

NASAL SEPTUM

MED. NASAL RIM

0.4

Fig. 18-3. Three-dimensional reconstruction of the face of No. 492, a typical representative of stage 18. By this time the nose and future upper jaw are definitely outlined. There is still a small gap between the right and left upper jaws, which will be smoothed out by the further enlargement and blending of the two premaxillary centers. When that occurs, the nasal septum will be closed off from the oral opening. It is still too early to speak of lips. The growth center marked *MAX'* is a subdivision of the maxillary center and is distinct from the lateral nasal process. Between the two is the nasomaxillary groove, which is commonly said to indicate the origin of the nasolacrimal duct, but Politzer (1936) disagreed. This figure forms a series with figures 15-3, 16-5, and 17-3. They are all enlarged to the same scale and hence are directly comparable. Drawing made by James F. Didusch. Reconstruction made by Osborne O. Heard.

from the external form. One can see, for instance, that the group of embryos shown in figure 18-2 is more advanced than the similar group of the preceding stage, shown in figure 17-2. The embryo of stage 18 is larger and has advanced in the coalescence of its body regions, which have now become more closely integrated in a common cuboidal bulk, no longer consisting of individual and obviously separable parts.

The hands in all specimens have distinct finger rays and interdigital notches on the rims. In the more advanced half of the group, one can begin to speak of an elbow. The feet in some specimens exhibit toe rays, but the rim is not definitely notched. Even in some of the more advanced members one can still find a trace of somitic elevations in the sacral region.

All the embryos illustrated in figures 18-1 and 18-2 have been serially sectioned and studied histologically, and all of them conform microscopically to the criteria arbitrarily set for stage 18. The two embryos in figure 18-1 are typical specimens taken respectively from

among less-advanced and more-advanced members of the group. The embryos in figure 18-2 illustrate such variations as are incident to differences in photography, methods of fixation, and variations in the degree of development encountered within this stage. The most advanced specimen (fig. 18-2, I) is on the borderline of the next stage.

Face

Above and below the eye one sees in more-advanced specimens of this stage the early rudiments of the eyelids (more marked in stage 19: Pearson, 1980) and the grooves initiating the conjunctival sacs. The thin outer lamina of the retina now contains considerable pigment, causing the retinal rim to be conspicuous. This is particularly true in formalin-preserved specimens, where the tissues are translucent. In embryos of stage 18 this pigmented rim of the optic cup is characteristically polygonal, partly because of the forward pro-jection of the upper margin of the retina and partly because of the retinal fissure. At the same time, white opaque zones of mesenchymal condensation spread progressively forward over the pigmented area, es-pecially above and lateral to it. These opaque thick-enings mark the laying down of the sclera and its muscular attachments.

In profile views of the nasal region one can begin to recognize the tip of the nose and the frontonasal angle, from which point the future bridge of the nose is to extend "forward." To see the face satisfactorily one must study either decapitated specimens or re-constructions of the facial region made from serial sections. Such a model of a representative embryo of stage 18 is illustrated in figure 18-3. The nose, nostrils, nasal tip or apex, nasal wings, and nasal septum (col-umella nasi) can be identified clearly. The nose at this time can be thought of as a raised window awning; later, as the bridge of the nose forms, the awning will be let down. What is now in a vertical plane will then be horizontal. The upper lip is not differentiated as a separate structure. It will be formed jointly and in segments by the premaxillary and maxillary centers of the two sides. In this same figure the auricular hillocks are visible, although they are seen better in profile views (figs. 18-1 and 18-2). These hillocks were prom-inent elevations in the preceding stage. Here they are merging with one another and the adjacent surfaces, thereby forming the primordia of definite parts of the auricle. Those rostral to the auditory cleft are more advanced than those caudal to it. Thus the two dorsal hillocks (Nos. 2 and 3) of the mandibular arch are losing their individuality in the process of fusing to form the crus helicis. In more-advanced specimens of the group, the two dorsal hillocks (Nos. 4 and 5) caudal to the cleft have similarly merged to become the helix. Hillocks 1 and 6 persist and become, respectively, the tragus and antitragus, with the lobule pendent from the latter.

Nasal Passages

The nostrils (fig. 18-4) are the rims of the right and left nasal depressions, that is, lines of junction of nasal disc and skin ectoderm. The depressed center of each disc takes the form of a deep pocket, and, as a result

of the growth of its own epithelium and the enveloping effect of the proliferating surrounding tissues, it be-comes a supplementary air passage. This passage at first ends blindly, but in the more advanced members of this stage its blind end opens through what had been the temporary bucconasal membrane and par-ticipates in the formation of the funnel-like transition into the pharynx. A communication between the re-spiratory system and the surface of the face is in this way provided. It by-passes the mouth, leaving the latter free to perform its own special functions.

Transverse serial sections through the nasal passages of two embryos belonging to this stage, one slightly less advanced than the other, are shown in figure 18-4. In the first one (No. 6524) it can already be seen that the walls of the passage are differentiated into regions, and that the ethmoidal epithelium (upper part of medial wall) is becoming distinct from the maxillary territory of the lateral wall. The shallow fold in the lower part of the medial wall marks the vomeronasal organ (fig. 18-14). These regional demarcations are still more evident in the second embryo (No. 4430). The epithelium, like that of the gut, is characterized by mosaic-like organ-forming regions, the boundaries of which are evident very early.

In these serial sections one can trace the fate of the nasal fin. In stage 17 it appeared as a plate of epithelium that maintains a connection between the nasal disc and the ordinary surface epithelium, in line with the groove between the maxillary and premaxillary growth cen-ters. In transverse sections the nasal fin has the ap-pearance of a ventral stem for the nasal passage. In the present stage, in the more rostral sections, it be-comes disconnected and is taken up by the overlying nasal epithelium. Caudally, this fin cleaves open to form part of the choanae. In doing so it becomes stretched to form the bucconasal membrane, and this in turn is detached and absorbed in the wall of the choana, leaving a free respiratory passage. The topo-graphical relations of the nasal passage are further clarified by sagittal sections.

Two embryos thus sectioned, a less advanced (No. 6525) and a more advanced one (No. 144), are shown in figure 18-4. Although in the more advanced of these two the respiratory by-pass is an open channel, its mature relations are not yet established. These will be attained through differential growth which is accom-

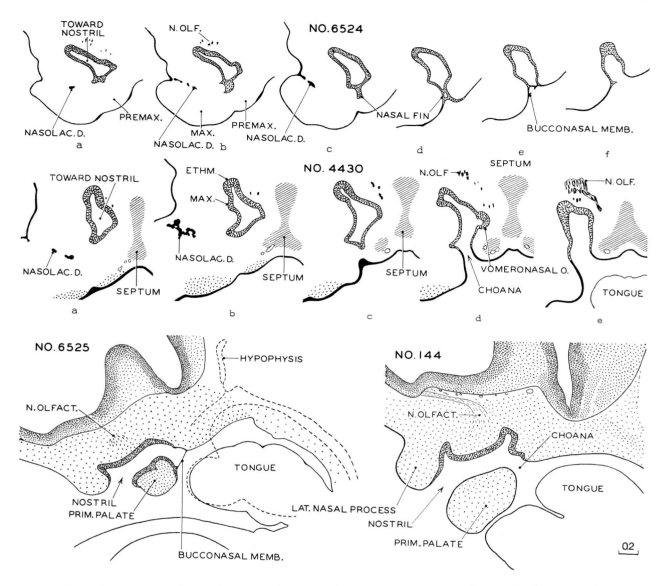

Fig. 18-4. Nasal passages in embryos of stage 18. The upper row shows transverse sections, at equal intervals, through the right nasal passage of a less advanced member of the group (No. 6524). Section a is the most rostral and f is the most caudal. In the caudal levels (d–f) the nasal epithelium, by means of its fin-like growth, has retained its continuity with the surface (oral) epithelium. Instead of remaining a solid plate, the nasal fin is now splitting to form the choana, its last remnants producing the bucconasal membrane.

The middle row (No. 4430) represents a more advanced member of the group, and the nasal epithelium shows specialized regions. The ethmoidal field is distinct from the maxillary field, and the choanal field differs from both of these. A definite vom-

eronasal organ is present (section d). The nasomaxillary groove is commonly said to indicate the origin of the nasolacrimal duct, but Politzer (1936) disagreed. A mesenchymal condensation now marks the primordium of the median cartilaginous septum of the nose.

The two sagittal sections of the lowest row show the final step in the establishment of a through nasal passage (the respiratory by-pass). On the drawing of No. 6525 is superimposed the outline of a median section, indicated by broken lines, showing the relative position of the tongue. The drawing of No. 144, a more advanced embryo, is a composite of two consecutive sections. All drawings are at the same scale.

panied by a relative shifting forward of the tongue and lower jaw.

The initiation of the nasolacrimal duct is shown in figure 18-4 (No. 6524 b and c, and No. 4430 a and b). An irregular lamina or strand of epithelium is seen sprouting from the under-surface of the nasomaxillary groove. This epithelial strand descends through the mesenchyme, and later joins the lateral wall of the inferior meatus of the nose. The transformation of this strand into a duct and the junction of its upper end by two small canals with the conjunctival sac occurs later in prenatal life. Politzer (1936) disagreed with the usual account of the early development of the naso-lacrimal duct.

CARDIOVASCULAR SYSTEM

Heart
(figs. 18-5 and 18-6)

An important feature is the appearance of septum secundum and hence the beginning of the foramen ovale at stages 18–21.

The heart is now a composite, four-chambered or-gan with separation of the pulmonary and aortic blood streams. In the more advanced members of the group the secondary interventricular foramen may already have closed, producing the future membranous part of the interventricular septum. The complete closure of the secondary interventricular foramen takes place during stages 18–21 (i.e., separating the cavity of the left ventricle from that of the right). The final bound-aries of the foramen are the conal septum (particularly the right conal ridge) and the fused atrioventricular cushions (Wenink, 1971).

The aortic and pulmonary valves have acquired in-creased definition and are becoming cup-shaped. The tricuspid and mitral valves are later in their differen-tiation, but one can now recognize the ridges of con-densed mesenchyme that are to form them. It is probable that they already have some valvular function.

Drawings of selected sagittal sections of a typical heart from one of the more advanced members of the group are shown in figure 18-5. In the condensing mesenchyme of the primary cardiac tube one sees, in such sections, sheets or areas of more-condensed tis-sue, shown in the figure by hatched lines, which un-derlie the endothelium and mark the proximity of cleavage and of adjustment of the walls.

From a coronal series of sections of another embryo at a similar level of development, a transparent recon-struction was made of the heart. Five study slabs (A–E) are illustrated in figure 18-6. The location of the front surface of each slab is indicated on the profile view of the heart, shown in the lower right corner. In this figure, as in the preceding one, the ventricular musculature is shown in solid black to distinguish it as a specialized tissue from the condensed mesen-chyme of the primary cardiac tube and the venous type of muscular wall of the atria. In slab A one sees the nature of the future membranous part of the interven-tricular septum separating the right and left ventricles. In slab B, directly behind it, is shown the fusion of the wall of the primary cardiac tube, which thereby sep-arates the tricuspid canal from the aortic corner of the left ventricle. In slab C is shown the complete sepa-ration of the aorta and pulmonary trunk, as far as the endothelium is concerned. Adjustments, however, are still in progress in the muscular and connective-tissue coats. The tricuspid and mitral passages are indicated. In slab D the sinus venosus is shown as it opens into the right atrium, immediately to the rear of the inferior vena cava. The two freely open at the same time, through the foramen ovale into the left atrium. In slab E is shown the manner of entrance of the superior vena cava. It is thus clear that from these three sources (sinus venosus, inferior vena cava, and superior vena cava) practically the whole of the incoming blood now ar-rives at the entrance of the foramen ovale.

Reconstructions of the heart at stage 18 have been illustrated by Kramer (1942, fig. 9) and by Vernall (1962).

DIGESTIVE SYSTEM

The esophagus shows distinct muscular and sub-mucous coats. The fundus of the stomach begins to develop at about stages 18 and 19.

RESPIRATORY SYSTEM

The vomeronasal organ is represented by a groove in the medial wall of the nasal cavity (fig. 18-14). Choanae are being produced by the breakdown of the bucco-nasal membrane. The larynx, which became definable

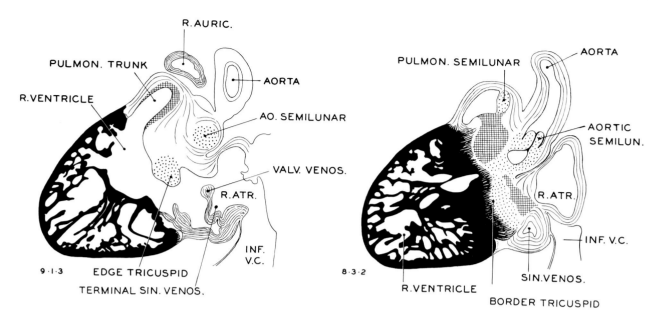

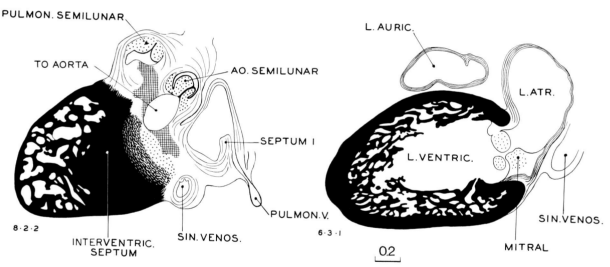

Fig. 18-5. Sagittal sections through a heart (No. 406) typical of stage 18. The interventricular septum is complete. The semilunar valves are now distinctly indicated. The tricuspid and mitral valves are scarcely more than rounded ridges of gelatinous reticular tissue. The latter tissue is last seen in these valves.

in the previous stage, is now undergoing specialization (O'Rahilly and Tucker, 1973).

The trachea possesses a dense connective-tissue coat (fig. 15-7D) and is markedly different from the esophagus in both its epithelium and its supporting wall.

The pattern of the bronchial tree is shown in figure 18-14. The segmental bronchi are well defined (Wells and Boyden, 1954, plate 2), and a few subsegmental

buds appear. In the embryonic period proper the left lung is said to lag behind the right lung in size and degree of development.

URINARY SYSTEM

Collecting tubules develop from the calices at stages 17 and 18 (fig. 18-14). They are surrounded by sharply

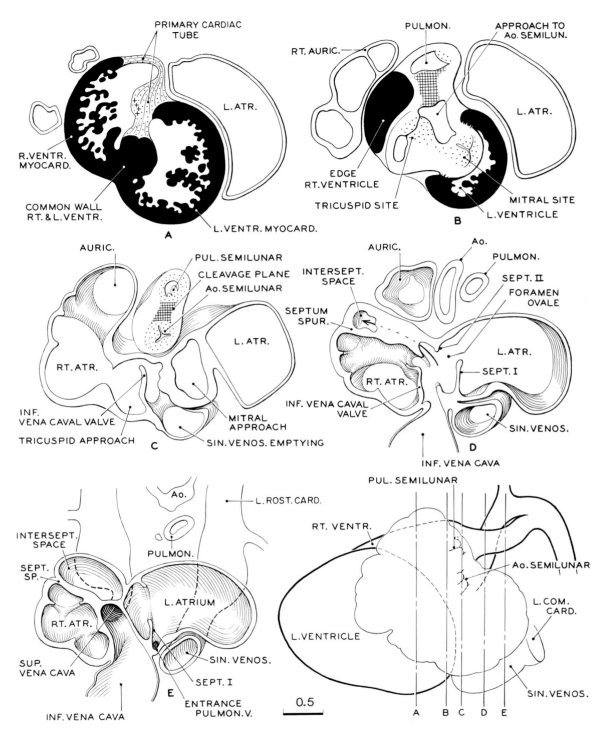

Fig. 18-6. Transparent reconstruction of a heart (No. 492) typical of stage 18. In the lower right-hand corner the heart is shown in left profile. The vertical lines through it indicate the front surface planes of the five transparent slabs shown separately as A–E. Each slab consists of a series of cellulose acetate sheets, properly oriented and spaced to give the correct third dimension. Tentative assembly showed that for reasons of clarity the slabs should not be thicker than is shown in the adopted levels.

It will be noted that, although the separation of aortic and pulmonary channels has been effected, the peri-endothelial coats are still more or less blended, from the semilunar valves proximally. Peripherally they are separate and have acquired their individual walls; no trace is left of the gelatinous reticulum. Ventricular myocardium is shown in solid black. Cleavage planes are shown by crossed lines.

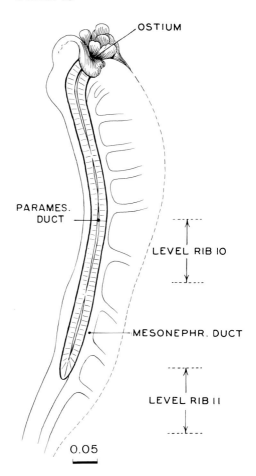

OSTIUM

PARAMES.
DUCT

LEVEL RIB 10

MESONEPHR. DUCT

LEVEL RIB 11

0.05

Fig. 18-7. Topography of the paramesonephric duct in a more advanced specimen (No. 406) of stage 18. The rib level refers to its free end and can be determined only approximately. Drawing made by James F. Didusch.

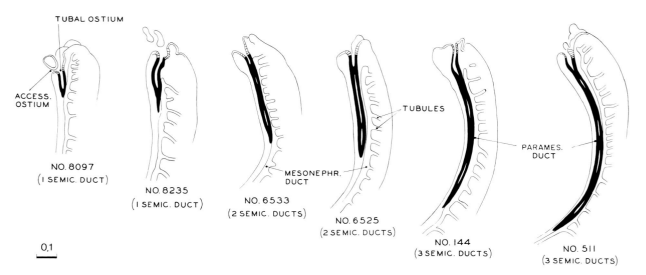

TUBAL OSTIUM

ACCESS.
OSTIUM

TUBULES

PARAMES.
DUCT

NO. 8097
(1 SEMIC. DUCT)

NO. 8235
(1 SEMIC. DUCT)

NO. 6533
(2 SEMIC. DUCTS)

MESONEPHR.
DUCT

NO. 6525
(2 SEMIC. DUCTS)

NO. 144
(3 SEMIC. DUCTS)

NO. 511
(3 SEMIC. DUCTS)

0.1

Fig. 18-8. The caudal extension of the paramesonephric duct occurring during stage 18. Less-advanced specimens are toward the left and more-advanced ones toward the right. Their order is based on the length of the duct, and this is found to correspond closely to other developmental characters. For example, in the less advanced ones only one semicircular duct is established in the inner ear, whereas the more advanced ones have the full complement of three semicircular ducts.

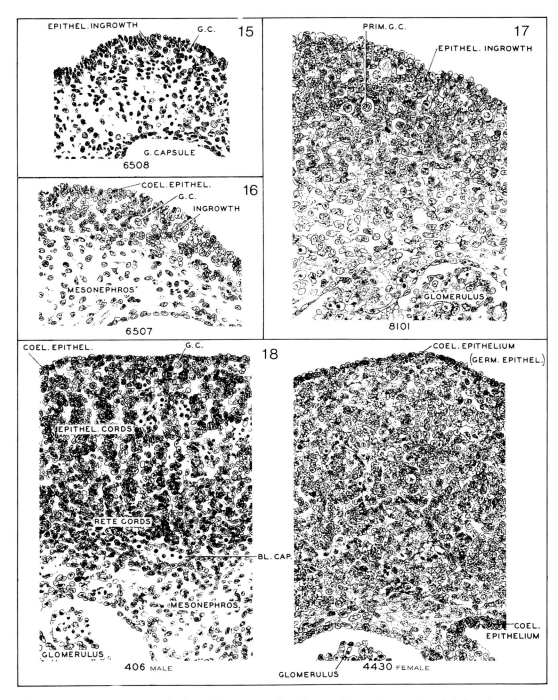

Fig. 18-9. Comparable sections passing transversely through the gonad in embryos selected as typical of stages 15–18. The first three stages show progressive phases of invasion and proliferation of the coelomic epithelium, providing the gonadal framework and follicular clusters around the primordial germ cells. Corresponding to the invasion, the surface is irregular, and one does not find a discrete surface layer of "germinal epithelium" before stage 18. Among the more advanced members of stage 18, one recognizes initial sexual differentiation. An example is shown of the male type of epithelial cords with active angiogenesis (No. 406) and of the female type (No. 4430). In both of these the surface of the gonad is smooth, and there is a distinctly marked-off layer of "germinal epithelium." Outlines were traced on photographic prints which were subsequently bleached. Section numbers are as follows: No. 6508, 35-2-5; No. 6507, 11-1-4; No. 8101, 29-4-6; No. 406, 41-1-4; No. 4430, 24-4-6. All are at the same magnification.

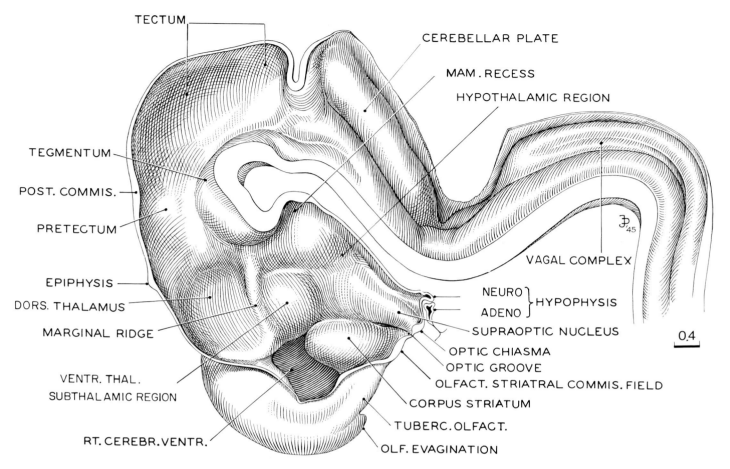

TECTUM

CEREBELLAR PLATE

MAM. RECESS

HYPOTHALAMIC REGION

TEGMENTUM

POST. COMMIS.

PRETECTUM

VAGAL COMPLEX

EPIPHYSIS

DORS. THALAMUS

MARGINAL RIDGE

NEURO ⎱
ADENO ⎰ HYPOPHYSIS

SUPRAOPTIC NUCLEUS

OPTIC CHIASMA

OPTIC GROOVE

VENTR. THAL.
SUBTHALAMIC REGION

OLFACT. STRIATRAL COMMIS. FIELD

CORPUS STRIATUM

RT. CEREBR. VENTR.

TUBERC. OLFACT.

OLF. EVAGINATION

0.4

Fig. 18-10. Reconstruction of right half of brain of embryo (No. 492) belonging among more-advanced members of stage 18. The basal plate continuing from the spinal cord and extending into the tegmentum has become thicker, and in transverse section the hypoglossal region begins to resemble sections of the mature hindbrain. The dorsal parts of midbrain and diencephalon are still backward compared with the basal structures that are situated below and rostral to the marginal ridge. The marginal ridge has become more prominent than in the preceding stage. The neurohypophysis is elongated and folded, and the adenohypophysis is characteristically expanded. The slender adenohypophysial stalk is still connected with the epithelium of the pharyngeal roof. The olfactory evagination has become prominent. Drawing made by James F. Didusch.

outlined condensed primordia in the process of forming secretory tubules. Renal corpuscles are not yet present. By stage 18 the mesonephric duct and the ureter open almost independently into the vesico-urethral canal (Shikinami, 1926): i.e., the common excretory duct is disappearing. The cloacal membrane is ready to rupture.

REPRODUCTIVE SYSTEM

In stage 15 the primordial germ cells are found sparsely distributed among the proliferating cells of

the coelomic epithelium (fig. 18-9). The coelomic epithelium provides the framework for the gonad. Ingrowth of the epithelium in stage 16 is sufficiently advanced to produce a crescentic strip of gonadal tissue that is fairly well demarcated from the mesonephros. In stage 17 the gonad has increased in size and is beginning to acquire an oval form. Its surface is still irregular. By stage 18 the gonad has become an elongated oval, distinctly set off from the mesonephros. The surface of the gonad is now smooth. Angiogenesis is commencing. The gonadal framework may begin to show sexual distinction by the presence of testicular

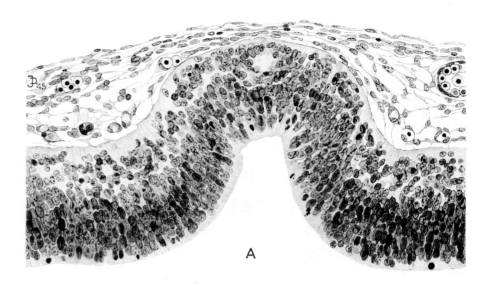

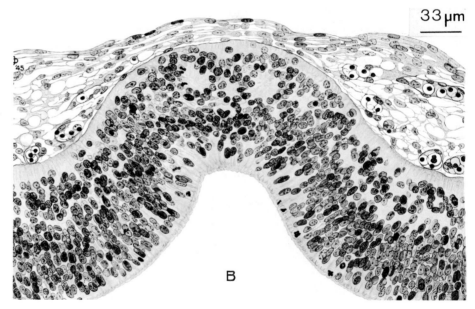

33 μm

Fig. 18-11. Sections through the roof of the third ventricle of two embryos belonging to stage 18, showing first steps in the formation of the "anterior lobe" of the epiphysis cerebri. Nuclei migrate externally from the ependymal stratum and form a mantle zone having a tendency to follicular arrangement of its cells. These minute follicles are not connected with the lumen of the evagination. The elongation of the epiphysial evagination into a duct is relatively backward, and follows rather than precedes the formation of the "anterior lobe." (A) No. 6527, section 11-3-4. (B) No. 7707, section 17-1-5. Drawing made by James F. Didusch.

Fig. 18-12 (facing page). (A–C) The retina at stages 16–18, showing the deposit of pigment granules in the external lamina as seen under a magnification of 1500. In A, only a few distinct granules and some refractive colorless droplets are visible. In B, the granules are more numerous and they show a tendency to cluster at the external surface. In C, a crust of granules is commonly visible on the external surface. In judging the amount of pigment, allowance must be made for section thickness. Angioblasts can be seen on the outer surface of the pigmented layer of the retina. At the bottom of the photographs is seen in each instance the inverted (neural) lamina of the retina. (A) No. 6507, 7-1-3, 10 μm. (B) No. 6520, 23-3-5, 10 μm. (C) No. 6528, 25-2-3, 8 μm.

(D) Section through an eye typical of stage 18. The migration to form the internal neuroblastic layer of the retina is now widespread. The cavity of the lens vesicle is reduced to a slit, with a corresponding building up of the body of lens fibers. One can see the characteristic distribution of lental nuclei and the fiber lines. It is to be noted that the mesenchyme has begun to invade the interval between lens epithelium and surface epithelium, a prelude to the formation of the cornea. Embryo No. 6527, section 19-3-5.

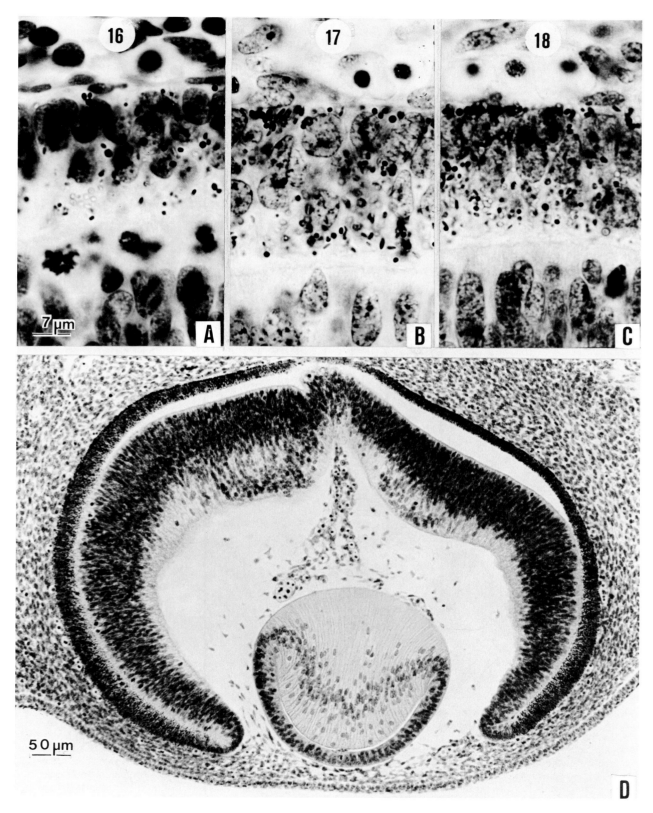

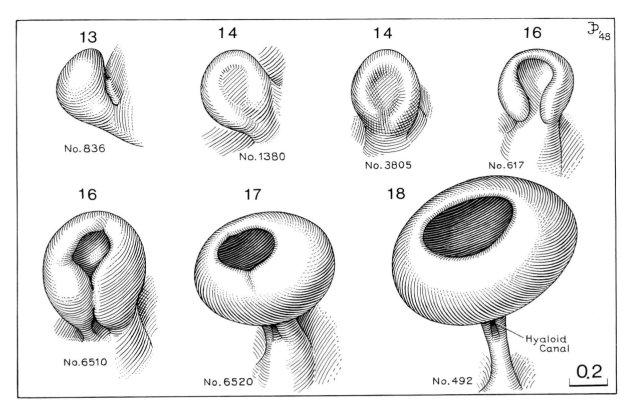

Fig. 18-13. Drawings of reconstructions of the optic vesicle and optic cup at stages 13–18. The drawings show steps in the growth and transformation of the optic vesicle into the optic cup, as well as the retinal fissure and the origin of the hyaloid canal. In the second specimen of stage 16, the rim of the optic cup can be seen to be polygonal.

cords. The presence of testicular cords in the gonadal blastema at stage 18 and of a tunica albuginea at stage 19 makes possible the determination of sexual differentiation in the male embryo.

A precise area of the coelomic epithelium, at the rostral end of the mesonephros, becomes thicker and invaginated to form the paramesonephric duct. The site of its infolding becomes the abdominal ostium of the uterine tube. In stage 18 the paramesonephric duct makes the principal part of its way down the front of the mesonephros, as a lateral companion to the mesonephric duct (fig. 18-7). The origin and rate of growth and elongation are precisely regulated, so that an additional clue to the level of development is provided. The duct tends to be straight, and its length can be calculated by multiplying the number of transverse sections by the thickness of each section. Alternatively, the length can be obtained by superimposing outlines of sagittal or coronal sections.

The paramesonephric ducts are present in all embryos of stage 18; their length was used by Streeter as an index of development within the stage. Of 35 specimens, a less advanced group of nineteen in which the length of the paramesonephric duct was 0.6 mm or less was distinguished from a more advanced group of sixteen specimens in which it was more than 0.6 mm. Most of the embryos in the first group range from 13 to 16.5 mm, whereas most of those in the second group are 14–17.2 mm in length.

In 34 embryos of stage 18, Streeter found that the length of the paramesonephric duct could be correlated with the level of development of other parts of the embryo. For example, in embryos in which only one semicircular duct had been pinched off in the membranous labyrinth, the paramesonephric duct ranged from 0.2 to 0.4 mm in length. Where two semicircular ducts were present, the range was 0.4–0.7 mm. Where three semicircular ducts were present, the range,

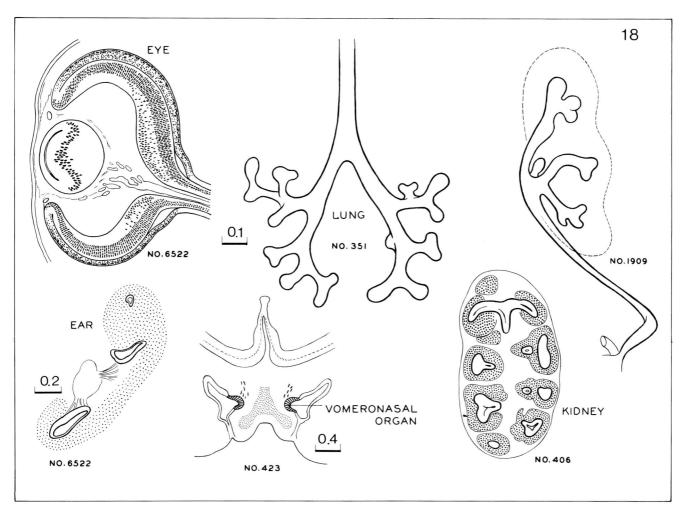

Fig. 18-14. Cluster of features characteristic of stage 18. In the eye the lens vesicle is reduced almost to a slit. The internal neuroblastic layer of the retina is widespread. The inner ear has from one to three semicircular ducts. A distinct vomeronasal organ is present. In the lung, some subsegmental buds are forming. In the kidney, the multiple calices have some sharply marked primordia of collecting tubules. As yet there are no definite glomeruli.

with but a few exceptions, was 0.8–1.1 mm in length (fig. 18-8). Hence, from the status of the paramesonephric duct, the degree of development of an organ as remote as the internal ear can be estimated.

NERVOUS SYSTEM
(fig. 18-10)

The most developed area of the brain is the rhombencephalon. The motor nuclei are better organized than the sensory. In the more advanced embryos the choroid plexus of the fourth ventricle begins to be identifiable by the presence of some villi. In the cerebellum, in addition to the inner cerebellar bulge present already in stage 17, an outer swelling appears and represents the future flocculus. Vestibulocerebellar fibers are present in great number at its surface. A clear distinction between auditory and optic colliculi in the midbrain as represented by Streeter has not been confirmed. In the diencephalon the neurohypophysis has folded walls. The adenohypophysis, open to the pharynx in stage 17, is now closed off from the pharyngeal cavity. An epithelial stalk, containing a faint lumen, is connected to the pharyngeal epithelium. The epiphysis, representing the "anterior lobe," is illustrated in figure 18-11. Sections of two specimens (A and B) belonging to the middle third of the embryos of stage 18 are shown. A pineal recess is forming for the first time, and a follicular arrangement of the cells may be encountered in some embryos. This "anterior lobe" of the epiphysis corresponds to Stadium III of Turkewitsch (O'Rahilly, 1968). The rostral part of the diencephalic roof is richly vascularized, and some ingrowth of the epithelial lamina at the level of the telencephalon indicates the first signs of a choroid plexus of the lateral ventricles. Approximately half of the length of the cerebral hemispheres now extends more rostrally than the lamina terminalis. A slight groove is developing in the corpus striatum, which has grown considerably and now reaches as far caudally as the preoptic sulcus. The olfactory bulb is better delimited and, in some embryos, contains an olfactory ventricle.

Eye
(figs. 18-12C,D, 18-13, and 18-14)

Mesenchyme invades the interval between the lens epithelium and the surface ectoderm (as may have already begun in the previous stage), and possibly the posterior epithelium of the cornea (the mesothelium of the anterior chamber) is forming. The cavity of the lens vesicle is becoming obliterated by primary lens fibers.

Reconstructions of the optic vesicle/optic cup at stages 13–18 are shown in figure 18-13.

Ear
(fig. 18-14)

The semicircular ducts form from thick epithelial areas of the membranous labyrinth. Adjacent epithelial layers fuse, lose their basement membrane, and disappear (O'Rahilly, 1963). From one to three semicircular ducts are formed during this stage, and the order is anterior, posterior, and lateral. The crus commune is evident from the beginning. The cochlear duct is L-shaped. The mesenchymal stapes (containing the stapedial artery) and the stapedius can be identified, and the bars of pharyngeal arches 1 and 2 may begin to chondrify.

INTRODUCTION TO STAGES 19–23

As the embryo advances into more-specialized levels, it becomes necessary to take into account the developmental status of various internal structures in order to assign the specimen precisely to a stage.

For stages 19–23, Streeter devised a system of rating the development of selected structures by "point scores." The eight features chosen were the cornea, optic nerve, cochlear duct, adenohypophysis, vomeronasal organ, submandibular gland, metanephros, and humerus. He regarded these as arbitrarily selected key structures that were readily recognizable under the microscope and that could be recorded by camera lucida sketches from serial sections.

The developmental points for a given embryo were added, and the resulting value was used to determine not only the stage (Table 19-1) but even the relative position within that stage.

Although Streeter's original data for the point scores for the various features of individual embryos are no longer available, the final score for each embryo that he studied at stages 19–23 is known and appears in the lists of embryos given here.

A detailed table showing the assignment of scoring

TABLE 19-1   Number of Developmental Points per Embryo

Stage	Range of Points
19	10–16.5
20	19–29.5
21	30–39
22	40.5–46
23	48–60.5

points is available in Streeter's work (1951, pp. 170 and 171) but is not reproduced here because of the considerable technical difficulty that would be involved in repeating Streeter's successful but rather personal procedure in a consistent manner. Moreover, some slight problems exist in the arrangement of the table, as it was printed. These may have been caused by the circumstance that the final version had to be prepared by others, namely Heuser and Corner.

It is to be stressed that considerable caution needs to be exercised in assigning a given embryo to stages 19–23, particularly in the absence of detailed studies of its internal structure. The external form of a new embryo should be compared in detail with Streeter's photographs (figs. 19-1, 20-1, etc.). The greatest length of the embryo should also be taken into account.

Stage 19 is not quite as difficult as the later stages to identify, because toe rays are prominent but interdigital notches have not yet appeared. The foot is still an important guide in later stages but difficulties may well be encountered in stages 20–22, such that it is frequently more prudent to conclude with a weak designation such as "approximately stage 20" or "stage 20–21" or "probably stage 22." Stage 23, at least at its full expression, is again less difficult to identify because of its more mature appearance. In addition, certain internal features, such as the status of the skeleton, are important guides for stages 19–23.

Some embryos from other laboratories have unfortunately been recorded in the literature as belonging to various specific stages without sufficiently detailed and careful examination of their structural features.

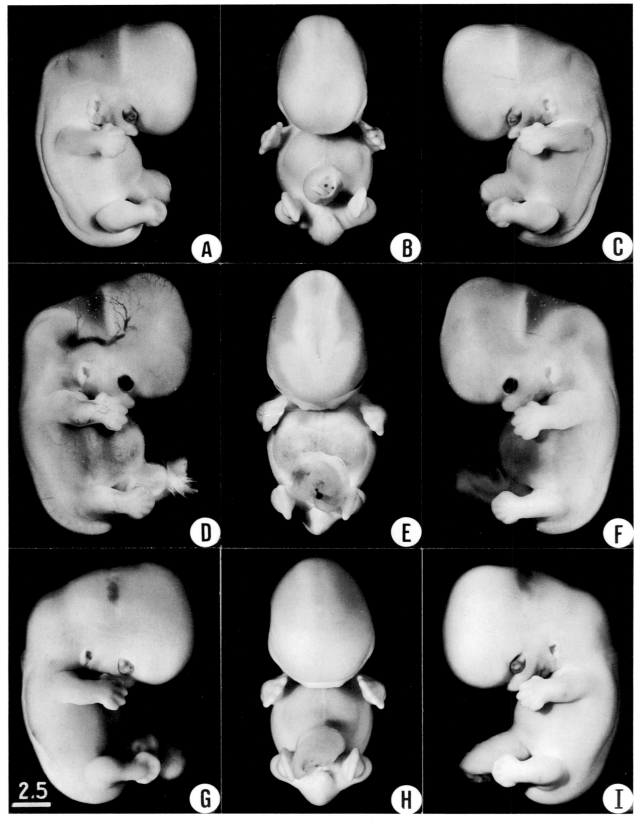

Fig. 19-1. Photographs of three embryos belonging to stage 19. The trunk is now beginning to straighten, and the cervical angulation is less acute. The coalescence of parts in the pharyngeal region has altered the appearance of the auricle, and the hillocks are less conspicuous. The longitudinal axes of the upper limbs are almost at a right angle to the dorsal contour of the body of the embryo, and the axes of the upper and lower limbs are more or less parallel, so that each limb has a pre-axial and a postaxial border. The transverse and sigmoid sinuses are prominent in D. The brain in E shows, from above downward, the mesencephalon, diencephalon, and cerebral hemispheres. Top row, No. 8092. Middle row, No. 6824. Bottom row, No. 4501. All views are at the same magnification.

STAGE 19

Most embryos of this stage measure 17–20 mm in length.

The age is believed to be approximately 47–48 post-ovulatory days. One embryo (No. 1390) is known to be "exactly 47 days" (Mall, 1918), although another appears to have been only 41 days (Moore, Hutchins, and O'Rahilly, 1981).

EXTERNAL FORM

The trunk has begun to elongate and straighten slightly, with the result that the head no longer forms a right angle with the line of the back of the embryo. The limbs extend nearly directly forward. The toe rays are more prominent, but interdigital notches have not yet appeared in the rim of the foot plate.

FEATURES FOR POINT SCORES

1. Cornea. A thin layer of mesenchyme crosses the summit of the cornea (Streeter, 1951, fig. 14). General views of the eye at stages 13–23 are shown in figures 19-2 and 19-3, and at stages 19–23 in figure 19-5.

2. Optic nerve. The optic nerve is slender (fig. 19-4). Nerve fibers can be traced for a short distance beyond the retina but have not yet reached the middle region of the stalk.

3. Cochlear duct. The tip of the L-shaped cochlear duct turns "upward" (fig. 19-6).

4. Adenohypophysis. The pars intermedia is beginning to be established, as well as the lateral lobes that will form the pars tuberalis (fig. 19-7). The stalk is relatively thick and contains the remains of the lumen of the hypophysial sac. Transverse views of the gland at stages 19–23 are shown in figure 19-8.

5. Vomeronasal organ. The vomeronasal organ is a thickening of the nasal epithelium that still bounds a shallow groove or pit (fig. 19-9).

6. Submandibular gland. The primordium of the submandibular gland is present in stage 18 as an epithelial thickening in the groove between the tongue and the future lower jaw. In stage 19, an area of condensed mesenchyme appears beneath the duct (fig. 19-10 and Streeter, 1951, fig. 24).

7. Metanephros. In many areas the metanephrogenic tissue around the ampullae of the collecting tubules remains undifferentiated but, in others, nodules become separated from the metanephrogenic mantle (fig. 19-11). In some of these, small cavities have appeared, transforming them into renal vesicles.

8. Humerus. Differentiation of chondrocytes had already progressed to phase 3 by stage 18, and phases 1–3 continue to be present in stages 19 and 20 (Streeter, 1949, fig. 3 and plate 2). The middle of the shaft is becoming clearer. Although no sign is present in the humerus, ossification begins in the clavicle and mandible in one of the stages from 18 to 20, and in the maxilla at stage 19 or stage 20 (O'Rahilly and Gardner, 1972).

ADDITIONAL FEATURES

Blood vascular system. The arterial system has been depicted by Evans in Keibel and Mall (1912, fig. 447). Excellent views of reconstructions of the aortic arches at stages 11–19 were published by Congdon (1922, figs. 29–40).

Heart. The ventricles are situated ventral to the atria, so that a horizontal section corresponds approximately to a coronal section of the adult organ. Such a section has been reproduced by Cooper and O'Rahilly (1971, fig. 1), who also provided an account of several features of the heart at stages 19–21. Fusion of the aortic and mitral endocardial cushion material occurs at stage 19

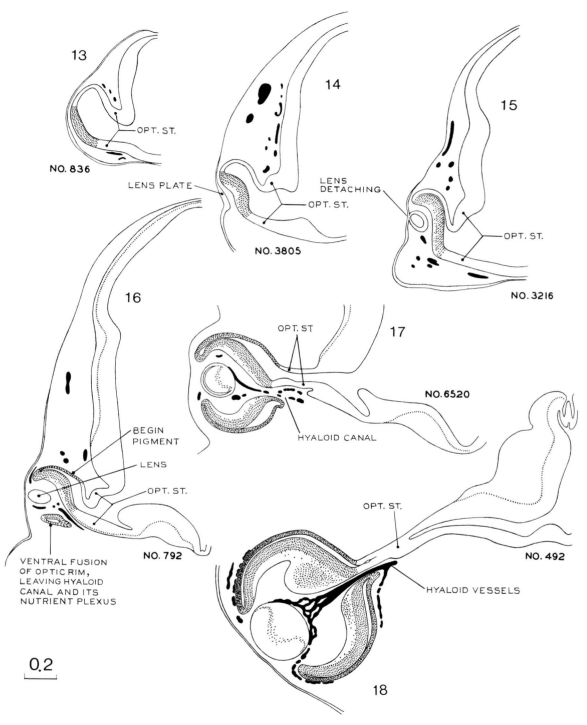

Fig. 19-2. Drawings of sections through the optic vesicle/cup and stalk at stages 13–18. As the optic vesicle is being transformed into the optic cup, the inverted (neural) lamina of the retina retains direct connection at all times with the wall of the brain. At stages 13–17 the optic ventricle communicates freely with the cavity of the diencephalon. The body of the lens is thickening and, in stage 18, the primary fibers fill the lumen of the lens.

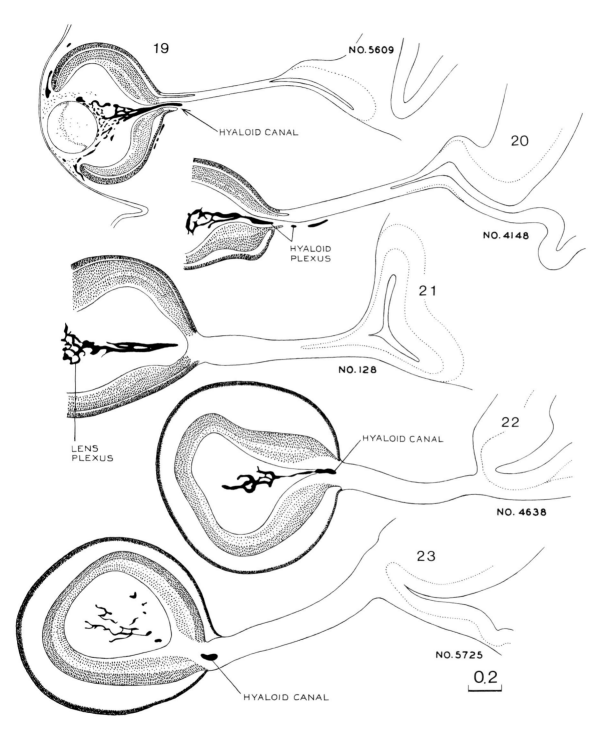

Fig. 19-3. A continuation of the previous illustration, showing the eye and optic nerve at stages 19–23. Several sections in each embryo were combined to show the form of the optic nerve. All drawings in this and in the previous figure are at the same scale.

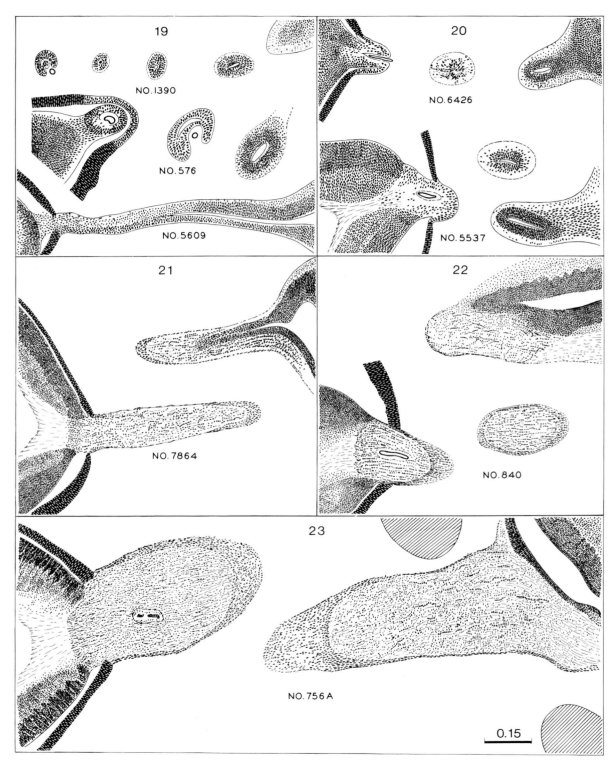

Fig. 19-4. Drawings of sections showing the form of the optic nerve and the progressive spread of nerve fibers from retina to brain. Some fibers have grown through the whole tract (which really is the so-called optic nerve) and are arriving at the brain at stage 20. In the more advanced stages many (neuro-ectodermal, including glial) cells are seen in longitudinal rows between bundles of nerve fibers. All drawings are at the same scale, which is slightly less than twice that of the previous two figures.

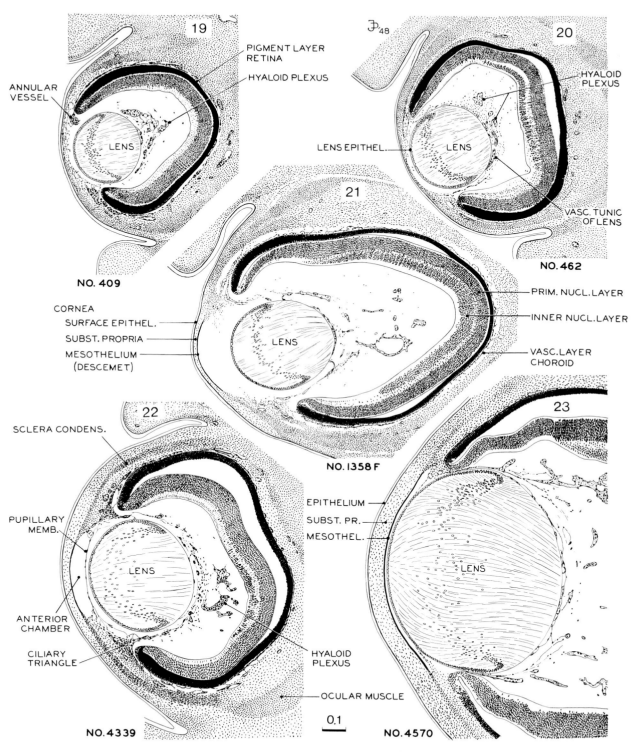

Fig. 19-5. Drawings of mid-sections of the eye at stages 19–23. The sections were selected to demonstrate the organization and relations of the various parts of the eye. The lens remains nearly spherical throughout this period and occupies a relatively large amount of the eye. The pupillary membrane is developing and the anterior chamber is emerging (stage 22). The hyaloid plexus partly fills the vitreous chamber and forms a network on the back of the lens. All drawings are at the same scale.

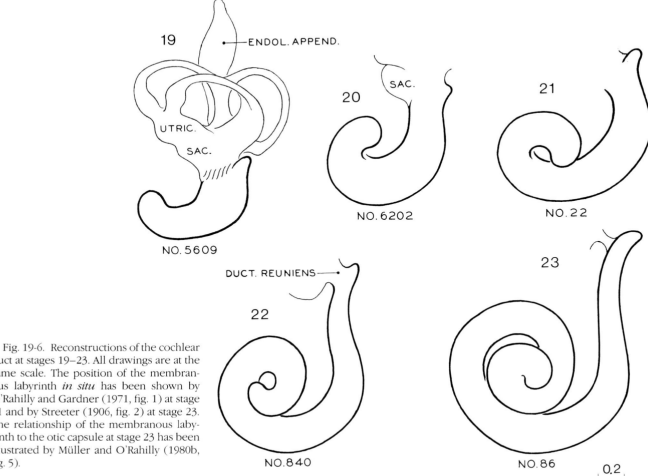

Fig. 19-6. Reconstructions of the cochlear duct at stages 19–23. All drawings are at the same scale. The position of the membranous labyrinth *in situ* has been shown by O'Rahilly and Gardner (1971, fig. 1) at stage 21 and by Streeter (1906, fig. 2) at stage 23. The relationship of the membranous labyrinth to the otic capsule at stage 23 has been illustrated by Müller and O'Rahilly (1980b, fig. 5).

(Teal, Moore, and Hutchins, 1986).

Lungs. The bronchial tree was reconstructed by Wells and Boyden (1954, plates 3 and 4). The first generation of subsegmental bronchi is now complete.

Cloacal region. The cloacal membrane ruptures from urinary pressure at stage 18 or stage 19, and the anal membrane becomes defined.

Gonads. The rete testis develops from the seminiferous cords at stages 19–23, and the tunica albuginea forms (Jirásek, 1971). Cords representing the rete ovarii are also developing (Wilson, 1926a).

Sternum. Right and left sternal bars, which are joined cranially to form the episternal cartilage, are present by stage 19 (Gasser, 1975, figs. 7-17 and 7-22).

Brain. A general view of the organ was given by Gilbert (1957, fig. 18), and certain internal details were provided by Hines (1922, figs. 15 and 16).

In the rhombencephalon the migration for the formation of the olivary and arcuate nuclei has begun. In most embryos the choroid plexus of the fourth ventricle is now present. In median sections the paraphysis marks the limit between diencephalic and telencephalic roof. A characteristic wedge appearance of the "anterior lobe" of the epiphysis is found (O'Rahilly, 1968). The stria medullaris thalami reaches the habenular nuclei. The habenular commissure may begin to develop. Half of the length of the cerebral hemispheres reaches further rostrally than the lamina terminalis, and half of the diencephalon is covered by them. The occipital pole of the hemisphere can be distinguished caudally and ventrolaterally. The internal capsule begins to develop.

EMBRYO OF STAGE 19 ALREADY DESCRIBED

Harvard No. 839, 17.8 mm G.L. Described and illustrated in monographic form by Thyng (1914).

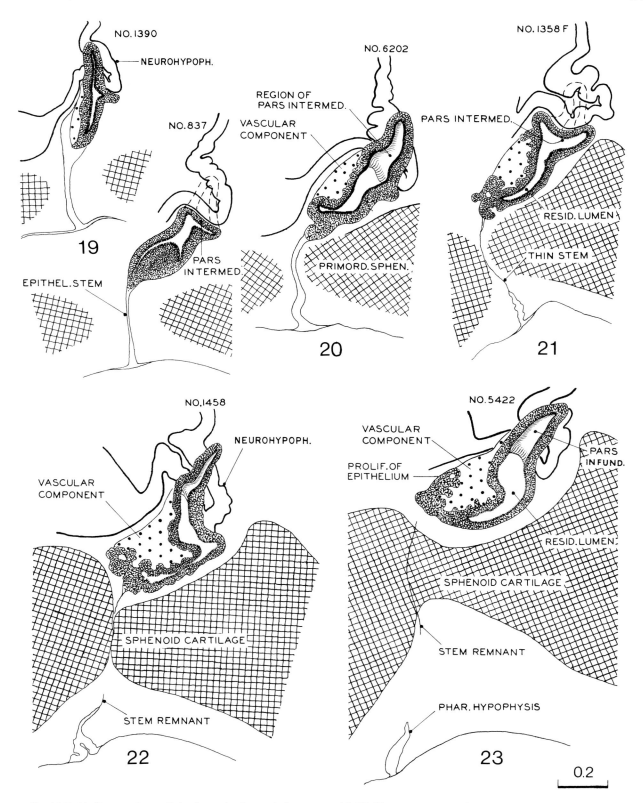

Fig. 19-7. Median sections of the hypophysis cerebri at stages 19–23. Two or more sections were combined in preparing the drawings. Several sections were used to represent the lateral processes of the pars intermedia, which grow dorsally around the sides of the infundibular stem to form the pars infundibularis (or tuberalis). All drawings are at the same scale.

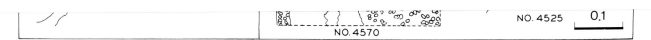

Fig. 19-9. Drawings from sections of the vomeronasal organ at stages 19–23. All drawings are at the same scale.

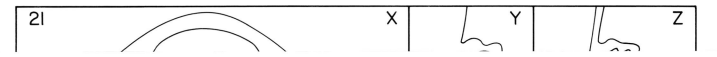

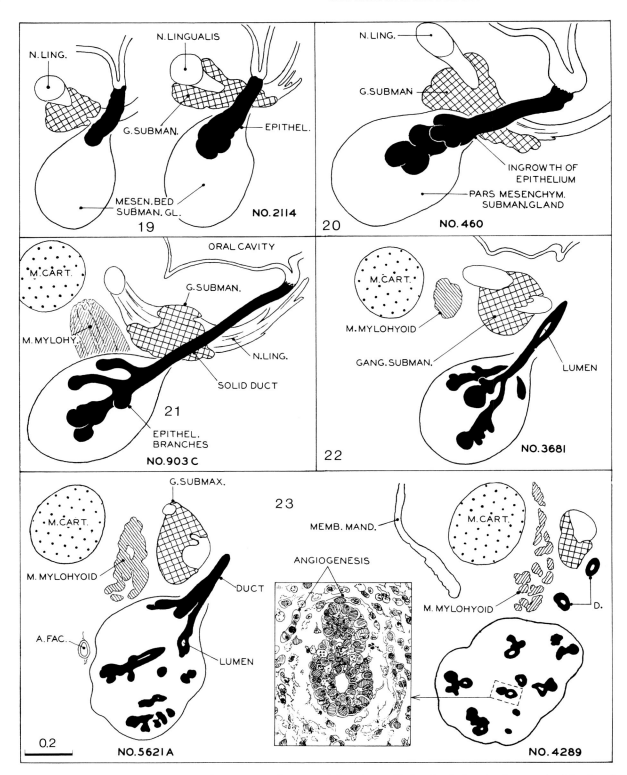

Fig. 19-10. Semidiagrammatic drawings of the submandibular gland, showing the growth of the ductal system into the mesodermal component at stages 19–23. All drawings (except the inset) are at the same scale.

Legends for Figs. 19-11 and 19-12 (printed on next two pages):

Fig. 19-11. Semidiagrammatic drawings showing the origin and development of the tubules in the metanephros at stages 19–21. Practically all the embryos of stage 19 show the beginning formation of renal vesicles. Most of the specimens of stage 20 have S-shaped lumina in the vesicles, and spoon-shaped capsules have appeared in a few of the more advanced members of the group. The tubules in stage 21 show a wider range of development because new ones are being added peripherally; at the same time, those first established continue to differentiate.

Fig. 19-12. A continuation of the previous illustration, showing the further development of the metanephros at stages 22 and 23. More large glomeruli have appeared, and short secretory tubules are present in nearly all specimens. By the end of the period, tubules of the fourth or fifth generation have formed. All drawings in this and in the previous figure are at the same scale.

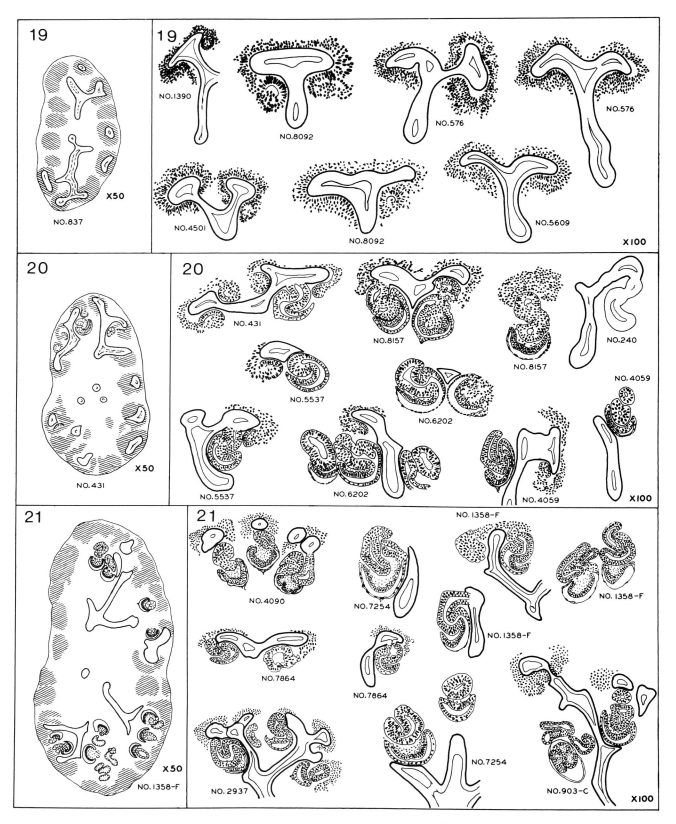

Figs. 19-11 and 19-12. Legends on preceding page.

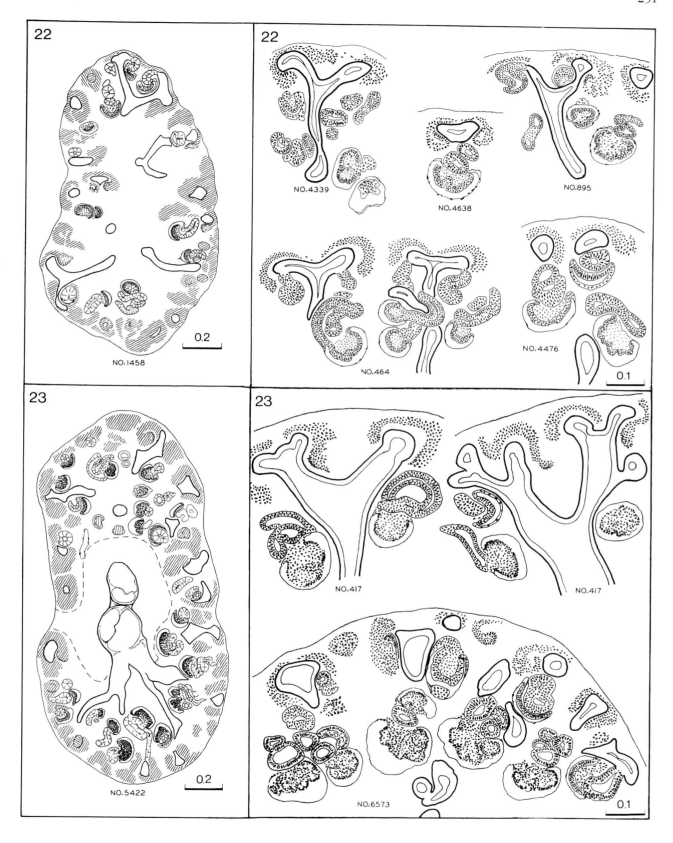

22

NO. 1458

0.2

22

NO.4339

NO.4638

NO.895

NO.464

NO.4476

0.1

23

NO.5422

0.2

23

NO.417

NO.417

NO.6573

0.1

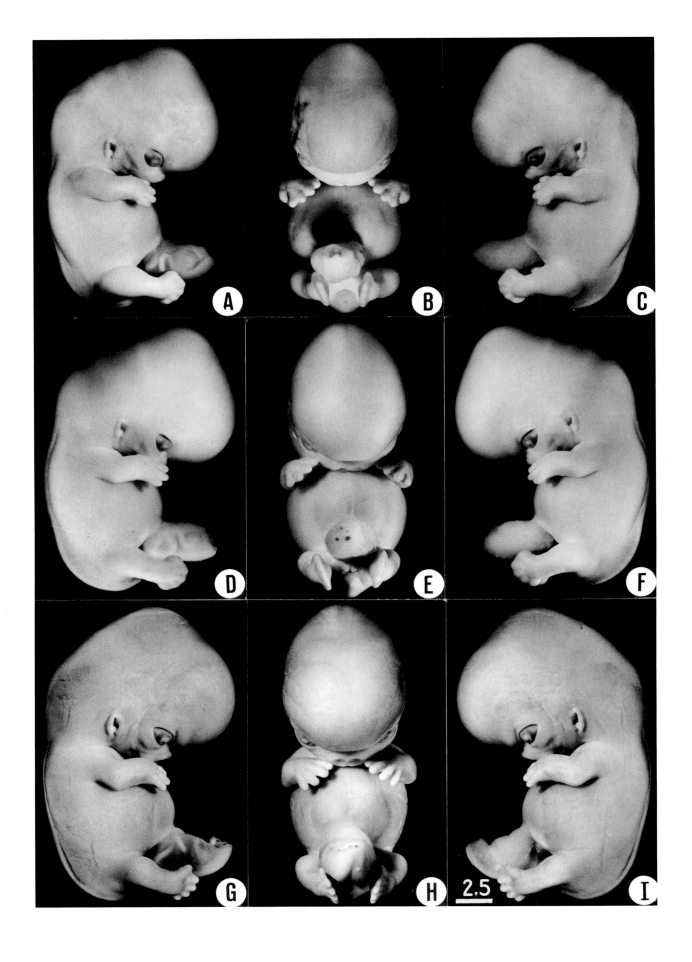

STAGE 20

SIZE AND AGE

Most embryos of stage 20 measure 21–23 mm in length.

The age is believed to be approximately 50–51 post-ovulatory days.

EXTERNAL FORM

Details of internal structures may now be obscured from surface view because of the thickening mesoderm, except in fresh or formalin-fixed specimens. Thus the cerebellum is no longer distinct as seen from the surface (fig. 20-1).

The upper limbs have increased in length and become slightly bent at the elbows (fig. 20-1). The hands with their short, stubby fingers are still far apart, but they are curving slightly over the cardiac region and approach the lateral margins of the nose.

A delicate, fringe-like vascular plexus now appears in the superficial tissues of the head (fig. 20-2). In the temporofrontal region a growth center arches over the eye, and in the occipital region a second growth center occurs above the ear. The edge of the plexus is approximately halfway between the eye-ear level and the vertex of the head.

FEATURES FOR POINT SCORES

1. Cornea. The developing cornea comprises the anterior epithelium, an acellular postepithelial layer (the future substantia propria), and the posterior epithelium.

2. Optic nerve. Few nerve fibers are present. A lumen may still extend along practically the whole length of the stalk, but it is becoming obliterated (O'Rahilly, 1966, fig. 49).

3. Cochlear duct. The tip of the duct, having grown "upward," now proceeds "horizontally" (fig. 19-6).

4. Adenohypophysis. The stalk is long and slender. Capillaries are appearing in the mesoderm at the rostral surface of the adenohypophysis.

5. Vomeronasal organ. The vomeronasal organ appears as a shallow, blind sac with a broad opening (fig. 19-9).

6. Submandibular gland. The duct is longer and knobby and is situated well within the gland (fig. 19-10).

7. Metanephros. The renal vesicles are developing S-shaped lumina (fig. 19-11).

8. Humerus. The appearances are transitional between those of stages 19 and 21 (Streeter, 1949, fig. 3).

ADDITIONAL FEATURES

Blood vascular system. The arteries and veins have been illustrated by Blechschmidt (1963, plate 37).

Digestive system. A reconstruction of the pharynx and adjacent endocrine glands was published by Weller (1933, plate 1), ones of the alimentary canal by Shikinami (1926, plate 3) and by Blechschmidt (1963, plate 44).

Larynx. Three photomicrographs were published by Tucker and O'Rahilly (1972, figs. 14–16).

Urinary system. A reconstruction of the urinary system has been published by Shikinami (1926, fig. 5).

Fig. 20-1 (facing page). Photographs of three embryos belonging to stage 20. A slight bend is present at the elbow, and the hands are curving medially over the cardiac region. Top row, No. 7274. Middle row, No. 7906. Bottom row, No. 8157. All views are at the same magnification.

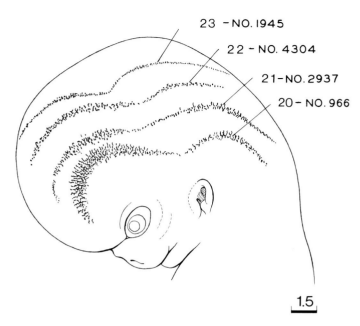

23 – NO. 1945
22 – NO. 4304
21 – NO. 2937
20 – NO. 966

1.5

Fig. 20-2. Composite drawing showing the edge of the superficial vascular plexus in the head at stages 20–23. A subcutaneous capillary plexus that spreads upward toward the vertex of the head is a conspicuous feature of specimens measuring from about 20–24 mm in length. The transition from vascular to avascular mesoderm is more gradual in earlier stages and becomes more abrupt later.

The external surface of the metanephros is said to be slightly lobulated.

Testis. From stage 20 onward the testis is said to be elliptical and have a smooth surface (Lee, 1971). It contains short, straight tubules surrounded by a darkly stained mesenchymal sheath and the rete testis. The tunica albuginea appears to be continuous with the coelomic epithelium.

Ovary. From stage 20 onward the ovary is said to be cylindrical and have a coarse surface (Lee, 1971). The presence of an ovary is first determined *per exclusionem* and not earlier than stage 20. Cord-like structures are absent from the cortex, and the surface epithelium shows no sign of development into a tunica albuginea. The ovary consists of "a mass of undifferentiated oogonia" (Wilson, 1926a) intermingled with fusiform mesenchymal cells and intermediate pre-granulosa cells (Lee, 1971), and covered by the surface epithelium.

Skeletal system. Skeletal development and the muscular system have been illustrated by Blechschmidt (1963, plates 36 and 38). The skull has been described and illustrated by Lewis (1920).

Brain. A general view of the organ can be seen in Lewis (1920, plate 3, fig. 8), and certain internal details were provided by Hines (1922, fig. 17). The nervous system as a whole was illustrated by Blechschmidt (1963, plate 35).

The hemispheres now cover two-thirds of the diencephalon. The inferior colliculus of the mesencephalon can be discerned (Bartelmez and Dekaban, 1962). Some optic fibers reach the optic chiasma. The choroid plexus of the lateral ventricles is present. The primordium of the falx cerebri begins to form (O'Rahilly and Müller, 1986b).

Eye. The lens cavity is obliterated and a lens suture begins to form.

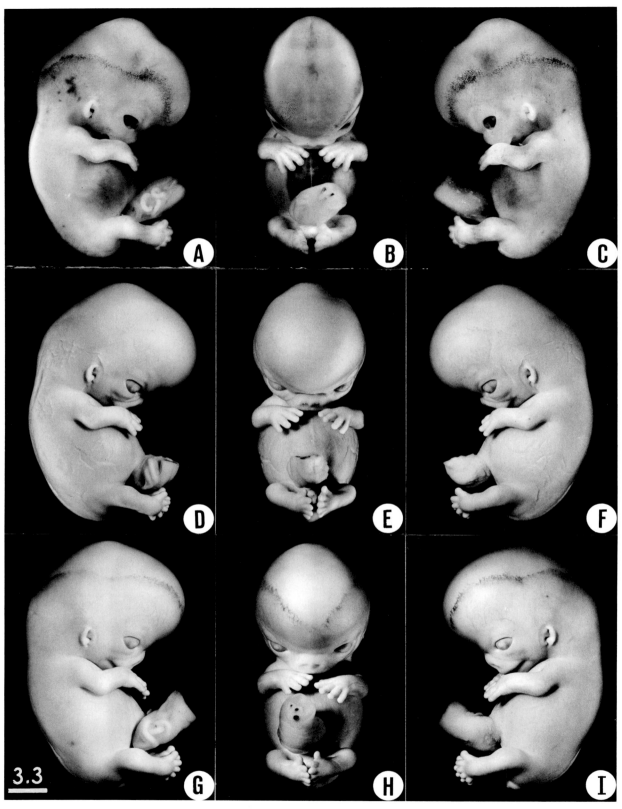

3.3

Fig. 21-1. Photographs of three embryos belonging to stage 21. The superficial vascular plexus of the head is plainly visible in several of these views, such as A. It has spread to a level more than halfway between an eye-ear line and the vertex of the head. The fingers are longer and show an early phase in the development of touch pads. These *Tastballen* are shown at higher magnification by Cummins (1929) at stage 20 (his fig. 7) and stage 22 (his fig. 8). The hands are flexed at the wrists and are approaching each other over the cardiac region. The lower limbs are curving toward the median plane, and toes of the two feet make contact with each other in some specimens. Top row, No. 4090. Middle row, No. 8553. Bottom row, No. 7392. All views are at the same magnification.

STAGE 21

Most embryos of this stage measure 22–24 mm.

The age is believed to be approximately 52 post-ovulatory days.

External Form

The superficial vascular plexus of the head has spread upward to form a line at somewhat more than half the distance from eye-ear level to the vertex.

The fingers are longer and extend further beyond the ventral body wall than they did in the previous stage. The distal phalangeal portions appear slightly swollen and show the beginning of tactile pads. The hands are slightly flexed at the wrists and nearly come together over the cardiac eminence. The feet are also approaching each other, and the toes of the two sides sometimes touch.

Features for Point Scores

1. Cornea. Cells are beginning to invade the post-epithelial layer, converting it into the substantia propria (Streeter, 1951, fig. 16).

2. Optic nerve. Remnants of ependyma are present and may extend along practically the whole length of the optic stalk. A hyaloid groove is visible at the bulbar end. A few nerve fibers are arriving at the brain.

3. Cochlear duct. The tip of the duct now points definitely "downward" (fig. 19-6).

4. Adenohypophysis. The thread-like stalk is beginning to be absorbed (fig. 19-7).

5. Vomeronasal organ. The opening of the sac is reduced in size, a short, narrow neck is present, and the end of the sac is expanded (fig. 19-9).

6. Submandibular gland. The duct has begun to form knob-like branches (fig. 19-10).

7. Metanephros. Spoon-shaped glomerular capsules are developing, but no large glomeruli are present yet (fig. 19-11).

8. Humerus. Cartilaginous phases 1–4 are present (Streeter, 1949, figs. 3, 19, and 20).

Additional Features

Heart. Some photomicrographs were reproduced by Cooper and O'Rahilly (1971, figs. 15–17).

Testis. The testis shows a flattened surface epithelium, an underlying tunica albuginea, and branching and anastomosing cords: "the forerunners of the seminiferous tubules" (Wilson, 1926a).

Brain. A general view of the organ was given by O'Rahilly and Gardner (1971, fig. 1).

The olivary nucleus is present in the rhombencephalon. Three-quarters of the surface of the diencephalon is covered by the cerebral hemispheres. The optic tract reaches approximately the site of the lateral geniculate body. The insula can now be recognized as a faint concavity at the surface of the hemisphere.

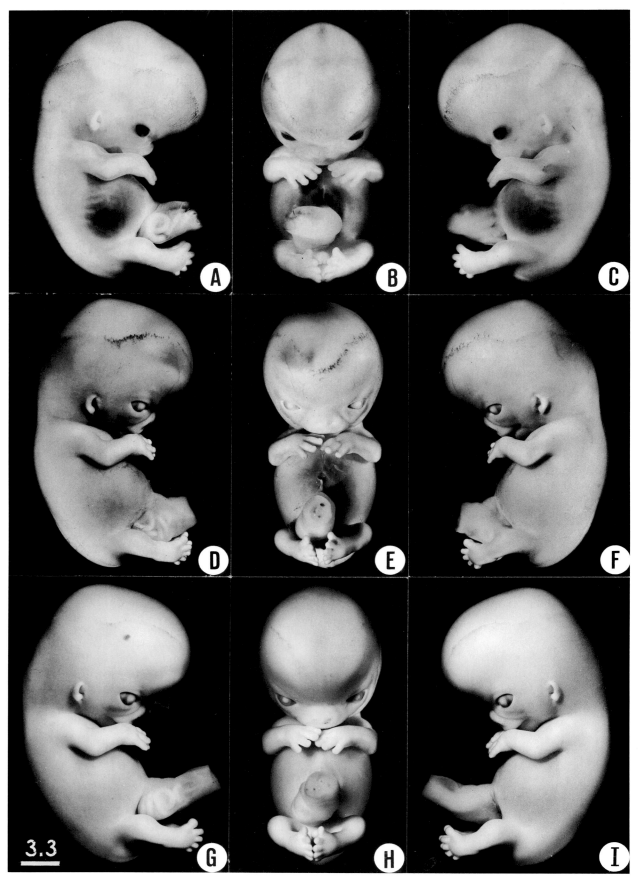

Fig. 22-1. Photographs of three embryos belonging to stage 22. The eyes are more than half covered by the eyelids. The limbs have increased in length, and the digits touch or overlap. Top row, No. 6701. Middle row, No. 6832. Bottom row, No. 8394. All views are at the same magnification.

STAGE 22

SIZE AND AGE

The middle group of embryos of this stage measure 25–27 mm in length.

The age is believed to be approximately 54 postovulatory days.

EXTERNAL FORM

The eyelids, which have been thickening gradually, are now rapidly encroaching upon the eyes. The formation of the auricle has progressed noticeably: the tragus and antitragus especially are assuming a more definite form. The superficial vascular plexus of the head extends upward about three-quarters of the way above the eye-ear level. The hands extend further out in front of the body of the embryo, and the fingers of one hand may overlap those of the other.

FEATURES FOR POINT SCORES

1. Cornea. The cellular invasion of the postepithelial layer is complete centrally in some eyes (Streeter, 1951, fig. 17). A scleral condensation is now definite (Gilbert, 1957).

2. Optic nerve. The mesenchyme surrounding the optic nerve forms a definite sheath.

3. Cochlear duct. The tip of the duct points "upward" for the second time (fig. 19-6).

4. Adenohypophysis. Remnants of the incomplete stalk are present at each end (fig. 19-7).

5. Vomeronasal organ. The appearances are intermediate between those of stages 21 and 23 (fig. 19-9).

6. Submandibular gland. The duct shows secondary branches. It is practically solid but a suggestion of a lumen can be found in its oral part (fig. 19-10).

7. Metanephros. A few large glomeruli are present (fig. 19-12).

8. Humerus. Cartilaginous phases 1–4 are still present (Streeter, 1949, figs. 3 and 15–17). The formation of osteoblasts is beginning. A bony collar appears in the humerus, radius, ulna, and femur and tibia during stages 22 and 23 (O'Rahilly and Gardner, 1972).

ADDITIONAL FEATURES

Blood vascular system. The aortic arch system has been illustrated by Boyd (1937, fig. 1).

Heart. Reconstructions of the atrial region were reproduced by Licata (1954, figs. 4 and 5). Chordae tendineae begin to form at stages 22 and 23 (Magovern, Moore, and Hutchins, 1986).

Paramesonephric ducts. The paramesonephric ducts lie side-by-side caudally and show rostral vertical, middle transverse, and caudal vertical portions.

Brain. A general view of the organ was given by Hochstetter (1919, fig. 42).

The superior and inferior colliculi of the midbrain are indicated by their lamination (Bartelmez and De-kaban, 1962). The epithalamus is individualized by the presence of the sulcus dorsalis. In the hemispheres the cortical plate begins to appear.

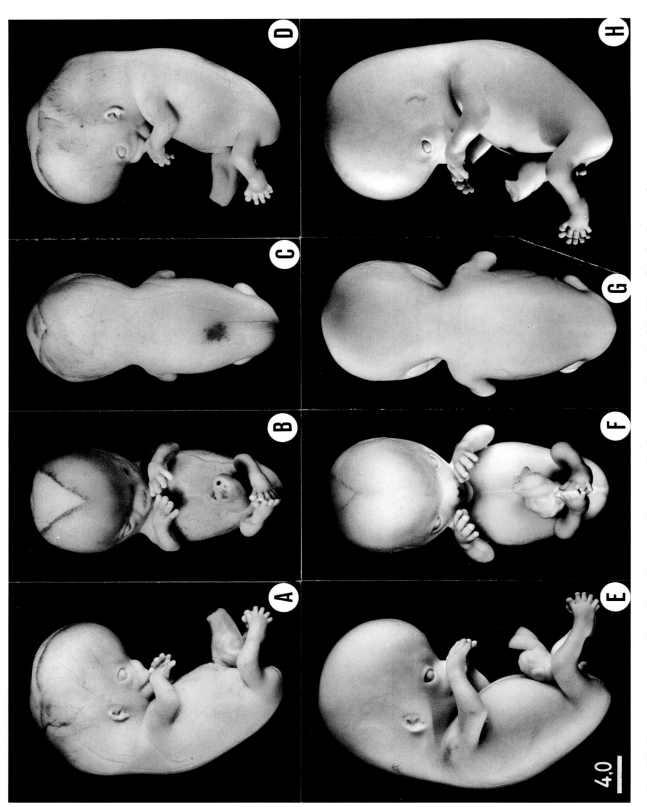

Fig. 23-1. Photographs of two embryos belonging to stage 23. The superficial vascular plexus of the head has spread nearly to the vertex. A considerable growth in length of the limbs has occurred during the past 2 days. The forearm is sometimes raised to a level above that of the shoulder (H), and the hands extend far out in front of the trunk. "Praying feet" are visible in B and F. Upper row, No. 7425. Lower row, No. 4570. All views are at the same magnification.

4.0

STAGE 23

SIZE AND AGE

The middle group of embryos of stage 23 measure 28–30 mm in length but the full range extends from 23 to 32 mm.

The age is believed to be approximately 56–57 post-ovulatory days (Olivier and Pineau, 1962), and not 47 days, as thought formerly on the basis of comparisons with the rhesus monkey. It should be emphasized that the ages of human embryos cannot be obtained "by matching the specimens against macaque embryos of known ovulation age having a similar degree of development" (Streeter, 1942). In point of fact, the rhesus monkey (*Macaca mulatta*) develops more rapidly during the embryonic period, such that stage 23 is reached at or before 7 weeks (Hendrickx and Sawyer, 1975; Gribnau and Geijsberts, 1981), compared to 8 weeks in the human. That a 30-mm human embryo may be expected to have an age of 8 postovulatory weeks has been confirmed ultrasonically *in vivo* (Drumm and O'Rahilly, 1977).

EXTERNAL FORM

The head has made rapid progress in its bending toward the erect position. The head is distinctly rounded out, and the cervical region and trunk are of a more mature shape. The eyelids may show some fusion laterally and medially, but the eyes may be largely open (fig. 23-1E). Streeter (1942) had originally intended to extend his staging system "up to fetuses between 32 and 38 mm long, the stage at which the eyelids have come together."

The limbs have increased markedly in length and show more-advanced differentiation of their subdivisions. The forearm ascends to or above the level of the shoulder.

The superficial vascular plexus is rapidly approaching the vertex of the head, leaving only a small non-vascular area that will soon become bridged by anastomosing branches.

The external genitalia are well developed but do not suffice for the detection of sex. In particular, some males tend to be diagnosed as females (Wilson, 1926b). Only in fetuses of about 50 mm is it safe to make an assessment.

FEATURES FOR POINT SCORES

1. Cornea. The cornea now comprises the anterior epithelium and its basement membrane, the substantia propria, and the posterior epithelium (Streeter, 1951, fig. 18, and O'Rahilly, 1966, figs. 51 and 59).

2. Optic nerve. The sheath is quite distinct, at least in the more advanced specimens (O'Rahilly, 1966, fig. 55). A vascular canal is present.

3. Cochlear duct. The tip of the duct, having proceeded "horizontally" again, now points "downward" for the second time (fig. 19-6). The duct is coiled to nearly its final extent of 2½ turns.

4. Adenohypophysis. Scant trace of the stalk remains (fig. 19-7). Lobules of epithelium project into the mesodermal component of the gland, and oriented epithelial follicles are present (Streeter, 1951, plate 2). Abundant angioblasts and capillaries are found.

5. Vomeronasal organ. A narrow canal is seen in the long, tapering duct. The sac is beginning to shrink and retrogress (fig. 19-9).

6. Submandibular gland. Lumina are found in many terminal branches of the duct (fig. 19-10). Orientation of the epithelial tree is beginning, and angiogenesis is commencing around the epithelium. A mesodermal sheath is beginning to form around the gland.

7. Metanephros. The secretory tubules are changing from short to long, and becoming more convoluted. The epithelium in some tubules is high. Renal tubules of fourth and fifth orders are present. Large glomeruli are numerous (fig. 19-12).

8. Humerus. All five cartilaginous phases are now present (Streeter, 1949, figs. 3 and 18).

Stage 23 marks the end of the embryonic period proper, as defined by Streeter. The arbitrary but useful criterion that he used was the replacement of the cartilage of the humerus by bone marrow. "If the onset can be recognized in a given specimen, that specimen is straightway classed as a fetus." A drawing of a photomicrograph showing this process in a 34-mm fetus was provided by Streeter (1949, fig. 6).

ADDITIONAL FEATURES

Blood vascular system. The left superior vena cava is obliterated during stages 21–23 (McBride, Moore, and Hutchins, 1981).

Heart. The heart has been described in some detail by Licata (1954), and the nerve supply and conducting system were investigated by Gardner and O'Rahilly (1976b).

Palate. The palate at stages 18–23 has been described and classified by Waterman and Meller (1974), and the palate at stages 19–23 has been studied by Diewert (1981). According to the latter, in half of embryos of stage 23 the palatal shelves have made contact and "epithelial adhesion in the midpalatal region" is present.

Intestine. Although nerves reach the extremity of the intestinal loop, fibers are not yet anchored to the visceral musculature (Bossy, 1981).

Larynx. The larynx has been reconstructed and described by Müller, O'Rahilly, and Tucker (1981, 1985).

Diaphragm. The diaphragm and adjacent abdominal organs have been illustrated by Wells (1954, fig. 33).

Mesonephros. A detailed study of, and comparison between, the mesonephros and the metanephros in staged embryos is unfortunately lacking.

Metanephros. The kidneys have ascended from a sacral level at stages 13–15 to a lumbar level at stages 17–23. At stage 23 they are generally at the level of lumbar vertebrae 1–3 (Müller and O'Rahilly, 1986a).

Suprarenal gland. The development of the suprarenal gland at stages 13–23 was studied in detail by Crowder (1957).

Testis. Testicular tubules are identifiable. The rete testis makes contact, but no actual union with the mesonephric elements has occurred yet (Wilson, 1926a).

Clusters of cells have started their differentiation into interstitial cells.

Ovary. The rete ovarii is closely related to but not united with the mesonephric elements (Wilson, 1926a).

Paramesonephric ducts. The paramesonephric ducts meet the urogenital sinus and fuse with each other in the median plane (Koff, 1933; Pillet, 1968). The sinusal tubercle has appeared.

Skull. The chondrocranium has been reconstructed and described in detail by Müller and O'Rahilly (1980b). In the more advanced specimens, ossification may commence in several skeletal elements of the skull, and also in the scapula and distal phalanges of the hand (O'Rahilly and Gardner, 1972).

Vertebrae. The vertebral column has been studied by O'Rahilly, Müller, and Meyer (1980, 1983). Either 33 or 34 cartilaginous vertebrae are present. Spinous processes have not yet developed, so that a general appearance of total spina bifida occulta is given.

Joints. Stages 22 and 23 were included in Moffett's (1957) study of the temporomandibular joint. In the more advanced embryos, cavitation may have begun in the shoulder, elbow, wrist, hip, knee, and ankle joints (O'Rahilly and Gardner, 1975).

Brain. A general view of the organ was given by Gilbert (1957, fig. 22), and the cranial nerves were included by Müller and O'Rahilly (1980b, fig. 10).

The rhombencephalon by now shows a very advanced organization, and it presents striking resemblances to that of the newborn. In the cerebellum the external granular layer begins to develop on the rostral surface. Some of the cerebellar commissures have appeared. In the diencephalon the thin roof represents tela choroidea of the third ventricle. The interventricular foramen is reduced to a dorsoventral slit. The cerebral hemispheres cover almost the whole lateral surface of the diencephalon. The brain is now surrounded by loose tissue that is the forerunner of the subarachnoid space (O'Rahilly and Müller, 1986b). Most of the cisternae of the adult are already present.

Spinal cord. The general appearance of the spinal cord and spinal ganglia as a whole has been illustrated by O'Rahilly, Müller, and Meyer (1980, figs. 3–5).

Cutaneous innervation of the limbs. The sequence follows the proximodistal development of the external form but with a delay of 1–2 stages. At stage 23, the exploratory buds have reached the tips of the fingers and almost those of the toes (Bossy, 1982).

Eye. The retina comprises the pigmented layer, external limiting membrane, proliferative zone, external neuroblastic layer, transient fiber layer, internal neuroblastic layer, nerve fiber layer, and internal limiting membrane (O'Rahilly, 1966, fig. 53). The secondary vitrous body and secondary lens fibers are forming.

Ear. A detailed account of the middle and internal ear in embryos at the later stages is unfortunately lacking. The otic capsule at stage 23 has been reconstructed by Müller and O'Rahilly (1980b, fig. 5).

EMBRYONIC VS. FETAL PERIOD

The distinction between the embryonic and the fetal periods at 8 postovulatory weeks has proved valuable. It is based primarily on the probability that more than 90 percent of the more than 4,500 named structures of the adult body have appeared by that time (O'Rahilly, 1979). Nevertheless, it is not to be denied that this useful distinction is arbitrary and that alternative divisions of prenatal life are feasible. For example, based largely on mathematical and hormonal criteria (teratogenetic data are totally unconvincing in this regard), it has been argued that *"la période embryonnaire paraît bien s'étendre de la fécondation à la fin du 3ème mois et qu'on peut y démarquer un premier sous-stade de 45j allant jusqu'à la 1ère ébauche typiquement humaine ([Carnegie stage] 18 ou 19C); et un second sous-stade de finition histogénétique, de réglage des proportions, lui-même exigeant aussi 45 jours"* (Guyot, 1985). The total, some 90 days, would result in a length of approximately 90 mm.

It has been considered preferable to retain Streeter's system here because (1) there is no really convincing reason to change it at this time, (2) to do so would cause endless confusion (as would adopting a different staging system, as certain authors have done), (3) external changes would probably be too slight to be useful in adding further stages, and (4) in practical terms, adequately detailed information is not yet available beyond 8 postovulatory weeks.

APPENDIX 1

EMBRYOS IN THE CARNEGIE COLLECTION

The Carnegie specimens of stages 2–23 are listed in the following tables.

In columns "Size" (stage 9 and later), E. is the greatest length of the embryo and Ch. is the mean diameter of the chorion. In stages 16–18, an asterisk indicates a corrected or an estimated length. The grade refers to the total grade of the specimen and includes both its original quality and the condition of the mounted sections. The embedding medium was either paraffin (P) or a combination of celloidin and paraffin (C-P).

In stages 9–12 the number of paired somites is provided. In stage 18 the number of semicircular ducts (1–3) is given for each embryo, and also the length of the paramesonephric duct. Both of these serve as indices of relative level of development. In stages 19–23 Streeter's point score, from which the position of a given Carnegie embryo within a stage can be determined, is included (see p. 237).

The donors of most of these valuable specimens were named by Streeter (1942–1951) and O'Rahilly (1973). All those of stages 2, 3, 5a, and 5b, most of those of stage 5c, and many of those of stages 6 and 7 were presented by Drs. Hertig and Rock, whose contribution has been of enormous value to early human embryology.

———

The specimens in the excellent embryological collection of Professor E. Blechschmidt were assigned Carnegie Nos. 10315–10434 in 1972 because Professor Blechschmidt's wish was and is to have his collection combined with the Carnegie Collection. The Blechschmidt Collection is at present housed temporarily in the Department of Anatomy of Louisiana State University, New Orleans, and is under the care of Dr. Raymond F. Gasser. The collection has served as the basis of two important atlases (Blechschmidt, 1963, 1973), and the appropriate three-dimensional reconstructions are housed in the Anatomisches Institut der Universität Göttingen. The staging of these embryos has not been completed and hence they are not included in the following lists.

APPENDIX I

STAGE 2

Serial No.	Normality	Number of Blasto- meres	Size of Fixed Specimen (μm)	Fixative	Embedding Medium	Thinness (μm)	Stain	Year	Notes
8190	abnormal	9	160 × 104	Alc. & Bouin	C-P	6	Iron h., or G	1943	Hertig *et al.* (1954)
8260	*in vitro*	2	50 × 75	Bouin	C-P	8	H.&E.	1944	Menkin and Rock (1948)
8450	abnormal	8	100 × 96	Alc. & Bouin	C-P	6	H.&E., phlox.	1947	Hertig *et al.* (1954)
8452	abnormal	12	110 × 93	Alc. & Bouin	C-P	6	H.&E., phlox.	1946	Hertig *et al.* (1954)
8500.1	*in vitro*	3	50 × 86	Bouin	C-P	8	H.&E.	1947	Menkin and Rock (1948)
8630	abnormal	5	104 × 94	Alc. & Bouin	C-P	6	H.&E.	1948	Hertig *et al.* (1954)
8698	normal	2	122 × 88	Alc. & Bouin	C-P	6	H.&E.	1949	Hertig *et al.* (1954)
8904	normal	12	115	Bouin	Specimen lost			1951	Hertig *et al.* (1954)

STAGE 3

Serial No.	Normality	Number of Blasto- meres	Size of Fixed Specimen (μm)	Fixative	Embedding Medium	Thinness (μm)	Stain	Year	Notes
8663	normal	107	103 × 80	Alc. & Bouin	C-P	6	H.&E.	1949	Hertig *et al.* (1954)
8794	normal	58	108 × 86	Alc. & Bouin	C-P	6	H.&E.	1950	Hertig *et al.* (1954)

STAGE 5

Note: Measurements are given in Table 5-1

Stage 5a

Serial No.	Grade	Fixative	Embedding Medium	Thinness (μm)	Stain	Year	Notes
8020	Exc.	Alc. & Bouin	C-P	6	H.&E.	1942	Hertig and Rock (1945a)
8155	Exc.	Bouin	C-P	6	H.&E.	1943	Hertig and Rock (1949)
8225	Exc.	Alc. & Bouin	C-P	6	H.&E.	1944	Hertig and Rock (1945b)

Stage 5b

Serial No.	Grade	Fixative	Embedding Medium	Thinness (μm)	Stain	Year	Notes
8004	Exc.	Alc. & Bouin	C-P	6	H.&E.	1942	Hertig and Rock (1945a)
8171	Exc.	Alc.	C-P	6	H.&E.	1943	Hertig and Rock (1949)
8215	Exc.	Alc. & Bouin	C-P	6	H.&E.	1944	Hertig and Rock (1945c)
9350	Exc.	Bouin	?	?	H.&E.	1955	Heuser (1956)

Stage 5c

Serial No.	Grade	Fixative	Embedding Medium	Thinness (μm)	Stain	Year	Notes
4900	Poor	?	P	10	?	1925	Incomplete. Streeter (1926)
7699	Exc.	Bouin	C-P	6	H.&E.	1939	Hertig and Rock (1941)
7700	Exc.	Bouin	C-P	6	H.&E.	1938	Hertig and Rock (1941)
7770	Exc.	Bouin	C-P	6 & 10	H.&E.	1940	Abnormal
7771	Exc.	Bouin	C-P	10	H.&E.	1940	Abnormal
7950	Exc.	Alc. & Bouin	C-P	6	H.&E.	1941	Hertig and Rock (1944)
8000	Poor	Alc. & Bouin	C-P	8	H.&E.	1942	Abnormal
8139	Exc.	?	C-P	6	H.&E.	1943	Incomplete. Marchetti (1945)
8299	Exc.	Alc. & Bouin	C-P	6	H.&E., phlox.	1945	Abnormal
8329	Exc.	Alc. & Bouin	C-P	6	H.&E., phlox.	1945	Abnormal
8330	Exc.	Alc. & Bouin	C-P	6	H.&E., phlox.	1945	
8370	Poor	Alc. & Bouin	C-P	6	H.&E., phlox.	1946	Abnormal
8558	Exc.	Alc. & Bouin	C-P	6	H.&E.	1947	

STAGE 6

Serial No.	Grade	Fixative	Embedding Medium	Thinness (μm)	Stain	Year	Notes
6026	Poor	?	?	6?	H.&E.	1929	Lockyer embryo. Abnormal. Ramsey (1937)
6734	Poor	Zenker-acetic	P	10	H.&E.	1934	Yale embryo. Ramsey (1938)
6900	Poor	Formol	P	15	H.&E.	1940	Linzenmeier (1914)
7634	Poor	Formol	P	10	H.&E. etc.	1940	Torpin embryo. Krafka (1941)
7762	Good	Zenker-formol	P	8	?	1940	Wilson (1945)
7800	Exc.	?	C-P	8	H.&E.	1940	Abnormal
7801	Exc.	Bouin	C-P	8	H.&E.	1940	Heuser *et al.* (1945)
7850	Exc.	Alc. & Bouin	C-P	6	H.&E.	1940	Abnormal
8290	Exc.	Bouin	C-P	8	H. phlox.	1944	
8360	Exc.	Alc. & Bouin	C-P	6	H.&E., phlox.	1944	
8362	Poor	?	C-P	6	H.&E., phlox	1944	
8672	Exc.	Alc. & Bouin	C-P	6	H.&E.	1949	
8819	Exc.	Formol-chrom. subl.	C-P	8	H.&E.	1951	Edwards-Jones-Brewer (H.1496). Brewer (1938)
8905	Poor	Alc.	P	6	H.&E., phlox.	1951	Abnormal
8910	Good	Formol	C-P	8	H.&E., phlox.	1951	
9222	Good	Bouin	C-P	6 & 10	Azan	1954	Abnormal. Possibly stage 7
9250	Exc.	Bouin	P	8	H.&E.	1954	
9595	Poor	?	P	8	H.&E.	1958	
10003	Good	Bouin	P	5	Various	1963	

STAGE 7

Serial No.	Grade	Fixative	Embedding Medium	Thinness (μm)	Stain	Year	Notes
7802	Exc.	Alc. & Bouin	C-P	6	H.&E.	1940	Heuser *et al.* (1945)
8206	Good	?	C-P	6	H.&E.	1943	
8361	Good	Bouin	C-P	10	?	1946	Abnormal
8602	Exc.	Alc.	C-P	8	H.&E.	1948	
8752	Exc.	?	C-P	10	H.&E.	1950	
8756	Exc.	Formol	C-P	10	H.&E.	1950	
9217	Exc.	?	P	10	H.&E.	1954	

STAGE 8

Serial No.	Grade	Fixative	Embedding Medium	Plane	Thinness (μm)	Stain	Year	Notes
1399	Poor	Formol	P	Trans.	10	H.&E. etc.	1916	"Mateer embryo" described by Streeter (1920a)
3412	Poor	Formol	P	Trans.	5–15	Al. coch. E. au., or. G	1921	
5960	Good	Kaiserling	P	Trans.	5	Al. coch. & eosin	1929	Heuser (1932b)
6630	Poor	Formol	P	Oblique	6	H.&E.	1932	
6815	Poor	Formol	P	Oblique	10	Al. coch., or. G	1933	
7170a and b	Poor	Alc.	C-P	Trans.	6	H.&E.	1935	Twins
7545	Exc.	Formol	C-P	Trans.	6	H.&E.	1938	
7568	Poor	Formol	C-P	Trans.	10	Al. coch.	1938	
7640	Good	Formol & Bouin	P	Trans.	10	H.&E.	1939	George (1942)
7666	Exc.	Formol-chrom. subl.	C-P	Trans.	6	H.&E.	1939	"H. 1515"
7701	Exc.	?	C-P	Trans.	8	H.&E.	1939	
7822	Good	Formol	C-P	Trans.	10	H.&E.	1940	
7949	Good	Zenker	P	Sag.	10	H.&E. etc.	1941	
7972	Good	Alc. & Bouin	C-P	Sag.	6	H.&E.	1942	
8255	Exc.	Bouin	C-P	Sag.	8	H.&E., phlox.	1944	Slides showing embryo returned to Dr. Patten in 1962
8320	Good	Formol	C-P	Sag.	8	H.&E., phlox.	1945	
8352	Good	Formol	C-P	Trans.	8	H.&E., phlox.	1946	
8371	Poor	Alc. & Bouin	C-P	Sag.	8	H.&E., phlox.	1946	
8671	Exc.	Alc. & Bouin	C-P	Sag.	6	H.&E., phlox.	1949	
8725	Exc.	Alc. & Bouin	C-P	Sag.	6	H.&E., phlox.	1949	
8727	Exc.	Alc. & Bouin	C-P	Trans.	8	H.&E., phlox.	1949	Germ disc folded, possibly double (Hertig, 1968, fig. 180)
8820	Good	Zenker-formol	?	Trans.	10	H.&E.	1951	"Jones-Brewer I" (H. 1459) described by Jones and Brewer (1941)
9009a and b	Good	Formol	C-P	Sag.	6	H.&E.	1952	Twins described briefly by Heuser (1954)
9123	Good	Formol	C-P	Sag.	6	H.&E.	1953	
9251	Good	?	C-P	Trans.	10–12	Azan, H. & phlox.	1954	
9286	Exc.	Formol	C-P	Trans.	8	Azan	1955	
10157	Exc.	Formol	P	Trans.	?	Cason	1967	
10174	Exc.	Bouin	P	Trans.	8	Cason	1967	

STAGE 9

Serial No.	Pairs of somites	Size(mm)	Grade	Fixative	Embedding Medium	Plane	Thin-ness (μm)	Stain	Year	Notes
1878	2–3	E., 1.38 Ch., 12 × 10.5 × 7.5	Good	Formol	P	Cor.	10	H.&E.	1917	Described by Ingalls (1920)
5080	1	E., 1.5 Ch., 14.5	Poor	Formol	P	Trans.	10	Al. coch.	1926	Studied by Davis (1927)
7650	2–3	E., 2–3	Good	Alc. & Bouin	C-P	Trans.	6	H.&E.	1939	Said to be female (Park, 1957)

STAGE 10

All sections at stage 10 are transverse

Serial No.	Paired somites	Size (mm)	Grade	Fixative	Embedding medium	Thinness (μm)	Stain	Year	Notes
391	8	E., 2 Ch., 14	Good	Formol	P	10	Al. coch.	1907	Monograph by Dandy (1910)
1201	7	E., 2 Ch., 14.4	Good	Formol	P	8	H. & or. G.	1915	Univ. Chicago No. H 87
2795	4–5	E., 2	Poor	Alc.	P	6	Al. coch., or. G.	1919	
3707	12	E., 1.5	Good	Formol	P	12.5	I. H.	1921	Univ. Calif. No. H 197
3709	4	E., 1.74 Ch., 14.8	Poor	Formol	P	10	Erythrosin	1921	Univ. Chicago No. H 279

(continued)

STAGE 10 (continued)

All sections at stage 10 are transverse

Serial No.	Paired somites	Size (mm)	Grade	Fixative	Embedding medium	Thinness (μm)	Stain	Year	Notes
3710	12	E., 3.6 Ch., 19.0	Good	Formol	C-P	10	H. & or. G.	1921	Univ. Chicago No. H 392
4216	8	E., 2 Ch., 9.8	Good	Formol	P	15	?	1923	Monograph by Payne (1925)
5074	10	E., 3.3 Ch., 10.8	Exc.	Bouin	P	10	Al. coch.	1925	Univ. Rochester No. H 10. Monograph by Corner (1929)
6330	7	E., 2.83	Good	?	C-P	5	Ehr. H.	1931	Univ. Chicago No. H 1404
6740	12	E., 2.2	Good	?	?	8	?	1933	Litzenberg embryo. Studied by Boyden (1940)
7251	8	E., 1.27	Good	Formol	C-P	10	H.&E.	1941	"Singapore embryo." Univ. Cambridge No. H 98. Studied by Wilson (1914)
8244	6	E., 1.55 Ch., 8.5	Good	Alc.	C-P	8	H.&E., phlox.	1944	
8970	12	Ch., ca. 8	Good	Zenker	P	5	Various, chiefly carmine	1952	Univ. Chicago. No. H 637. Dicephaly

STAGE 11

Serial No.	Paired somites	Size (mm)	Grade	Fixative	Embedding medium	Plane	Thin-ness (μm)	Stain	Year	Notes
12	14	E., 2.1 Ch., 13	Poor		P	Trans.	10	Al. carm.	1893	
164	18	E., 3.5 Ch., 14	Good	Formol	P	Trans.	20	Al. coch.	1913	
318	13/14	E., 2.5 Ch., 16	Good		P	Trans.	25	Al. coch.	1905	
470	17	E., 4.3 Ch., 16	Good	Formol	P	Trans.	10	Al. coch.	1910	
779	14	E., 2.75 Ch., 16 × 14 × 12	Good	?	C	Trans.	15	Al. coch.	1913	Complete dysraphia. Studied by Dekaban and Bartelmez (1964)
1182b		E., 3 Ch., 15 × 12 × 5	Good	Formol	?	Trans.	20	Al. coch.	1915	
2053	20	E., 3.1 Ch., 12	Exc.	Formol	P	Trans.	10	Al. coch.	1918	Most advanced in group. Monograph by Davis (1923). Ag added to slide 2
4315	17	E., 4.7 Ch., 23 × 10.4 × 11	Exc.	?	C-P	Trans.	10	I.H. & E.	1923	Univ. Chicago No. 951. Studied by Wen (1928)
4529	14	E., 2.4 Ch., 21	Exc.	Formol	P	Trans.	10	Al. coch., or. G.	1924	Monograph by Heuser (1930)
4783	13	E., 2.3	Fair	?	?	Trans.	5	I.H.	1924	Monograph by Wallin (1913)
4877	13	E., 2 Ch., 15	Good	Formol	P	Trans.	15	Al. coch.	1925	
5072	17	E., 3	Good	Formol	P	Trans.	10	H.&E.	1925	Tubal. Type specimen. Monograph by Atwell (1930)
6050	19/21	E., 3 Ch., 10	Good	Formol	C-P	Cor.	10	Al. coch.	1930	Advanced
6344	13	E., 2.5 Ch., 17	Exc.	Formol	C-P	Trans.	6	Al. coch.	1931	Least advanced in group
6784	17	E., 5 Ch., 16	Exc.	Formol	C-P	Trans.	6	I.H., or. G.	1933	
7358	16	E., ? Ch., 15	Poor	Alc., formol	P	Oblique	25	H.&E.	1936	
7611	16	E., 2.4 Ch., 12	Exc.	Bouin	C-P	Trans.	8	H.&E.	1938	
7665	19	E., 4.36	Exc.	?	C-P	Trans.	6	?	1939	Univ. Chicago No. H 1516
7702	17	E., 3.7 Ch., 14	Good	Formol	C-P	Trans.	10	Al. coch.	1940	Returned to B.M. Patten
7851	13	E., 4.3 Ch., 18	Exc.	Formol	C-P	Trans.	8	H.&E.	1940	Slightly injured
8005	16/17	E., 3	Exc.	Bouin	C-P	Trans.	8	H.&E.	1942	Tubal
8116	17	E., 1.4 Ch., 17	Good	Formol	P	Sag.	8	Azan	1953	
8962	15	E., 1.55	Good	?	?	Sag.	?	?	1952	Tubal. Univ. Chicago No. H 810

STAGE 12

Serial No.	Paired somites	Size (mm)	Grade	Fixative	Embedding medium	Plane	Thin-ness (μm)	Stain	Year	Notes
209	ca. 24	E., 3 Ch., 15	Poor	Alc.	P	Cor.	50	Al. coch.	1902	
250	19?	E., 2 Ch., 10×9×9	Poor	?	?	Sag.	20	Al. coch.	?	
384	?	E., 2.5 Ch., 13	Poor	Formol	P	Trans.	10	H.&E.	1907	Macerated. Narrow yolk stalk
486	21	E., 4 Ch., 22	Good	Corros. acetic	P	Trans.	10	Al. coch.	1911	
1062	29	E., 4.5 Ch., 20	Good	Formol	P	Trans.	20	Al. coch.	1915	Transitional to next stage
2197	?	E., 5.3 Ch., 19.5	Poor	Formol	P	Trans.	10	Al. coch., or. G.	1918	
4245-7	ca. 24	E., 3.5 Ch., 24	Good	Alc., formol	P	Trans.	10	Al. coch.	1923	Caudal neuropore widely open
4479	?	E., 5.8 Ch., 17	Poor	Formol	P	Trans.	40	Al. coch.	1923	Macerated. Upper limb buds not visible
4736	26	E., 3.0 Ch., 20	Good	Formol	P	Cor.	10	Al. coch.	1924	No upper limb buds. Caudal neuropore closed
4759	?	E., 4.5 Ch., 15	Good	Formol	P	Trans.	15	H.&E.	1924	Neural tube folded
4784	23	E., 3	Good	?	P	Trans.	10	?	1924	
5035	25–28	E., 3.8 Ch., 18	Good	Formol	C-P	Trans.	10	Al. coch.	1925	
5048	ca. 25	E., 3.5	Good	Formol	C-P	Trans.	10	Al. coch.	1925	Tubal. Injured
5056	25	E., 3 Ch., 12	Good	Formol	P	Trans.	10	Al. Coch.	1925	
5206	?	E., 4 Ch., 51×31×30	Poor	?	?	Trans.	20	Al. coch.	1926	Tubal
5300	?	E., 4.5 Ch., 16.5	Poor	Formol	P	Trans.	20	Al. coch.	1926	Autopsy. Partly macerated
5923	28	E., 4 Ch., 15	Exc.	Formol	P	Trans.	10	Al. coch.	1929	
6097	25	E., 3.4 Ch., 12.5	Exc.	Formol	C-P	Trans.	10	Al. coch., eosin	1930	Tubal. Ag added to slides 1–3
6144	27	E., 3.3 Ch., 11	Good	Lysol-Zenker	C-P	Trans.	10	Al. coch.	1930	
6488	28	E., 3.2 Ch., 22	Good	Formol	C-P	Trans.	10	Al. coch.	1932	
6937	26	E., 3 Ch., 12	Poor	Formol	C-P	Cor.	10	I. H., or. G.	1934	Tubal. Caudal neuropore closed
7724	ca. 29	E., 3.5 Ch., 18	Good	Formol	C-P	Sag.	8	H.&E.	1940	Caudal end broken
7852	25	E., 3.7 Ch., 26	Exc.	Formol	C-P	Trans.	10	H.&E.	1940	Typical for stage 12
7999	ca. 28	E., 3.2 Ch., 15	Exc.	Bouin	C-P	Trans.	10	H.&E.	1942	Caudal defect
8505a	24	Ch., 23.5	Exc.	Formol	C-P	Trans.	?	H. Phlox.	1947	Twins
b	23	Ch., 24	Exc.	Formol	C-P	Sag.	?	Azan		
8941	28	E., 4.9 Ch., 35	Exc.	Zenker	C-P	Trans.	6	I.H.	1927	Univ. Chicago No. H 1261
8942	25	E., 3.8 Ch., 35	Exc.	Zenker	C-P	Cor.	5	I.H.	1930	Univ. Chicago No. H 1382
8943	22	E., 3.9 Ch., 20.4	Exc.	Formol-Zenker	C-P	Trans.	8	H.&E.	1934	Univ. Chicago No. H 1481
8944	25	E., 4 Ch., 25	Exc.	Formol-Zenker	C-P	Sag.	8	I.H.	1936	Univ. Chicago No. H 1514
8963	22	E., 3.8 Ch., 14.5	Fair	Formol	C-P	Trans.	10	I.H.	1928	Univ. Chicago. No. H 1093. Studied by Wen (1928)
8964	23	E., 2.8 Ch., 26.7	Poor	Formol	P	Trans.	8	I.H.	1928	Univ. Chicago No. H 984. Studied by Wen (1928)
9154	24	E., 5.4	Exc.	Formol	C-P	Trans.	8&6	I.H. & phlox.	1953	

STAGE 13

Serial No.	Size (mm)	Grade	Fixative	Embedding medium	Plane	Thinness (μm)	Stain	Year	Notes
1	E., 4.5 Ch., 30×30	Poor	Salicylic acid	P	Trans.	10	Hemat.	1887	Obtained by Mall while student
19	E., 5.5 Ch., 18×14	Poor	?	?	Trans.	20	Al. coch.	1895	
87	E., 4 Ch., 24×16×9	Poor	?	?	Trans.	20	Al. coch.	1896	
76	E., 4.5 Ch., 22×20	Poor	Alc.	P	Trans.	20	Al. coch.	1897	
112	E., 4	Poor	?	?	Sag.	10	Al. coch.	?	
116	E., 5	Poor	?	?	Sag.	?	Al. coch.	1898	
148	E., 4.3 Ch., 17×14×10	Poor	Alc.	P	Cor.	10	H.&E.	1899	Abnormal. Nasal discs fused
186	E., 3.5 Ch., 25×20×15	Poor	Alc.	P	Trans.	20	Al. coch.	1901	
239	E., 3.0	Poor	Formol	P	Trans.	10	H.&E.	1903	
248	E., 4.5 Ch., 30×23×15	Poor	?	?	Cor.	50	Al. coch.	1904	
407	E., 4 Ch., 14×13×7	Poor	Formol	?	Trans.	40	Al. coch.	1907	
463	E., 3.9 Ch., 17×12×7	Good	Formol	P	Cor.	10	Al. coch.	1910	
523	E., 5 Ch., 25×25×15	Fair	Formol	?	Trans.	?	Al. coch.	1911	
588	E., 4.0 Ch., 19×15×8	Good	Corros. acetic	P	Cor.	15	H.&E.	1912	Advanced
786	E., 4.5 Ch., 19×10×10	Poor	Alc.	P	Sag.	15	Al. coch.	1913	
800	E., 6.0	Good	Corros. acetic	P	Trans.	10	H.	1913	Curettage. Anencephaly
808	E., 4.0	Poor	Corros. acetic	P	Trans.	15	Al. coch.	1914	Tubal. Incomplete
826	E., 5.0 Ch., 13×13×9	Good	Formol	P	Trans.	20	Al. coch.	1914	Shrunken
836	E., 4.0 Ch., 22×18×11	Exc.	Corros. acetic	P	Trans.	15	Al. coch.	1914	Less advanced
963	E., 4.0 Ch., 23×18×16	Good	Formol	P	Cor.	20	Al. coch.	1914	
1075	E., 6.0 Ch., 46×32×20	Exc.	Corros. acetic	P	Cor.	20	H.&E., or. G.	1915	Most advanced in group
3956	E., 4.0	Poor	Formol	P	Trans.	20	Al. coch.	1922	Tubal. Incomplete
4046	E., 5 Ch., 22×20×20	Poor	Formol	P	Trans.	50	Al. coch.	1922	
5541	E., 6.0 Ch., 35×30×20	Good	Formol	P	Trans.	10	Al. coch., eosin	1927	
5682	E., 5.3 Ch., 29×25×13	Poor	Formol	P	Cor.	20	Al. coch.	1928	
5874	E., 4.8	Exc.	Bouin	P	Trans.	10	H.&E.	1929	Hysterotomy. Bromides only
6032	E., 5.8 Ch., 30×24×13	Poor	Formol	?	?	?	?	1929	Not good enough to cut
6469	E., 5.0 Ch., 25×18×18	Poor	Formol	?	?	?	?	1932	Fragmented on cutting. Not saved
6473	E., 5.0 Ch., 30×30×15	Exc.	Formol	C-P	Cor.	6	Al. coch.	1932	Less advanced. Ag added
7433	E., 5.2 Ch., 15×13×13	Exc.	Formol	C-P	Cor.	8	H.&E.	1937	Tubal
7618	E., 4.8 Ch., 18×15×15	Exc.	Bouin	C-P	Cor.	10	H.&E.	1939	Hysterectomy. Advanced. Ag added
7669	E., 5.0 Ch., 23×16×14	Good	Formol	C-P	Cor.	6	H.&E.	1939	Hysterectomy. Least advanced in group. Ag added
7889	E., 4.2	Exc.	Bouin	C-P	Cor.	6	H.&E.	1941	Hysterectomy
8066	E., 5.3 Ch., 20×18×15	Exc.	Bouin	C-P	Trans.	8	H.&E.	1942	Hysterectomy. Ag added to slide 2

(continued)

STAGE 13 (continued)

Serial No.	Size (mm)	Grade	Fixative	Embedding medium	Plane	Thin-ness (μm)	Stain	Year	Notes
8119	E., 5.3 Ch., 32 × 28 × 6.5	Exc.	Bouin	C-P	Trans.	8	H.&E.	1943	Hysterectomy
8147	E., 5.2 Ch., 27 × 21 × 19	Poor	Formol	?	?	?	?	1943	Tubal. Not cut
8239	E., 4.3	Exc.	Bouin	C-P	Sag.	8	H. phlox.	1944	
8372	E., 5.6	Exc.	Alc. & Bouin	P	Trans.	10	Azan	1946	
8581	E., 4.8	Good	Kaiserling	C-P	Sag.	8	Azan	1948	Most-advanced third
8967	E., 5.7	Exc.	Acetic Zenker	C-P	Trans.	6	H.&E.	1931	Head injured. Univ. Chicago No. H 1426
9296	E., 4.5	Exc.	?	C-P	Cor.	8	Azan	1955	
9297	E., 4.5	Exc.	?	C-P	Sag.	8	Azan	1955	
9697	E., 5.5		Bouin					1956	Not cut

STAGE 14

Serial No.	Size (mm)	Grade	Fixative	Embedding medium	Plane	Thin-ness (μm)	Stain	Year	Notes
4	E., 7	Poor	?	?	Trans.	10	Al. coch.	1892	
18	E., 7 Ch., 18 × 18	Poor	?	?	Trans.	20	Al. coch.	1895	
80	E., 5.0 Ch., 24 × 18 × 8	Good	Alc.	P	Trans.	20	Al. coch.	1897	
187	E., 7 Ch., 35 × 30 × 25	Poor	?	?	Sag.	20	Al. coch.	1902	
208	E., 7 Ch., 22 × 11 × 11	Poor	?	?	Sag.	20	Al. coch.	1902	
245	E., 6 Ch., 13 × 12 × 10	Poor	Formol, Zenker	?	Trans.	5	H.&E.	1904	
372	E., 7	Fair	?	?	Trans.	10	H.-Congo red	1902	
380	E., 6 Ch., 20 × 20 × 14	Poor	?	?	Sag.	20	H.&E.	1906	
387	E., 7 Ch., 45 × 40 × 50	Good	Formol	P	Trans.	20	H.&E.	1907	
442	E., 6 Ch., 25 × 20	Poor	Formol	?	Cor.?	50	Al. coch.	1908	
552	E., 6 Ch., 40 × 28 × 28	Poor	?	P	Sag.	40	Al. coch.	1911	Possible anencephaly
560	E., 7.0 Ch., 24 × 24	Poor	Formol	P	Cor.	40	Al. coch.	1912	
676	E., 6.0 Ch., 35 × 20 × 17	Good	Carnoy	P	Tr.-Cor.	20	H.&E.	1913	Possible spina bifida
873	E., 6.0 Ch., 35 × 28 × 16	Poor	Formol	P	Sag.	20	Al. coch.	1914	
988	E., 6.0 Ch., 38 × 30 × 23	Good	Formol-corros. acetic	P	Trans.	20	Al. coch.	1914	
1380	E., 5.7 Ch., 36 × 24 × 24	Exc.	Formol	P	Cor.	20	Al. coch.	1916	
1620	E., 6.6 Ch., 35 × 30 × 8	Good	Formol	P	Sag.	20	Al. coch.	1916	
2796	E., 6.68	Fair	?	?	Trans.	6	Al. coch., or. G.	1919	
2841	E., 5.3* Ch., 35 × 21	Good	Alc.	P	Trans.	20	H.&E., or. G.	1920	
3360	E., 6.0	Good	Formol	C	Trans.	20	H.&E., or. G.	1920	In myomatous uterus. Advanced.

(continued)

STAGE 14 (continued)

Serial No.	Size (mm)	Grade	Fixative	Embedding medium	Plane	Thin-ness (μm)	Stain	Year	Notes
3805	E., 5.9	Exc.	Bouin	P	Trans.	15	H.&E.	1921	Evans embryo No. 168. Serial bromides only
3960	E., 5.5	Good	Formol	C-P	Cor.	20	Al. coch.	1922	Blood vessels naturally injected
4154	E., 6.8 Ch., 33 × 31 × 20	Poor	Alc.	C-P	Trans.	8	H.&E.	1923	
4245-6	E., 7.0	Good	Formol	P	Trans.	15	Al. coch.	1923	Univ. Pennsylvania No. 40. Ag added
4629	E., 6.5 Ch., 32 × 23	Good	Formol	C-P	Sag.	10	H.&E.	1924	
4672	E., 8.2 Ch., 40 × 34 × 25	Good	Formol	P	Trans.	20	Al. coch.	1924	Advanced
4805	E., 7.3 Ch., 15 × 8 × 9	Good	Formol	C-P	Trans.	10	H.&E.	1924	Tubal
5437	E., 7.0	Good	Formol	C-P	Trans.	8	H.&E.	1927	Advanced
5654	E., 5.0 Ch., 30 × 23 × 17	Good	Formol	P	Trans.	10	Al. coch., eosin	1928	Less advanced
5787	E., 6.8 Ch., 32 × 30 × 23	Good	Formol	P	Sag.	10	Al. coch.	1928	
6428	E., 7.0 Ch., 30 × 28 × 25	Good	Formol	C-P	Cor.	6, 10	Al. coch.	1931	Advanced
6500	E., 4.9*	Good	Souza?	C-P	Sag.	10	Al. coch.	1931	E. Leitz, Berlin
6502	E., 6.7*	Exc.	Souza?	C-P	Trans.	5, 10	H.&E.	1931	E. Leitz, Berlin. Ag added to slides 1–25
6503	E., 6.3*	Exc.	Souza?	C-P	Cor.	10	Al. coch.	1931	E. Leitz, Berlin
6739	E., 8	Poor	Formol	C-P	Sag.	20	H.&E.	1933	
6830	E., 5.5 Ch., 47 × 23 × 15	Exc.	Formol	C-P	Cor.	8	H.&E.	1933	
6848	E., 7.8	Good	Formol	C-P	Cor.	10	H.&E.	1934	Tubal
7324	E., 6.6 Ch., 17 × 13 × 10	Good	Formol	C-P	Trans.	8	H.&E.	1936	Low implantation
7333	E., 6.3	Good	Formol	C-P	Trans.	8	H.&E.	1936	
7394	E., 7.2 Ch., 45 × 20 × 20	Exc.	Formol	C-P	Trans.	8	H.&E.	1937	
7400	E., 6.3 Ch., 35 × 25 × 20	Good	Formol	C-P	Cor.	10	H.&E.	1937	
7522	E., 7.7 Ch., 33 × 16 × 16	Good	Formol	C-P	Trans.	8	H.&E.	1938	Natural blood injection
7598	E., 7.0 Ch., 30 × 30 × 25	Poor	Alc.	C-P	Trans.	10	H.&E.	1938	Macerated
7667	E., 5 Ch., 16 × 14 × 12	Fair	Formol	P	Trans.	8	H.&E., phlox.	1939	
7829	E., 7.0	Exc.	Bouin	C-P	Trans.	8	H.&E.	1940	Advanced
7870	E., 7.2 Ch., 25 × 20 × 13	Exc.	Bouin	C-P	Trans.	8	H.&E.	1941	On borderline of next stage. Ag added
8141	E., 7.3 Ch., 33 × 28	Exc.	Formol	C-P	Cor.	8	H.&E.	1943	Shrinkage cracks in brain
8306	E., 5.3 Ch., 27	Exc.	Bouin	C-P	Trans.	10&20	H.&E., phlox.	1945	
8308	E., 5.85 Ch., 27 × 18 × 18	Exc.	Formol & Bouin	C-P	Sag.	8	Azan	1945	
8314	E., 8 Ch., 23 × 22	Exc.	Formol	C-P	Trans.	8	Azan	1945	
8357	E., 6.5	Good	Formol	C-P	Sag.	8	Azan	1946	
8552	E., 6.5	Exc.	Alc. & Bouin	C-P	Trans.	8	Azan	1947	
8999	E., 6 Ch., 16 × 15	Exc.	Alc. & Bouin	C-P	Sag.	8	Azan	1952	
9695	E., 8.5		?					1955	Not cut

STAGE 15

Serial No.	Size (mm)	Grade	Fixative	Embedding medium	Plane	Thin-ness (μm)	Stain	Year	Notes
2	E., 7.0 Ch., 25 × 25 × 25	Good	Alc.	P	Trans.	15	Al. carm.	1888	Least-advanced third
88	E., 8 Ch., 30 × 28 × 15	Poor	Alc.	?	Cor.	?	Al. coch.	1897	
113	E., 8	Poor	?	?	Sag.	10	Borax carmine	?	
241	E., 6.0	Good	Formol	P	Trans.	10	H. & Congo red	1904	
371	E., 6.6	Good	Formol	P	Sag.	10	Al. coch.	1913	Shrunken and cracked
389	E., 9	Poor	?	?	Sag.	20	H.&E.	1907	Tubal
721	E., 9.0 Ch., 30 × 20 × 10	Exc.	Zenker formol	P	Trans.	15	H.&E.	1913	Median in group
810	E., 7.0 Ch., 30 × 25 × 15	Good	Alc.	P	Sag.	20	Al. coch	1913	
855	E., 7.5	Poor	Formol	P	Trans.	100	Al. coch.	1914	Pathological between limbs
1006	E., 9.0 Ch., 37 × 26 × 22	Poor	Formol	P	Cor.	20	H.&E., or. G.	1914	Operative. Most-advanced third
1091	E., 7.2 Ch., 28 × 26 × 20	Poor	Formol	P	Cor.	20	Al. coch.	1915	Macerated
1354	E., 7.8 Ch., 35 × 30 × 25	Good	Formol	P	Sag.	20	Al. coch.	1916	Least-advanced third
1767	E., 11.0 Ch., 41 × 23 × 5	Good	Formol	P	Sag.	40	H.&E., or. G.	1917	Most-advanced third
2743	E., 7.2 Ch., 19 × 18 × 14	Poor	Formol	P	Trans.	20	Al. coch.	1919	Macerated. Least-advanced third
3216	E., 6.5 Ch., 30 × 30 × 5	Good	Formol	P	Trans.	20	Al. coch.	1920	Hysterectomy. Least-advanced third
3385	E., 8.3 Ch., 25 × 20 × 16	Exc.	Corros. acetic	P	Trans.	20	H.&E., or. G.	1921	Some sections lost. Most-advanced third. Ag added
3441	E., 8.0 Ch., 25 × 24 × 20	Good	Formol	P	Sag.	10	Al. coch.	1921	
3512	E., 8.5 Ch., 33 × 28 × 25	Good	Formol	P	Trans.	10	Al. coch.	1921	
3952	E., 6.7 Ch., 30 × 25 × 15	Good	Formol	P	Cor.	15	Al. coch.	1922	Median in group
4602	E., 9.3 Ch., 33 × 30 × 26	Good	Formol	P	Sag.	15	Al. coch.	1924	Medical abortion
4782	E., 9.0 Ch., 14 × 13 × 11	Poor	Formol	P	Cor.	20	Al. coch.	1924	
5772	E., 8	Poor	?	P	Cor.	15	Al. coch., eosin	1928	
5892	E., 7.3	Good	Corros. acetic	C-P	Cor.	10	Al. coch., phlox.	1929	Transitional to next stage
6223	E., 6.7	Poor	Alc.	C-P	Sag.	8	Or. G.	1930	Fragmented sections. Not saved
6504	E., 7.5*	Exc.	. . .	C-P	Sag.	6	Al. coch.	?	Least-advanced third. Ag added
6506	E., 7.5*	Exc.	. . .	C-P	Cor.	10	Al. coch.	?	Most-advanced third. Ag added
6508	E., 7.3*	Good	Corros. acetic	C-P	Trans.	6	Al. coch.	?	Many sections lost. Advanced
6595	E., 8.0	Good	Formol	C-P	Sag.	10	H.&E.	1932	
7199	E., 8.4	Good	Formol	C-P	Cor.	10	Al. coch., phlox.	1935	Operative. Good fixation
7364	E., 9.5 Ch., 35 × 30 × 25	Poor	Formol	C-P	Cor.	8	H.&E.	1936	Macerated. Median in group
8929	E., 6.35 Ch., 13.8 × 10.1 × 9	Exc.	Alc. & Bouin	C-P	Trans.	10	Azan	1951	Most-advanced third
8966	E., 7.1 Ch., 37 × 29 × 12	Good	Zenker	C-P	Sag.	10	H.&E.	1932	Less advanced. Univ. Chicago No. H 1454
8968	E., 8.8	Exc.	Zenker	C-P	Trans.	6	H.&E.	1928	Univ. Chicago No. H 1324
8997	E., 9.0	Exc.	Formol & Bouin	P	Cor. & Sag.	8	Azan	1952	Caudal quarter embedded separately
9140	E., 7.0	Good	Bouin	P	Cor.	8	Azan	1953	Mechanically distorted

STAGE 16

Serial No.	Size (mm)	Grade	Fixative	Embedding medium	Plane	Thin-ness (μm)	Stain	Year	Notes
163	E., 9.0 Ch., 35 × 35 × 20	Good	Formol	P	Trans.	20	Al. coch.	1899	Used by Bardeen and Lewis
221	E., 7.5 Ch., 40 × 33 × 33	Poor	Formol	P	Sag.	20	Al. coch.	1903	Macerated
383	E., 7.0 Ch., 15 × 15 × 15	Poor	Formol	P	Trans.	10	Al. carm., H. & Congo red	1904	
397	E., 8.0 Ch., 15 × 15 × 15	Poor	Formol	P	Trans.	10	H.&E.	1907	
422	E., 9.0 Ch., 30 × 30 × 30	Poor	Alc.	P	Trans.	40	Al. coch.	1910	Tubal. Partly macerated
559	E., 8.6 CH., 20 × 15 × 12	Good	Formol	P	Trans.	20	H. & Congo red	1911	Cyclopia. Formerly listed as stage 17
589	E., 11 Ch., 30 × 13 × 13	Poor	?	P	Sag.	50	Al. coch.	1912	
617	E., 7.0 Ch., 18 × 14 × 12	Good	Formol	P	Trans.	15	Al. coch.	1912	Median in group
636	E., 10 Ch., 28 × 28 × 22	Poor	Formol	P	Trans.	50	Al. coch.	1913	Macerated
651f	E., 7 Ch., 25 × 20 × 15	Poor	?	?	?	?	?	1913	Spina bifida
675	E., 10 Ch., 50 × 30 × 25	Poor	Formol	P	Sag.	100	Carmine	1915	Abnormal head and limbs
792	E., 8.0 Ch., 40 × 30 × 30	Good	Formol	P	Trans.	20	Al. coch.	1913	Advanced
887	E., 9.0 Ch., 31 × 28 × 17	Good	Formol	P	Trans.	40	Al. coch.	1914	Near next stage
1121	E., 11.8	Good	Corros. acetic	P	Cor.	40	Al. coch.	1915	Operative. Median in group
1197	E., 10.0 Ch., 23 × 19 × 15	Good	Formol	C	Sag.	20	H.&E., or. G.	1915	Advanced
1544	E., 7.2	Good	Zenker	P	Sag.	20	Al. coch.	1916	Tubal. Mechanical injury
1836	E., 11.0	Good	Formol	P	Trans.	20	H.&E.	1917	Most-advanced third
4677	E., 9.5 Ch., 48 × 36 × 30	Good	Formol	P	Trans.	10	Al. coch.	1924	Median in group
5515	E., 12.0 Ch., 47 × 37 × 25	Good	Formol	C-P	Trans.	10	H.&E.	1927	Near next stage
6054	E., 7.0 Ch., 21 × 17 × 12	Good	Formol	C-P	Trans.	8	H.&E.	1930	Least-advanced third
6507	E., 9.0*	Exc.	Corros. acetic	C-P	Cor.	10&8	Al. coch.	?	Middle or most-advanced third
6509	E., 8.1*	Exc.	Corros. acetic	C-P	Cor.	10	Al. coch.	?	Least-advanced or middle third
6510	E., 10.1*	Exc.	Corros. acetic	C-P	Cor.	10	Al. coch.	?	Close to No. 6507. Ag added
6511	E., 8.1*	Good	Corros. acetic	C-P	Sag.	10	Al. coch., iron H.	?	Surface injured by fixative. Most-advanced third
6512	E., 7.0*	Exc.	Corros. acetic	C-P	Trans.	10	Al. coch.	?	Least-advanced third. Borderline
6513	E., 7.2*	Good	Corros. acetic	C-P	Cor.	10	Al. coch	?	Surface injured by fixative. Least advanced in group
6514	E., 9.0*	Poor	Corros. acetic	C-P	Sag.	10	Al. coch.	?	Most-advanced third
6516	E., 10.5*	Good	Corros. acetic	C-P	Sag.	8	Al. coch.	?	Most-advanced third. Double left kidney and ureter
6517	E., 10.5*	Exc.	Corros. acetic	C-P	Trans.	8	Al. coch.	?	Close to No. 6516
6686	E., 11.0 Ch., 17 × 17 × 17	Poor	Formol	C-P	Cor.	20	Al. coch.	1933	Tubal. Partly macerated
6750	E., 10.0	Good	Formol	C-P	Trans.	10	H. & phlox.	1933	Tubal. Advanced
6909	E., 11.0	Good	Bouin	C-P	Cor.	10	H.&E.	1934	Tubal. Advanced
6931	E., 8.8 Ch., 37 × 33 × 16	Good	Formol	C-P	Cor.	10	Al. coch., phlox.	1934	Least-advanced third. Type specimen
6950	E., 9.0 Ch., 31 × 20 × 18	Good	Formol	C-P	Trans.	10	H.&E.	1934	Tubal. Partly fragmented
7115	E., 9.7 Ch., 30 × 23 × 15	Exc.	Bouin	C-P	Cor.	10	H. & phlox.	1935	Operative. Less advanced

(continued)

STAGE 16 (continued)

Serial No.	Size (mm)	Grade	Fixative	Embedding medium	Plane	Thin-ness (μm)	Stain	Year	Notes
7629	E., 11.5 Ch., 31 × 31	Good	Formol	C-P	Cor.	10	Al. coch., phlox.	1939	Hysterectomy. Most advanced in group
7804	E., 9.5 Ch., 26 × 21 × 16	Good	Formol	C-P	Trans.	10	H.&E.	1940	Least-advanced third
7897	E., 12.2 Ch., 31 × 24 × 23	Good	Formol	C-P	Trans.	10	H.&E.	1941	Tubal. Advanced
8098	E., 10.0 Ch., 30	Good	Formol	C-P	Cor.	6	H.&E.	1942	Tubal. Median in group
8112	E., 10.9	Exc.	Bouin	C-P	Cor.	8	H.&E.	1943	Most-advanced third
8179	E., 11.9 Ch., 23 × 18 × 17	Good	Formol	C-P	Cor.	10	H.&E.	1943	Tubal
8436	E., 10.9 Ch., 13 × 15 × 17	Good	Formol	P	Cor.	10	Azan	1946	Advanced
8692	E., 10	Good	Bouin	P	Trans.	10	H.&E.	1949	Rubella. Medical abortion. Mechanically damaged
8697	E., 11.3	Poor	Formol	C-P	Trans.	10	H.&E.	1949	Perhaps stage 17
8773	E., 11	Exc.	Bouin	P	Cor.	10	Azan	1950	
8971	E., 10 Ch., 20.5 × 14.5 × 13.7	Poor	Formol		Trans.	15	H.&E.	1932	Synophthalmia. Univ. Chicago No. H 1439
9055	E., ca. 10	Exc.	Bouin	P	Trans.	20	Azan & Ag	1953	Damaged
9229	E., 9.5	Exc.	Formol	P	Trans.	6	Ag & H.&E.	1954	Stage 15, 16, or 17? Mislaid

STAGE 17

Serial No.	Size (mm)	Grade	Fixative	Embedding medium	Plane	Thin-ness (μm)	Stain	Year	Notes
353	E., 11.0 Ch., 40 × 35 × 20	Good	Formol	P	Cor.	10	H.&E.	1906	Very advanced
485	E., 13.0 Ch., 33 × 25	Exc.	Formol	P	Cor.	40	Al. coch.	1911	Injected (India ink)
544	E., 11.5 Ch., 30	Good	Zenker-formol	P	Sag.	40	Al. coch.	1911	Operative. Injected (India ink)
562	E., 13.0 Ch., 28 × 17 × 17	Poor	Formol	P	Sag.	100	Al. coch.	1912	Advanced
623	E., 10.1	Good	Alc.	P	Trans.	20	H. & Congo red	1912	Operative. Median in group
695	E., 13.5 Ch., 40 × 40 × 17	Poor	Formol	P	Trans.	10	H. & Congo red	1913	Macerated
916	E., 11.0 Ch., 30 × 30 × 16	Good	Bouin	C	Trans.	40	H.&E., or. G.	1915	Most-advanced third
940	E., 14.0 Ch., 28 × 23 × 21	Good	Formol	C	Trans.	40	H.&E., or. G.	1914	Advanced
1232	E., 14.5 Ch., 35 × 35 × 30	Poor	Formol	P	Cor.	40	Al. coch.	1915	Close to No. 1267A
1267A	E., 14.5 Ch., 35 × 30 × 26	Good	Formol	C	Sag.	20 40	H.&E., or. G	1915	Excellent C.N.S.
1771	E., 12.5	Good	Formol	P	Sag.	20	H.&E.	1917	Tubal
5642	E., 11.5 Ch., 33 × 30 × 17	Good	Formol	P	Trans.	15	Al. coch.	1928	Right upper limb injured
5893	E., 13.2	Good	Formol	C-P	Trans.	20	Al. coch.	1929	Most advanced in group
6258	E., 14.0 Ch., 48 × 35 × 25	Good	Formol	C-P	Trans.	10	H.&E.	1930	Median in group
6519	E., 10.8*	Exc.	Corros. acetic	C-P	Sag.	8	Al. coch.	?	Least-advanced or middle third

(continued)

STAGE 17 (continued)

Serial No.	Size (mm)	Grade	Fixative	Embedding medium	Plane	Thin-ness (μm)	Stain	Year	Notes
6520	E., 14.2*	Exc.	Corros. acetic	C-P	Trans.	10	Al. coch.	?	Median in group. Ag added to slides 1–25
6521	E., 13.2*	Exc.	Corros. acetic	C-P	Trans.	8–18	Al. coch.	?	Sections vary in thinness
6631	E., 13.0	Good	Formol	C-P	Cor.	10	H.&E.	1932	Tubal. Advanced
6742	E., 11.0 Ch., 50×40×15	Good	Formol	C-P	Trans.	12	H. & phlox.	1933	Good primary germ cells
6758	E., 12.8	Good	Formol	C-P	Trans.	10	H. & phlox.	1933	Least-advanced third
7317	E., 10.0*	Good		P	Cor.	10	H.&E.	1936	His embryo "Ru." Every third section
7436	E., 13.0	Good	Formol	C-P	Cor.	30	Al. coch.	1937	Most-advanced third
8101	E., 13.0	Exc.	Bouin	C-P	Trans.	10	H.&E.	1943	Operative
8118	E., 12.6	Exc.	Bouin	C-P	Cor.	10	H.&E.	1943	Middle third
8253	E., 11.2 Ch., 30×20×10	Good	Bouin	C-P	Cor.	10	Al. coch., phlox.	1944	Operative. Least advanced in group
8789	E., 11.7	Exc.	Bouin	C-P	Sag.	10	Azan	1950	
8969	E., 11.2	Exc.	?	?	Trans.	15	Azan	1919	Univ. Chicago No. H 566
8998	E., 11.0	Exc.	?	C-P	Cor.	10	Azan	1952	
9100	E., 12.0 Ch., 12×13×10	Exc.	Formol-chrom. subl.	C-P	Sag.	10	Azan	1933	Univ. Chicago No. H 1475
9282	E., 12.0 Ch., 16	Good	Alc.	P	Trans.	15	Ag	1955	Mislaid

STAGE 18

Serial No.	Size (mm)	Grade	Fixative	Embedding medium	Plane	Thin-ness (μm)	Stain	Semic. ducts	P.-M. duct (mm)	Year	Notes
109	E., 12.0* Ch., 30	Poor	Alc.	P	Trans.	20	Al. coch.	1	0.4	1897	Tubal. Least-advanced third
144	E., 16.0* Ch., 40×30×30	Good	Formol	P	Sag.	40	Al. coch.	3	0.85	1899	Most-advanced third
175	E., 13.0 Ch., 30×25×25	Poor	Alc.	P	Trans.	20	Al. coch.	2	0.6	1900	Tubal. Partly macerated
296	E., 17.0	Poor	Alc.	P	Cor.	20	Various	3	0.85	1905	Most-advanced third
317	E., 16.0	Good	Formol	P	Cor.	20	H. & or. G.	2	0.7	1905	Middle third
351	E., 14.0*	Good	Formol	P	Cor.	250	Slightly car-mine	2	0.38	1904	Injected (Berlin blue)
406	E., 16.0 Ch., 40×40×40	Good	Formol	P	Sag.	20	H.&E.	3	0.7	1907	Operative. Most-advanced third
423	E., 15.2	Good	Formol-Zenker	P	Trans.	50	Carmine	3	0.85	1904	
424	E., 17.2	Good	Formol	P	Trans.	50	Carmine	3	1.0	1904	Double injection. Advanced
492	E., 16.8 Ch., 40×40	Exc.	Zenker	P	Cor.	40	Al. coch.	3	0.7	1911	Injected (India ink)
511	E., 16.0* Ch., 38×32×32	Good	Alc.	P	Sag.	40	Al. coch.	3	1.1	1911	Head injured. Most advanced in group
670	E., 12.5	Poor	Alc.	P	Sag.	50	H.&E.	3	1.0	1913	Tubal. Advanced
719	E., 15.0 Ch., 50×30×30	Good	Formol	P	Trans.	40	Al. coch.	2	0.6	1913	Median in group
733	E., 15.0 Ch., 45×40×25	Poor	Formol	P	Sag.	50	Al. coch.	2	0.6	1913	Median in group
841	E., 15.0 Ch., 18×16×9	Good	Formol	P	Cor.& Trans.	10 20	H.&E., car-mine	2	0.32	1914	Operative. Head cut separately
899	E., 16.0* Ch., 30×18×15	Good	Bouin	P	Sag.	50	Al. coch.	3	0.65	1914	Tubal. Head injured
991	E., 17.0	Good	Formol	P	Sag.	50	H., V. Gieson	3	0.9	1914	Advanced

(continued)

STAGE 18 (continued)

Serial No.	Size (mm)	Grade	Fixative	Embedding medium	Plane	Thinness (μm)	Stain	Semic. ducts	P.-M. duct (mm)	Year	Notes
1909	E., 14.6	Good	Formol	P	Cor.	20	Al. coch., or. G.	1	0.3	1917	Less advanced
2673	E., 15.5	Good	Formol	P	Trans.	40	Al. coch.	2	0.52	1919	Median in group
4430	E., 14.0 Ch., 51×40×21	Exc.	Corros. acetic	P	Trans.	15	Al. coch., or. G.	3	0.9	1923	Most-advanced third
5542B	E., 16.0 Ch., 37×32×25	Good	Formol	P	Trans.	40	Al. coch.	2	0.7	1927	Other twin abnormal
5747	E., 15.2 Ch., 32×27×25	Poor	Alc.-formol	P	Sag.	25	Al. coch.	2	0.25	1928	Least-advanced or middle third
5935A	E., 13.5 Ch., 40×30×30	Good	Formol	P	Cor.	40	Al. coch.	1	0.38	1929	Other twin stunted
6522	E., 13.2*	Good	Corros. acetic	C-P	Cor.	10	Al. coch.	3	0.8	?	Middle or most-advanced third
6524	E., 11.7*	Exc.	Corros. acetic	C-P	Trans.	10	Al. coch.	1	0.4	?	Least-advanced third
6525	E., 13.8*	Exc.	Corros. acetic	C-P	Sag.	8	Al. coch.	2	0.42	?	Weak staining
6527	E., 14.4*	Exc.	Corros. acetic	C-P	Trans.	15	Al. coch.	2	0.67	?	Mechanical damage
6528	E., 13.4*	Exc.	Corros. acetic	C-P	Cor.	8	Al. coch.	1	0.33	?	Least-advanced third
6529	E., 15.6*	Good	Corros. acetic	C-P	Cor.	10	Al. coch.	2	0.4	?	Middle third
6533	E., 12.5*	Good	Corros. acetic	C-P	Sag.	6, 8, 10	Al. coch.	2	0.45	?	Middle third
6551	E., 18.0	Poor	Formol	P	Cor.	40	H.&E.	3	0.8	1932	Tubal
7707	E., 14.5 Ch., 37×32	Exc.	Bouin	C-P	Trans.	10	H.&E., phlox.	2	0.54	1939	Operative. Middle third
8097	E., 15.5 Ch., 37×25×21	Good	Formol	C-P	Trans.	10	H.&E.	1	0.19	1942	Least advanced in group
8172	E., 16.5	Exc.	Bouin	C-P	Trans.	20	H.&E.	3	0.58	1943	Operative. Very advanced
8235	E., 14.0*	Good	Bouin	C-P	Sag.	10	H.&E., Mallory	2	0.25	1944	Tubal
8355	E., 15.0 Ch., 23	Exc.	Formol	C-P	Cor.	10	Azan			1946	Tubal. Duplicated spinal cord caudally
8812	E., 12.9	Exc.	Formol	C-P	Trans.	10	H.&E.			1950	Rubella. Medical abortion. Midbrain punctured
8945	E., 13.9	Good	Zenker	P	Trans.	8	Borax, carm.			1952	Univ. Chicago No. H 1254
9107	E., 17.0 Ch., 38×28×22	Good	Bouin	P	Trans.	15	Borax, carm.			1918	Univ. Chicago No. H 516
9247	E., 15.0	Exc.	Bouin	C-P	Sag.	8	Azan			1954	Tubal

STAGE 19

Serial No.	Size (mm)	Grade	Fixative	Embedding medium	Plane	Thinness (μm)	Stain	Point score	Sex	Year	Notes
17	E., 18 Ch., 40×30×20	Poor	Alc.	P	Sag.	50, 100	Al. carm.	16.5	♀	1894	
43	E., 16	Good	Alc.	P	Sag.	50	Al. coch.	10	♀	1894	
293	E., 19	Poor	Alc.	P	Sag.	50	Coch.	16.5	♀	1905	
390	E., 19	Good	Formol?	P	Sag.	20, 50	H.&E.	11.5	♀	1906	Tubal. Injected
409	E., 18 Ch., 50×40×40	Good	Formol	P	Trans.	20	Copper, iron H. & erythrosin	14.5	♀	1907	
432	E., 18.5 Ch., 45×35×20	Good	Formol	P	Sag.	20	H. & Congo red	13.5	♀	1910	Tubal
576	E., 17 Ch., 60×40	Good	Formol	P	Sag.	15, 20	H.&E.	14.5	♂	1912	Tubal
626	E., 21.5 Ch., 40×30×21	Good	Formol	P	Trans.	100	Al. coch.	14.5	♂	1913	
678	E., 20 Ch., ca. 30	Poor	Formol	P	Sag.	50	Al. coch.	12	♀	1913	Head damaged
709	E., 19 Ch., 40×35×25	Poor	Alc.	P	Cor.	40	Al. coch., Lyons blue	15	?♀	1913	
837	E., 21 Ch., 65×45×38	Good	Formol	P	Sag.	40	Al. coch.	14.5	♀	1914	

(continued)

STAGE 19 (continued)

Serial No.	Size (mm)	Grade	Fixative	Embedding medium	Plane	Thinness (μm)	Stain	Point score	Sex	Year	Notes
1324	E., 18 Ch., 50×30×18	Good	Formol	C	Cor.	40	H.&E. aur., or. G.	12.5	?♀	1915	Tubal
1332	E., 19 Ch., 40×43×22	Poor	Formol	C	Cor.	40	H.&E. aur., or. G.	15	♀	1915	
1390	E., 18 Ch., 40×38×15	Good	Formol	P	Sag.	20	Al. coch.	10.5	♀	1916	Tubal
1584	E., 18 Ch., 35×31×25	Good	Formol	P	Sag.	50	Al. coch.	13.5	♂	1916	Protruding midbrain
2114	E., 19.3 Ch., 49×42×33	Good	Formol	P	Trans.	40	Al. coch.	12	♀	1918	
4405	E., 15.5	Good	Formol	P	Trans.	10	Coch., Mallory	13.5	♂	1923	Midbrain injured
4501	E., 18	Exc.	Bouin	P	Trans.	15	Coch., or. G.	14	♂	1924	Cystic left kidney
5609	E., 18	Exc.	Formol	P	Cor.	25	Al. coch.	13.5	♂	1927	
6150	E., 17 Ch., 40×39×30	Good	Bouin	C-P	Trans.	15	H.&E.	16.5	♀	1930	Tubal
6824	E., 18.5 Ch., 45×40×25	Good	Formol	C-P	Sag.	12	H.&E.	14.5	♂	1933	
7900	E., 16.5	Good	Bouin	C-P	Sag.	20	H.&E., phlox.	11.5	...	1941	Tubal
8092	E., 16.3 Ch., 52×47	Exc.	Bouin	C-P	Trans.	20	H.&E., phlox.	13	♀	1942	
8913	E., ? Ch., 34	Poor	Formol	P	Trans.	10	Azan	?	?	1951	Rubella. Medical abortion. Isolated head damaged
8965	E., 19.1 Ch., 42×32×19	Good	Formol-Zenker	C-P	Trans.	10	Borax, carm., or. G.	?	?	1952	Univ. Chicago No. H 173
9097	E., 21	Exc.	Formol-glucose	C-P	Cor.	10	Azan	?	?	1930	Univ. Chicago No. H 1380
9113	E., 18.5 Ch., 24	Exc.	Formol	C-P	Trans.	10	Azan	?	♂	1953	Rubella. Medical abortion
9325	E., 17.0 Ch., 32×28×20	Good	Formol-acetic	P	Trans.	15 & 8-10	Azan & Ag	?	?	1955	Tubal

STAGE 20

Serial No.	Size (mm)	Grade	Fixative	Embedding medium	Plane	Thinness (μm)	Stain	Point score	Sex	Year	Notes
240	E., 20 Ch., 50×40×30	Poor	Formol	P	Cor.	20	Iron H.	27	♂	1904	
256	E., 21	Poor	Alc.	P	Sag.	25	Coch.	23	♀	1904	Tubal. Partial anencephaly
368	E., 20	Poor	Alc.	P	Sag.	20	H. & Congo red	22.5	♀	1906	
431	E., 19 Ch., 30×25×25	Good	Formol	P	Sag.	20	H. & Congo red	25.5	♀	1908	Tubal
437	E., 23 Ch., 80×60×50	Poor	Formol	P	Sag.	50	Coch.	24	?	1909	
453	E., 23 Ch., 60×40×30	Poor	Formol	P	Sag.	20	H. & Congo red	23.5	?	1910	
460	E., 21	Exc.	Bichlor. acetic	P	Trans.	40	H.&E., coch.	24.5	♀	1910	Injected
462	E., 20 Ch., 50×40×30	Exc.	Formol	P	Trans.	40	Al. coch.	23.5	♂	1910	
635B	E., 22	Poor	Alc.	P	Trans.	50	Al. coch.	26.5	♀	1913	
657	E., 25 Ch., 35×20×15	Poor	Formol	C	Sag.	40	H.&E. aur., or. G.	25	♀	1913	Tubal
966	E., 23 Ch., 51×38×13	Exc.	Bichlor. acetic	P	Cor.	40	Al. coch.	27	♀	1914	
1108	E., 19.8 Ch., 30×25×18	Poor	Bichlor.	C	Trans.	40	H.&E. aur., or. G.	21.5	?	1915	
1134E	E., 21.3	Good	Formol	P	Sag.	100	Al. coch.	22	?	1915	
1266	E., 23	Poor	Formol	P	Sag.	100	Al. coch.	20.5	?	1915	
2393	E., 23.1 Ch., 61.5×50×35	Poor	Formol	C-P	Sag.	25	H.&E. aur., or. G.	26.5	♂	1919	

(continued)

STAGE 20 (continued)

Serial No.	Size (mm)	Grade	Fixative	Embedding medium	Plane	Thinness (μm)	Stain	Point score	Sex	Year	Notes
3527	E., 22 Ch., 32×30×10	Good	Formol	P	Sag.	25	Al. coch.	28	♀	1921	
4059	E., 21.6	Good	Formol	P	Cor.	15	Al. coch., Mallory	29.5	♀	1922	
4148	E., 21 Ch., 45×34×30	Good	Formol	P	Cor.	15	Al. coch., Mallory	19	♀	1922	
4361	E., 22 Ch., 52×42×23	Poor	Formol	P	Trans.	20	Coch.	24	♂	1923	
5537	E., 22	Exc.	Bouin	P	Trans.	20	Al. coch.	21	♂	1927	
6202	E., 21 Ch., 35×35×22	Exc.	Bouin	P	Sag.	20	H.&E.	20.5	♂	1930	Tubal
6426	E., 21.5	Good	Formol	C-P	Trans.	20	H.&E.	21	♂	1931	
7274	E., 18.5 Ch., 48×44×35	Exc.	Bouin	C-P	Trans.	20	H.&E., phlox.	20	♀	1936	
7906	E., 19.5	Exc.	Bouin	C-P	Cor.	20	H.&E.	22	♂	1941	Left renal agenesis
8157	E., 20.8	Exc.	Bouin	C-P	Cor.	20	H.&E.	24	♂	1943	
8226	E., 18.0	Exc.	Bouin	C-P	Sag.	10	Azan	?	♂	1944	

STAGE 21

Serial No.	Size (mm)	Grade	Fixative	Embedding medium	Plane	Thinness (μm)	Stain	Point score	Sex	Year	Notes
22	E., 20 Ch., 35×30×30	Good	Alc.	P	Trans.	50	Al. carm.	34.5	♂	1895	
57	E., 23 Ch., ca. 30	Poor	Alc.	P	Sag.	50	Al. coch.	36	♂	1896	
128	E., 20 Ch., 50×43	Good	Formol	P	Cor.	50	Al. coch.	33	♂	1898	
229	E., 19	Poor	Alc.	P	Sag.	50	Al. coch.	33	♀	1903	
349	E., 24	Good	Zenker	C	Cor.	250	Unstained	36	?	1905	Double vascular injection
455	E., 24 Ch., 42×34×20	Good	Alc.	P	Trans.	30	H.&E.	36.5	♂	1910	
632	E., 24 Ch., 60×50×30	Good	Bichlor. acetic	P	Sag.	40, 100, 250	Al. coch.	33	♀	1913	Injected
903C	E., 23.5	Good	Formol	P	Trans.	40	Al. coch.	38.5	♀	1914	
1008	E., 26.4	Good	Formol	P	Sag.	40	Al. coch.	39	♂	1914	
1358F	E., 23	Good	Formol	P	Sag.	40	Al. coch.	37.5	♀	1916	
2937	E., 24.2	Good	Bouin	P	Trans.	50	H.&E. aur., or. G.	39	♀	1920	
3167	E., 24.5 Ch., 60×50×40	Poor	Bichlor. acetic, formol	P	Trans.	20	Al. coch.	32	♂	1920	
4090	E., 22.2 Ch., 66×46×30	Good	Formol	P	Trans.	40	Al. coch.	30	♀	1922	
4160	E., 25	Poor	Formol	P	Sag.	25	H.&E.	39	♂	1923	Tubal
4960	E., 22 Ch., 47×42×28	Good	Formol	P	Trans.	15	Al. coch., Mallory	31.5	♀	1925	
5596	E., 21.5	Good	Formol	P	Sag.	50	Al. coch.	34	♀	1927	
6531	E., 22	Poor	Glacial acetic, abs. alc.	C-P	Trans.	10	H.&E.	31.5	♀	1931	Leitz Collection
7254	E., 22.5	Exc.	Bouin	C-P	Trans.	20	H.&E.	33.5	♂	1936	
7392	E., 22.7	Exc.	Bouin	C-P	Trans.	20	H.&E.	36	♂	1937	
7864	E., 24	Exc.	Formol	C-P	Frontal	20	H.&E.	32.5	♂	1941	
8553	E., 22	Exc.	Bouin	C-P	Trans.	12	H.&E.	38	♀	1947	
9614	E., 22.5	Exc.	Bouin	P	Cor.	10 & 15	Azan	?	♂	1958	Rubella. Hysterectomy

STAGE 22

Serial No.	Size (mm)	Grade	Fixative	Embedding medium	Plane	Thinness (μm)	Stain	Point score	Sex	Year	Notes
392	E., 23 Ch., 45 × 45 × 25	Poor	...	P	Sag.	50	Al. coch.	42	♀	1907	Brödel Collection. Injected
405	E., 26	Good	Formol	C	Sag.	40	Carmine	42.5	♂	1907	
464	E., 26 Ch., 45 × 40 × 30	Good	Formol?, alc.?	P	Sag.	100	Al. coch.	44.5	♂	1910	
584A	E., 25 Ch., 50 × 42 × 40	Poor	Formol	P	Sag.	50	Al. coch.	41	?	1913	
630	E., 25	Poor	Formol	P	Trans.	100	Al. coch.	46	♂	1913	
840	E., 24.8	Good	Formol	P	Trans.	50	Al. coch.	44.5	♀	1914	
875	E., 27 Ch., 40 × 28 × 22	Good	Formol	P	Sag.	40	Al. coch.	45	♂	1914	
895	E., 26 Ch., 67 × 62 × 54	Good	Formol	P	Trans.	25	Al. coch.	46.5	♀	1914	
1315	E., 25	Good	Formol	P	Sag.	50	Al. coch.	40.5	♀	1915	Spina bifida and anencephaly
1458	E., 27.5 Ch., 45 × 45 × 30	Exc.	Formol	C	Sag.	50	H.&E. aur., or. G.	45.5	♂	1916	
1894	E., 24.6	Good	Formol	C	Sag.	40,80	H.&E. aur., or. G.	41	♀	1917	
2206	E., 27 Ch., 50 × 30 × 18	Poor	Formol	P	Trans.	40	H.&E.	44.5	♂	1918	
3681	E., 26.3 Ch., 36 × 36 × 34	Good	Formol	P	Trans.	25	Al. coch.	44.5	♂	1921	
4304	E., 25 Ch., 66 × 45 × 45	Good	Bouin	P	Trans.	20	H.&E.	44.5	♀	1923	Injected
4339	E., 24.5	Good	Formol	P	Trans.	15	Al. coch., Mallory	46.5	♀	1923	
4476	E., 26.2	Good	Bouin	P	Trans.	40	H.&E.	46	♀	1923	Tubal
4638	E., 23.4	Exc.	Bouin	P	Trans.	15,20	Al. coch., or. G.	41.5	♂	1924	
6701	E., 24	Poor	Formol	P	Cor.	20	H.&E.	41	♀	1933	
6832	E., 25.8	Exc.	Bouin	C-P	Cor.	20	H.&E.	42	♀	1934	
8394	E., 25.3 Ch., 48 × 50 × 34	Exc.	Bouin	C-P	Trans.	20	H.&E., Masson	44.5	♀	1946	
8948	E., 26.7 Ch., 61 × 51 × 50	Poor	Formol-Zenker	?	Trans.	15	Ag	?	?	1952	

STAGE 23

Serial No.	Size (mm)	Grade	Fixative	Embedding medium	Plane	Thinness (μm)	Stain	Point score	Sex	Year	Notes
45	E., 28 Ch., 40 × 35 × 20	Poor	?	P	Cor. trans.	50	Al. coch.	51.5	♀	1895	
75	E., 30	Good	Alc.	P	Sag.	50	Coch.	57	♂	1897	
86	E., 30	Good	?	?	Cor.	50	Coch.	?	♂	1897	May be an early fetus
100	E., 27	Poor	?	P	Sag.	50	Al. coch.	57.5	?	1897	
108	E., 28 (est.)	Poor	Picro-sulph. acid	P	Sag.	45	Borax carm.	52.5	♂	1897	
227	E., 30 Ch., 60 × 40 × 20	Poor	Formol	P	Sag.	50, 100	Al. coch.	54	♂	1903	
417	E., 32 Ch., 70 × 60 × 40	Good	Formol	P	Trans.	100	Al. coch.	58.5	♀	1907	
756A	E., 27 Ch., 60 × 45 × 35	Good	Formol	P	Cor.	50	Al. coch.	56	♂	1913	
782	E., 28 Ch., 80 × 80 × 70	Good	Formol	P	Trans.	40	Multiple	53	♂	1913	
950	E., 29	Good	Formol	P	Trans.	50	Al. coch.	54	♂	1914	
1199	E., 26 Ch., 60 × 40 × 30	Good	Formol	C	Cor.	40	H.&E. aur., or. G.	54.5	♂	1915	
1535	E., 28 Ch., 50 × 45 × 15	Poor	Formol	P	Trans.	40	H.&E.	49.5	♂	1916	

(continued)

STAGE 23 (continued)

Serial No.	Size (mm)	Grade	Fixative	Embedding medium	Plane	Thinness (μm)	Stain	Point score	Sex	Year	Notes
1945	E., 27.3 Ch., 83 × 53 × 22.5	Good	Formol	C-P	Trans.	50	H.&E. aur., or. G.	48	♀	1917	
2561	E., 27.5	Good	Formol	C-P	Trans.	25	H.&E. aur., or. G.	48.5	♂	1919	
4205	E., 29.5	Good	Bouin	P	Trans.	50	Al. coch.	55.5	♀	1923	
4289	E., 32.2 Ch., 52 × 35 × 25	Good	Formol	P	Trans.	15,20	Al. coch., Mallory	59	♀	1923	
4525	E., 30	Good	Formol	P	Sag.	20	H.&E.	57	♂	1924	
4570	E., 30.7 Ch., 52 × 50 × 28	Exc.	Bouin	P	Trans.	15	H.&E., phlox.	55	♂	1924	
5154	E., 32	Good	Bouin	P	Trans.	20	H.&E.	59.5	♂	1926	
5422	E., 27	Good	Formol	P	Sag.	40	H.&E.	52.5	♀	1927	
5621A	E., 27.5	Good	Formol	P	Trans.	20	H.&E.	52.5	♂	1927	Other twin has spina bifida and fused kidneys
5725	E., 23	Good	Formol	P	Cor.	25	H.&E. aur., or. G.	50.5	♀	1928	
6573	E., 31.5	Good	Bouin	C	Trans.	20	H.&E.	58.5	♀	1932	
7425	E., 27	Exc.	Bouin	C-P	Cor.	20	H.&E.	47	♀	1937	Ag added
9226	E., 31	Exc.	Formol	C-P	Trans.	12	Azan	?	♂	1954	
D.122	E., 27	Exc.	?	?	Trans.	19	Ag	?	?	1976	Yntema and Truex

APPENDIX II

INDEX OF SPECIMENS OF STAGES 1–9

The following is an alphabetical list of named and numbered specimens that have been described or cited in the literature. Their authors have also been included in the list. In the case of each specimen, the stage to which it is believed to belong is indicated, and further details will be found in the text under the heading of the appropriate stage.

Specimen or Author	Stage
Am. 10	6b
Andô	6b
Bagiński and Borsuk, 1967	9
Bandler, 1912	5
Barnes	5c
Bayer	6b
Beitler (No. 763)	8?
Beneke	6b
Bi I	6b
Bi 24	7
Biggart	7(6?)
Boerner-Patzelt and Schwarzacher, 1923	8
Brewer, 1937, 1938 (Edwards-Jones-Brewer)	6b
Broman, 1936	8
Bryce, 1924 (M'Intyre)	8
(Teacher-Bryce I)	5
(Teacher-Bryce II)	6b
Carnegie No. 763	8?
1399	7
1878	9
4900	5c
5080	9
5960	8
5981	8
5982	9
6026 (path.)	6b?
6027	8?
6630	8
6706	6–8?
6734	6a
6815	8
6900	6a
7634	6a
7640	8
7699	5c
7700	5c
7762	6b
7770 (path.)	5c
7771 (path.)	5c
7800 (path.)	7
7801	6b
7802	7
7850 (path.)	5–6
7950	5c
8000 (path.)	5c

Specimen or Author	Stage
8004	5b
8020	5a
8139	5c
8155	5a
8171	5b
8190 (path.)	2
8215	5b
8225	5a
8260	2
8290 (path.)	6?
8299 (path.)	5c
8329 (path.)	5c
8330	5c
8360	6a
8370 (path.)	5c
8450 (path.)	2
8452 (path.)	2
8500.1	2
8558	5c
8602	7
8630 (path.)	2
8663	3
8671	8
8672	6a
8698	2
8727	8
8794	3
8819	6b
8820	8
8904	2
8905	6
9009	8
9250	6
9350	5b
Da 1 (No. 5982)	9
Dankmeijer and Wielenga, 1968	5
D'Arrigo, 1971	7?
Davies, 1944 (Davies-Harding)	5c
Debeyre, 1912	7
Dible and West, 1941	5c
Dickmann et al., 1965	1
Dobbin	8
Doyle et al., 1966	2
Dy	8
E.B.	6a
Edwards and Fowler, 1970	2,3

Specimen or Author	Stage
Edwards et al., 1966	2
1969	1
1970	2
Edwards-Jones-Brewer (No. 8819)	6b
Eternod, 1899b, 1909 (Vulliet)	8
Faber, 1940 (E.B.)	6a
Fahrenholz, 1927 (Ho)	7
Falkiner	7
Fetzer, 1910	6b
Fife-Richter	6b
Fitzgerald	7
Fitzgerald-Brewer I	8
II	7
Florian. See Bi I, Manchester 1285, T.F., etc.	
Frassi, 1908	8
Fruhling et al., 1954	5a
Gar	7
George, 1942 (No. 7640)	8
Gladstone and Hamilton, 1941 (Shaw)	8
Gläveke	8
Gle. See Gläveke	
Goodwin	7
Graf Spee (Gläveke)	8
Greenhill, 1927	6?
Grosser, 1913 (Kl. 13)	8
1922 (Kleinhans)	5c
1931a (H. Schm. 10)	7
1931b (Wa 17)	8
Guá	7(8?)
Gv (Madrid)	9
H3	9
H381	6
H.R. 1	6b(8?)
H. Schm. 10	7
Häggström, 1922	2
Hamilton, 1946, 1949	1
Hamilton and Boyd, 1960 (Missen)	7
Hamilton et al., 1943 (Barnes)	5c
1967	6?
Harrison and Jeffcoate, 1953 (Liverpool I)	6b
Harvard No. 55	6a
825	6b

Specimen or Author	Stage
HEB-18	6b
HEB-37	7
HEB-42	8
Herranz and Vásquez, 1964	2
Hertig and Rock. See specimen numbers under Carnegie	8
Hertig *et al.*, 1958 ("No. 55")	6a
Herzog, 1909 (Manila)	6
Heuser, 1932b (No. 5960)	8
1954 (No. 9009)	8
Heuser. See also specimen numbers under Carnegie	
Hill. See Bi 24, Dobbin, etc.	
Hiramatsu, 1936 (Andô)	6b
His embryo E	9–10
Ho	7
Hugo	7
Ingalls, 1918 (Western Reserve No. 1)	8
1920 (No. 1878)	9
Jahnke and Stegner, 1964	6
Jiménez Collado and Ruano Gil (Gv)	9
Johnston, 1940 (H.R.1)	6b(8?)
Johnstone, 1914	6
Jones and Brewer, 1941 (Jones-Brewer I; No. 8820)	8
Jones and Brewer II	7
Jung, 1908	6
Keibel, 1890 (Bayer)	6b
1907 (Frassi)	8
Keller and Keller, 1954	5
Khvatov, 1959	1
1967	3
1968	2
Kindred, 1933 (Goodwin)	7
Kistner, 1953	6
Kl. 13	8
Kleinhans	5c
Knorre (VMA-1)	6a
Krafka, 1939	2
1941 (Torpin)	6a
1942	3(2?)
Krause, 1952 (Am. 10)	6b
Krukenberg, 1922	8
Lbg	6b
Lewis and Harrison, 1966 (Liverpool II)	6b
Linzenmeier, 1914 (Stöckel)	6a
Liverpool I	6b
Liverpool II	6b
Lockyer (No. 6026)	6b?

Specimen or Author	Stage
Lordy, 1931 (Guá)	7(8?)
Lqt	8
Ludwig, 1928 (Da 1)	9
Macafee	5
M'Intyre, 1926	8
Mal	7
Manchester No. 1285	7
Manila	6
Marchetti, 1945 (No. 8139)	5c
Martin and Falkiner, 1938	7
Mateer (No. 1399)	7
Mazanec, 1960 (HEB-18)	6b
Mazanec and Musilovà, 1959 (HEB-42)	8
Menkin and Rock, 1948 (No. 8260)	2
(No. 8500.1)	2
Merrill	6
Meyer, 1924 (P.M.)	7
Miller (No. 4900)	5c
Minot (Harvard No. 825)	6b
Missen	7
Morton, 1949 (Biggart)	7(6?)
(Macafee)	5
Müller, 1930	5
Noback *et al.*, 1968	6
Normentafel 1 (Frassi)	8
2 (Gläveke)	8
Noyes *et al.*, 1965	1
Odgers, 1937 (Thomson)	6b
1941 (R.S.)	8
Op	6b
P.M.	7
Peh.1-Hochstetter	8
Penkert, 1910	6b?
Peters, 1899	6a
Petrov, 1958	2
Pha I	7
Pha II	7
Pha XVII	8
Piersol, 1938 (T439)	9
Pommerenke, 1958	5
R.S.	8
Ramsey, 1937 (Lockyer)	6b?
1938 (Yale)	6a
Richter, 1952 (Fife-Richter)	6b
Robertson *et al.*, 1948	7(8?)
Rochester (No. 7762)	6b
Rossenbeck, 1923 (Peh.1-Hochstetter)	8

Specimen or Author	Stage
Sch	5
Schlagenhaufer and Verocay, 1916	6
Schö	8
Scipiades, 1938	5(6?)
Shaw	8
Shettles, 1956, 1957, 1960	3
1958, 1960	2
Stieve, 1926 (Hugo)	7
1936 (Werner)	5c
Stöckel (No. 6900)	6a
Strahl, 1916	8
Strahl-Beneke	6b
Streeter, 1920a (Mateer)	7
1926 (Miller)	5c
Stump, 1929 (H 381)	6
Swett (No. 6815)	8
T439 (Toronto)	9
T.F.	6b
Teacher-Bryce I	5
Teacher-Bryce II	6b
Thomas and van Campenhout, 1953	6
1963	5?
Thompson and Brash, 1923	8
Thomson	6b
Thyng (No. 6026)	6b?
Torpin (No. 7634)	6a
Triepel, 1916 (Dy)	8
v. H. (von Herff)	6
VMA-1 (Knorre)	6a
von Möllendorff, 1921b (Op)	6b
1921a (Sch.)	5
1925 (Wo)	6b
von Spee, 1889, 1896 (Gläveke)	8
1896 (v. H.)	6
Vuill. See Vulliet	
Vulliet	8
Wa17	8
Waldeyer, 1929a (Schö)	8
Way and Dawson, 1959	2
Werner	5c
West 1952 (Gar)	7
1952 (Mal)	7
Western Reserve No. 1	8
Wharton (No. 6706)	6–8?
Wilson, 1914 (H3)	9
1945 (Rochester)	6b
1954	5c
Wo	6b
Yale (No. 6734)	6a
Zamboni *et al.*, 1966	1

BIBLIOGRAPHY

Aasar, Y. H. 1931. The history of the prochordal plate in the rabbit. *J. Anat., 46*, 14–45.

Adams, W. E. 1960. Early human development. *N. Z. Med. J., 59*, 7–17.

Adelmann, H. B. 1922. The significance of the prechordal plate: an interpretative study. *Amer. J. Anat., 31*, 54–101.

Allan, F. D. 1963. Observations on the organizer areas of the human pre-somite embryo. *Anat. Rec., 145*, 199.

Allen, E., Pratt, J. P., Newell, Q. U., and Bland, L. J. 1930. Human tubal ova; related early corpora lutea and uterine tubes. *Carnegie Instn. Wash. Publ. 414, Contrib. Embryol., 22*, 45–76.

Allen, M. S., and Turner, U. G. 1971. Twin birth—identical or fraternal twins? *Obstet. Gynecol., 37*, 538–542.

Andersen, H., Ehlers, N., and Matthiessen, M. E. 1965. Histochemistry and development of the human eylids. *Acta ophthalmol., 43*, 642–668.

Andersen, H., Ehlers, N., Matthiessen, M. E., and Claesson, M. H. 1967. Histochemistry and development of the human eyelids II. *Acta ophthalmol., 45*, 288–298.

Anderson, R. H. 1973. An investigation of bulboventricular morphogenesis in the human heart. *Proc. Anat. Soc. Great Britain and Ireland*, p. 12 (abstract).

Anderson, R. H., Wilkinson, J. L., and Becker, A. E. 1978. The bulbus cordis—A misunderstood region of the developing human heart. *In* Rosenquist, G. C., and Bergsma, D. (ed.). *Morphogenesis and Malformation of the Cardiovascular System.* Liss, New York, pp. 1–28.

Anson, B. J., and Black, W. T. 1934. The early relation of the auditory vesicle to the ectoderm in human embryos. *Anat. Rec., 58*, 127–137.

Arey, L. B. 1938. The history of the first somite in human embryos. *Carnegie Instn. Wash. Publ. 496, Contrib. Embryol., 27*, 233–269.

Arey, L. B., and Henderson, J. W. 1943. The Huber six-somite human embryo (No. 71). *Anat. Rec., 85*, 295.

Ashley, D. J. B. 1959. Are ovarian pregnancies parthenogenetic? *Amer. J. Hum. Genet., 11*, 305–310.

Atwell, W. J. 1926. The prechordal plate in a human embryo with small neuropore. *Anat. Rec., 32*, 200 (Abstr.).

Atwell, W. J. 1930. A human embryo with seventeen pairs of somites. *Carnegie Instn. Wash. Publ. 407, Contrib. Embryol., 21*, 1–24.

Avila Fredes, W. 1970. Caracteristicas morfologicas del corazon del embrion humano de 4, 5 mm. (Horizontes XII y XIII, de Streeter). *An. Desarrollo, 15*, 173–182.

Avendaño, S., Croxatto, H.D., Pereda, J., and Croxatto, H.B. 1975. A seven-cell human egg recovered from the oviduct. *Fertil. Steril., 26*, 1167–1172.

Baca, M., and Zamboni, L. 1967. The fine structure of human follicular oocytes. *J. Ultrastruct. Res., 19*, 354–381.

Bagiński, S., and Borsuk, I. 1967. (Micromorphology of the human fetus in the third week of tubal pregnancy). *Folia Morphol.* (Warszawa), *26*, 153–160.

Bandler. 1912. The earliest recorded case of ectopic gestation. *Amer. J. Obstet. Gynecol., 66*, 454.

Barniville, H. L. 1915. The morphology and histology of a human embryo of 8.5 mm. *J. Anat. Physiol., 49*, 1–71.

Bartelmez, G. W. 1922. The origin of the otic and optic primordia in man. *J. Comp. Neurol., 34*, 201–232.

Bartelmez, G. W. 1923. The subdivisions of the neural folds in man. *J. Comp. Neurol., 35*, 231–247.

Bartelmez, G. W., and Blount, M. P. 1954. The formation of neural crest from the primary optic vesicle in man. *Carnegie Instn. Wash. Publ. 603, Contrib. Embryol., 35*, 55–71.

Bartelmez, G. W., and Dekaban, A. S. 1962. The early development of the human brain. *Carnegie Instn. Wash. Publ. 621, Contrib. Embryol., 37*, 13–32.

Bartelmez, G. W., and Evans, H. M. 1926. Development of the human embryo during the period of somite formation, including embryos with 2 to 16 pairs of somites. *Carnegie Instn. Wash. Publ. 362, Contrib. Embryol., 17*, 1–67.

Baxter, J. S., and Boyd, J. D. 1939. Observations on the neural crest of a ten-somite human embryo. *J. Anat., 73*, 318–326.

Bellairs, R. 1986. The primitive streak. *Anat. Embryol., 174*, 1–14.

Bergquist, H. 1952. Formation of neuromeres in Homo. *Acta Societatis Medicorum Upaliensis, 57*, 23–32.

Blandau, R. J. (ed.). 1971. *The Biology of the Blastocyst.* University of Chicago Press, Chicago.

Blechschmidt, E. 1948. *Funktionsentwicklung. I. Mechan-*

ische Genwirkungen. Musterschmidt, Göttingen.

Blechschmidt, E. 1963. *Der menschliche Embryo. Dokumentationen zur kinetischen Anatomie.* Schattauer, Stuttgart.

Blechschmidt, E. 1968. *Vom Ei zum Embryo.* Deutsche Verlags-Anstalt, Stuttgart.

Blechschmidt, E. 1972. Die ersten drei Wochen nach der Befruchtung. *Image Roche*, Basel, *47*, 17–24.

Blechschmidt, E. 1973. *Die pränatalen Organsysteme des Menschen.* Hippokrates, Stuttgart.

Bloom, W., and Bartelmez, G. W. 1940. Hematopoiesis in young human embryos. *Amer. J. Anat., 67*, 21–53.

Boerner-Patzelt, D., and Schwarzacher, W. 1923. Ein junges menschliches Ei in situ. *Z. Anat. Entw., 68*, 204–229.

Bonnot, E., and Severs, R. 1906. On the structure of a human embryo eleven millimeters in length. *Anat. Anz., 29*, 452–459.

Born, G. 1883. Die Plattenmodelliermethode. *Arch. mikr. Anat., 22*, 584–599.

Bossy, J. 1980a. Development of olfactory and related structures in staged human embryos. *Anat. Embryol., 161*, 225–236.

Bossy, J. 1980b. Développement séquential de la glande mammaire primitive pendant la période embryonnaire vraie. *Senelogia, 5*, 325–328.

Bossy, J. 1980c. Développement des branches dorsales des nerfs spinaux durant la période embryonnaire vraie. *Bull. Ass. Anat., 64*, 199–206.

Bossy, J. 1981. Innervation séquentielle de l'anse intestinale chez l'embryon humain. *Bull. Ass. Anat., 65*, 245–251.

Bossy, J. 1982. Séquence du développement de l'innervation cutanée des membres chez l'embryon humain. *Bull. Ass. Anat., 66*, 57–61.

Böving, B. G. 1963. Implantation Mechanisms. Ch. 7 in C. G. Hartman (ed.), *Conference on Physiological Mechanisms Concerned with Conception.* Pergamon, Oxford.

Böving, B. G. 1965. Anatomy of Reproduction. Ch. 1 in J. P. Greenhill, *Obstetrics.* 13th edition, Saunders, Philadelphia.

Böving, B. G. 1981. Vascular relations of implanting human conceptuses. *Anat. Rec., 199*, 33A–34A.

Boyd, J. D. 1937. The development of the human carotid body. *Carnegie Instn. Wash. Publ. 479, Contrib. Embryol., 26*, 1–31.

Boyd, J. D., and Hamilton, W. J. 1966. Electron microscopic observations on the cytotrophoblast contribution to the syncytium in the human placenta. *J. Anat., 100*, 535–548.

Boyd, J. D., and Hamilton, W. J. 1970. *The Human Placenta.* Heffer, Cambridge.

Boyden, E. A. 1940. A volumetric analysis of young human embryos of the 10- and 12-somite stage. *Carnegie Instn.*

Wash. Publ. 518, Contrib. Embryol., 28, 157–191.

Boyden, E. A. 1955. *A Laboratory Atlas of the 13-mm. Pig Embryo.* Wistar Institute, Philadelphia, 3rd edition.

Boyden, E. A., Cope, J. G., and Bill, A. H. 1967. Anatomy and embryology of congenital intrinsic obstruction of the duodenum. *Amer. J. Surg., 114*, 190–202.

Brackett, B. G., Seitz, H. M., Rocha, G., and Mastroianni, L. 1972. The mammalian fertilization process. *In* Moghissi, K. S., and Hafez, E. S. E. (ed.). *Biology of Mammalian Fertilization and Implantation.* Thomas, Springfield, Illinois. Ch. 6 (pp. 165–184).

Bremer, J. L. 1906. Description of a 4-mm. human embryo. *Amer. J. Anat., 5*, 459–480.

Bremer, J. L. 1914. The earliest blood-vessels in man. *Amer. J. Anat., 16*, 447–475.

Brewer, J. I. 1937. A normal human ovum in a stage preceding the primitive streak (The Edwards-Jones-Brewer ovum). *Amer. J. Anat., 61*, 429–481.

Brewer, J. I. 1938. A human embryo in the bilaminar blastodisc stage (The Edwards-Jones-Brewer ovum). *Carnegie Instn. Wash. Publ. 496, Contrib. Embryol., 27*, 85–93.

Brewer, J. I., and Fitzgerald, J. E. 1937. Six normal and complete presomite human ova. *Amer. J. Obstet. Gynecol., 34*, 210–224.

Broman, I. 1896. Beschreibung eines menschlichen Embryos von beinahe 3-mm. Länge. *Morphol. Arbeit., 5.* Cited by Streeter (1945).

Broman, I. 1936. Ein frühembryonales (etwa 20 Tage altes) menschliches Monstrum. *Morphol. Jahrb., 78*, 421–444.

Bryce, T. H. 1924. Observations on the early development of the human embryo. *Trans. Roy. Soc. Edinburgh, 53*, 533–567.

Bujard, E. 1913–1914. Description d'un embryon humain (Eternod-Delaf), de 20 somites, avec flexion dorsale. *Internat. Monatschr. Anat. Physiol., 31*, 238–266.

Bulmer, M. G. 1970. *The Biology of Twinning in Man.* Clarendon Press, Oxford.

Burow, W. S. 1928. A human embryo in the first month of embryonic life. *Med. J. Irkutsk* [In Russian; no illustrations], *6*, 71–79. Cited by Heuser and Corner (1957).

Butler, H. and Juurlink, B.H.J. 1987. *An Atlas for Staging Mammalian and Chick Embryos.* CRC. Boca Raton, Florida.

Buxton, B. H. 1899. Photographs of a series of sections of an early human embryo. *J. Anat. Physiol., 33*, 381–385.

Congdon, E. D. 1922. Transformation of the aortic arch system during the development of the human embryo. *Carnegie Instn. Wash. Publ. 277, Contrib. Embryol., 14*, 47–110.

Cooper, M. H., and O'Rahilly, R. 1971. The human heart at

seven postovulatory weeks. *Acta anat., 79,* 280–299.

Cordier, G., and Coujard, R. 1939. Sur un embryon humain de 1-mm.05. *Ann. Anat. path., 16,* 239–253.

Corner, G. W. 1929. A well-preserved human embryo of 10 somites. *Carnegie Instn. Wash. Publ. 394, Contrib. Embryol., 20,* 81–102.

Corner G. W. 1955. The observed embryology of human single-ovum twins and other multiple births. *Amer. J. Obstet. Gynecol., 70,* 933–951.

Coste, M. 1849. *Histoire générale et particulière du développement des corps organisés.* Paris. Cited by Streeter (1942).

Crowder, R. E. 1957. The development of the adrenal gland in man, with special reference to origin and ultimate location of cell types and evidence in favor of the "cell migration" theory. *Carnegie Instn. Wash. Publ. 611, Contrib. Embryol., 36,* 193–210.

Croxatto, H. B., Díaz, S., Fuentealba, B., Croxatto, H. D., Carrillo, D., and Fabres, C. 1972. Studies on the duration of egg transport in the human oviduct. I. The time interval between ovulation and egg recovery from the uterus in normal women. *Fertil. Steril., 23,* 447–458.

Cummins, H. 1929. The topographic history of the volar pads (walking pads; Tastballen) in the human embryo. *Carnegie Instn. Wash. Publ. 394, Contrib. Embryol., 20,* 105–126.

Dandy, W. E. 1910. A human embryo with seven pairs of somites, measuring about 2-mm. in length. *Amer. J. Anat., 10,* 85–109.

Daniel, J. C., and Olson, J. D. 1966. Cell movement, proliferation and death in the formation of the embryonic axis of the rabbit. *Anat. Rec., 156,* 123–127.

Dankmeijer, J., and Wielenga, G. 1968. Observation d'un oeuf humain d'environ dix jours. *Bull. Ass. Anat., 53,* 793–796.

D'Arrigo, S. 1961. Illustrazione di un embrione umano al principio della terza settimana di sviluppo. *Riv. Patol. Clin. Sper., 2,* 1–15.

Davies, F. 1944. A previllous human ovum, aged nine to ten days (the Davies-Harding ovum). *Trans. Roy. Soc. Edinburgh, 61,* 315–326.

Davis, C. L. 1923. Description of a human embryo having twenty paired somites. *Carnegie Instn. Wash. Publ. 332, Contrib. Embryol., 15,* 1–51.

Davis, C. L. 1927. Development of the human heart from its first appearance to the stage found in embryos of twenty paired somites. *Carnegie Instn. Wash. Publ. 380, Contrib. Embryol., 19,* 245–284.

Daya, S., and Clark, D. A. 1986. Production of immunosuppressor factor(s) by preimplantation human embryos. *Amer. J. Reprod. Immunol. Microbiol., 11,* 98–101.

deBeer, G. 1958. *Embryos and Ancestors.* 3rd edition, Clarendon Press, Oxford.

Debeyre, A. 1912. Description d'un embryon humain de 0-mm.9. *J. Anat. Physiol.,* Paris, *48,* 448–515.

Debeyre, A. 1933. Sur la présence de gonocytes chez un embryon humain au stade de la ligne primitive. *C. R. Ass. Anat., 28,* 240–250.

Dekaban, A. S. 1963. Anencephaly in early human embryos *J. Neuropathol. Exp. Neurol., 22,* 533–548.

Dekaban, A. S., and Bartelmez, G. W. 1964. Complete dysraphism in 14 somite human embryo. A contribution to normal and abnormal morphogenesis. *Amer. J. Anat., 115,* 27–41.

Delmas, A. 1939. Les ébauches pancréatiques dorsales et ventrales. Leurs rapports dans la constitution du pancréas définitif. *Ann. Anat. pathol., 16,* 253–266.

Dénes, J., Honti J., and Lèb, J. 1967. Dorsal herniation of the gut: a rare manifestation of the split notochord syndrome. *J. Pediat. Surg., 2,* 359–363.

Denker, H. -W. 1983. Basic aspects of ovoimplantation. *Obstet. Gynecol. Annual, 12,* 15–42.

de Vries, P. A. 1981. Evolution of precardiac and splanchnic mesoderm in relationship to the infundibulum and truncus. *In* Pexieder, T. (ed.). *Perspectives in Cardiovascular Research. 5. Mechanisms of Cardiac Morphogenesis and Teratogenesis.* Raven, New York.

de Vries, P. A., and Friedland, G. W. 1974. The staged sequential development of the anus and rectum in human embryos and fetuses. *J. Pediat. Surg., 9,* 755–769.

de Vries, P. A., and Saunders, J. B. de C. H. 1962. Development of the ventricles and spiral outflow tract in the human heart. *Carnegie Instn. Wash. Publ. 621, Contrib. Embryol., 37,* 87–114.

Dible, J. H., and West, C. M. 1941. A human ovum at the previllous stage. *J. Anat., 75,* 269–281.

Dickmann, Z., Chewe [Clewe], T. H., Bonney, W. A., and Noyes, R. W. 1965. The human egg in the pronuclear stage. *Anat. Rec., 152,* 293–302.

Diewert, V. M. 1981. Active contributions of differential craniofacial growth to secondary palate development in man. *Anat. Rec., 199,* 69A–70A.

Dodds, G. S. 1941. Anterior and posterior rhachischisis. *Amer. J. Pathol., 17,* 861–872.

Döderlein. 1915. *Handbuch der Geburtshilfe.* Wiesbaden. Cited by Streeter (1942).

Dorland, W. A. N., and Bartelmez, G. W. 1922. Clinical and embryologic report of an extremely early tubal pregnancy; together with a study of decidual reaction, intra-uterine and ectopic. *Amer. J. Obst. Gynecol., 4,* 215–227 and 372–386.

Doyle, L. L., Lippes, J., Winters, H. S., and Margolis, A. J. 1966. Human ova in the fallopian tube. *Amer. J. Obstet. Gynecol., 95,* 115–117.

Drumm, J. E., and O'Rahilly, R. 1977. The assessment of pre-natal age from the crown-rump length determined ultra-sonically. *Amer. J. Anat. 148*, 555–560.

Dvořák, M., Tesařík, J., Pilka, L., and Trávník, P. 1982. Fine structure of human 2-cell ova fertilized and cleaved in vitro. *Fertil. Steril. 37*, 661–667.

Edwards, R. G. 1972. Fertilization and cleavage *in vitro* of human ova. *In* Moghissi, K. S., and Hafez, E. S. E. (ed.). *Biology of Mammalian Fertilization and Implantation.* Thomas, Springfield, Illinois. Ch. 9 (pp. 263–278).

Edwards, R. G., Bavister, B. D., and Steptoe, P. C. 1969. Early stages of fertilization *in vitro* of human oocytes matured *in vitro. Nature, 221*, 632–635.

Edwards, R. G., Donahue, R. P., Baranki, T. A., and Jones, H. W. 1966. Preliminary attempts to fertilize human oocytes ma-tured in vitro. *Amer. J. Obstet. Gynecol., 96*, 192–200.

Edwards, R. G., and Fowler, R. E. 1970. Human embryos in the laboratory. *Sci. Amer., 223*, 44–54.

Edwards, R. G., Mettler, L., and Walters, D. E. 1986. Identical twins and in vitro fertilization. *J. in vitro Fertiliz. Emb. Transfer, 3*, 114–117.

Edwards, R. G., and Steptoe, P. C. (ed.). 1985. *Implantation of the Human Embryo.* Academic Press, London.

Edwards, R. G., Steptoe, P. C., and Purdy, J. M. 1970. Fertil-ization and cleavage *in vitro* of preovulator[y] human oocytes. *Nature, 227*, 1307–1309.

Elze, C. 1907. Beschreibung eines menschlichen Embryo von zirka 7 mm grösster Länge unter besonderer Berück-sichtigung der Frage nach der Entwickelung der Extrem-itätenarterien und nach der morphologischen Bedeutung der lateralen Schilddrüsenanlage. *Anat. Hefte, 106*, 411–492.

Enders, A. C. 1965. Formation of syncytium from cytotro-phoblast in the human placenta. *Obstet. Gynecol., 25*, 378–386.

Enders, A. C. 1976. Cytology of human early implantation. *Res. Reprod., 8*, 1–4.

Enders, A. C., Hendrickx, A. G., and Schlafke, S. 1983. Im-plantation in the rhesus monkey: initial penetration of endometrium. *Amer. J. Anat., 167*, 275–298.

Enders, A. C., and Schlafke, S. 1981. Differentiation of the blastocyst of the rhesus monkey. *Amer. J. Anat., 162*, 1–21.

Enders. A. C., Schlafke, S., and Hendrickx, A. G. 1986. Differ-entiation of the embryonic disc, amnion, and yolk sac in the rhesus monkey. *Amer. J. Anat., 177*, 161–185.

Eternod, A. C. F. 1896. Sur un œuf humain de 16.3 mm. avec embryon de 2.11 mm. (utérus et annexes). *Actes Soc. hel-vet. sci. nat., 79*, 164–169.

Eternod, A. C. F. 1899a. Premiers stades de la circulation san-guine dans l'oeuf et l'embryon humains. *Anat. Anz., 15*, 181–189.

Eternod, A. C. F. 1899b. Il y a un canal notochordal dans l'embryon humain. *Anat. Anz., 16*, 131–143.

Eternod, A. C. F. 1909. *L'oeuf humain.* Georg, Geneva.

Evans, H. M. 1912. The development of the vascular system. *In* Keibel, F., and Mall, F. P. (ed.). *Manual of Human Embryology.* Lippincott, Philadelphia. *2*, 570–708.

Evans, H. M., and Bartelmez, G. W. 1917. A human embryo of 7 to 8 somites. *Anat. Rec., 2*, 355–356.

Faber, V. 1940. Beobachtungen an einem etwa 2 Wochen alten menschlichen Ei. *Z. mikr.-anat. Forsch., 48*, 375–386.

Fahrenholz, C. 1927. Ein junges menschliches Abortivei. *Z. mikr.-anat. Forsch., 8*, 250–324.

Felix, W. 1912. The development of the urinogenital organs. *In* Keibel, F., and Mall, F. P., (ed.). *Manual of Human Embryology.* Lippincott, Philadelphia. *2*, 752–979.

Ferner, H. 1939. Zur Differenzierung der Rumpf-Schwanz-knospe beim Menschen. *Z. mikr.-anat. Forsch., 45*, 555–562.

Fetzer, M. 1910. Über ein durch Operation gewonnenes men-schliches Ei, das in seiner Entwickelung etwa dem Pe-tersschen Ei entspricht. *Verh. Anat. Ges., Erg. Heft. Anat. Anz., 37*, 116–126.

Fetzer, M., and Florian, J. 1929. Der jüngste menschliche Embryo (Embryo "Fetzer") mit bereits entwickelter Kloak-enmembran. *Anat. Anz., 67*, 481–492.

Fetzer, M., and Florian, J. 1930. Der Embryo "Fetzer" mit beginnender Axialmesodermbildung und bereits angeleg-ter Kloakenmembran. *Z. mikr.-anat. Forsch., 21*, 351–461.

Florian, J. 1927. Über zwei junge menschliche Embryonen. *Verh. Anat. Ges., Erg. Heft Anat. Anz., 63*, 184–192.

Florian, J. 1928a. Ein junges menschliches Ei in situ (Embryo T. F. mit Primitivstreifen ohne Kopfforsatz). *Z. mikr.-anat. Forsch., 13*, 500–590.

Florian, J. 1928b. Grafická rekonstrukce velmi mladých lid-ských zárodků (Graphische Rekonstruktion sehr junger menschlicher Embryonen). *Spisy Lékařské Fakulty Masa-rykovy University v Brně*, ČSR (Publications de la Faculté de Médecine, Brno, Répub. Tchécosl.), *6*, 1–64.

Florian, J. 1928c. La gouttière primitive, le canal de Lieber-kühn et la plaque chordale chez deux embryons humains (Bi II Bi III) avec quatre somites. *C. R. Ass. Anat., 23*, 154–162.

Florian, J. 1930a. The formation of the connecting stalk and the extension of the amniotic cavity towards the tissue of the connecting stalk in young human embryos. *J. Anat., 64*, 454–476.

Florian, J. 1930b. Über den Verlauf der Schnittebene bei einigen bisher beschriebenen jungen menschlichen Em-bryonen. *Anat. Anz., 71*, 54–61.

Florian, J. 1931. "Urkeimzellen" bei einem 625 μ langen menschlichen Embryo. *Verb. Anat. Ges., Erg. Heft Anat. Anz., 72*, 286.

Florian, J. 1933. The early development of man, with special reference to the development of the mesoderm and the cloacal membrane. *J. Anat., 67*, 263–276.

Florian, J. 1934a. Über die Existenz von zwei verschiedenen Typen junger menschlicher Embryonen. *Biol. Gen., 10*, 521–532.

Florian, J. 1934b. Ein Schema der Entwicklung der Axialgebilde des menschlichen Embryos bis in das Stadium von 10 Urwirbelpaaren. *Biol. Gen., 10*, 533–544.

Florian, J. 1934c. Über einige bisher unkorrigiert gebliebene fehlerhafte Angaben der junge menschliche Embryonen beschreibenden Arbeiten. *Anat. Anz., 78*, 445–450.

Florian, J. 1945. Gastrulace a notogenese obratlovců, zuláště člověka (La gastrulation et la notogénèse des vertébrés, surtout de l'homme). *Věstník Královské České Společnosti Nauk Třída Matematicko-Přírodovědecká*, Ročník, 1–26.

Florian J., and Beneke, R. 1931. Neue Befunde am Embryo "Beneke." *Verb. Anat. Ges., Erg. Heft Anat. Anz., 71*, 229–232.

Florian, J., and Hill, J. P. 1935. An early human embryo (No. 1285, Manchester Collection), with capsular attachment of the connecting stalk. *J. Anat., 69*, 399–411.

Florian, J., and Völker, O. 1929. Über die Entwicklung des Primitivstreifens, der Kloakenmembran und der Allantois beim Menschen. *Z. mikr.-anat. Forsch., 16*, 75–100.

Fol, H. 1884. L'anatomie d'un embryon humain d'un peu plus de trois semaines. *Rev. méd. Suisse romande, 4*, 177–201.

Fol., H. 1884. Description d'un embryon humain de cinq millimètres et six dixièmes. *Rec. zool. suisse, 1*, 357–401.

Forssner, H. 1907. Die angeborenen Darm- und Oesophagusatresien. *Anat. Hefte, 34*, Abt. I, 1–163. Cited by Streeter (1942).

Franchi, L. L. 1970. The ovary. *In* Philipp, E. E., Barnes, J., and Newton, M. (ed.). *Scientific Foundations of Obstetrics and Gynaecology*. Davis, Philadelphia.

Frassi, L. 1908. Weitere Ergebnisse des Studiums eines jungen menschlichen Eies in situ. *Arch. mikr.-anat. Entwicklungsgesch., 71*, 667–695.

Frazer, J. E. 1923. The nomenclature of disease states caused by certain vestigial structures in the neck. *Brit. J. Surg., 11*, 131–136.

Frazer, J. E. 1926. The disappearance of the precervical sinus. *J. Anat., 61*, 132–143.

Frazier, C. H., and Whitehead, E. 1925. The morphology of the Gasserian ganglion. *Brain, 48*, 458–475.

Fruhling, L., Ginglinger, A., and Gandar, R. 1954. Oeuf humain âgé de 8 jours. *Bull. Féd. Gynécol. Obstét. franç., 6*, 110–111.

Gage, S. P. 1905. A three weeks' human embryo, with especial reference to the brain and nephric system. *Amer. J. Anat., 4*, 409–443.

Gardner, E., and O'Rahilly, R. 1976a. Neural crest, limb development, and Thalidomide embryopathy. *Lancet, 1*, 635–637.

Gardner, E., and O'Rahilly, R. 1976b. The nerve supply and conducting system of the human heart at the end of the embryonic period proper. *J. Anat., 121*, 571–587.

Gasser, R. L. 1975. *Atlas of Human Embryos*. Harper & Row, Hagerstown, Maryland.

Gaunt, P. N., and Gaunt, W. A. 1978. *Three Dimensional Reconstruction in Biology*. Pitman, Tunbridge Wells, Kent.

Gedda, L. 1961. *Twins in History and Science*. Thomas, Springfield, Illinois.

George, W. C. 1942. A presomite human embryo with chorda canal and prochordal plate. *Carnegie Instn. Wash. Publ. 541, Contrib. Embryol., 30*, 1–7.

Giacomini, C. 1898. Un oeuf humain de 11 jours. *Arch. ital. Biol., 29*, 1–22.

Giglio-Tos, E. 1902. Sulle cellule germinative del tubo midollare embrionale dell'uomo. *Anat. Anz., 20*, 472–480. Cited by Streeter (1942).

Gilbert, P. W. 1957. The origin and development of the human extrinsic ocular muscles. *Carnegie Instn. Wash. Publ. 611, Contrib. Embryol., 36*, 59–78.

Gilbert, C., and Heuser, C. H. 1954. Studies in the development of the baboon (Papio ursinus). *Carnegie Instn. Wash. Publ. 603, Contrib. Embryol, 35*, 11–54.

Gilmour, J. R. 1941. Normal haemopoiesis in intra-uterine and neonatal life. *J. Pathol. Bacteriol, 52*, 25–55.

Girgis, A. 1926. Description of a human embryo of 22 paired somites. *J. Anat., 60*, 382–411.

Gitlin, G. 1968. Mode of union of right and left coelomic channels during development of the peritoneal cavity in the human embryo. *Acta anat., 71*, 45–52.

Gladstone, R. J., and Hamilton, W. J. 1941. A presomite human embryo (Shaw) with primitive streak and chorda canal, with special reference to the development of the vascular system. *J. Anat., 76*, 9–44.

Goedbloed, J. F. 1960. De vroege ontwikkeling van het middenoor. Thesis, Leiden, pp. 1–116.

Goor, D. A., and Lillehei, C. W. 1975. *Congenital Malformations of the Heart*. Grune & Stratton, New York.

Greenhill, J. P. 1927. A young human ovum in situ. *Amer. J. Anat., 40*, 315–354.

Gribnau, A. A. M., and Geijsberts, L. G. M. 1981. Developmental stages in the rhesus monkey (Macaca mulatta). *Adv. Anat. Embryol. Cell Biol., 68*, 1–84.

Grosser, O. 1913. Ein menschlicher Embryo mit Chordakanal. *Anat. Hefte, 47*, 649–686.

Grosser, O. 1922. Zur Kenntnis der Trophoblastschale bei jungen menschlichen Eiern. *Z. Anat. Entw., 66*, 179–198.

Grosser, O. 1926. Trophoblastschwache und zottenarme menschliche Eier. *Z. mikr.-anat. Forsch., 5*, 197–220.

Grosser, O. 1931a. Primitivstreifen und Kopffortsatz beim Menschen. *Verh. Anat. Ges., Erg. Heft Anat. Anz., 71*, 135–139.

Grosser. O. 1931b. Der Kopffortsatz des Primitivstreifens beim Menschen. Seine Differenzierung bei dem Embryo Wa 17. *Z. Anat. Entw., 94*, 275–292.

Grosser, O. 1931c. Weiteres über den Primitivstreifen des Menschen. *Verh. Anat. Ges., Erg. Heft Anat. Anz., 72*, 42–44.

Grosser, O. 1934. Über Variabilität in der menschlichen Embryonalentwicklung. *Z. Morphol. Anthropol. 34*, 108–112.

Gruber, G. B. 1926. Zur Frage der neurenterischen Oeffnung bei Früchten mit vollkommener Wirbelspaltung. *Z. Anat. Entw., 80*, 433–453.

Gruenwald, P. 1941a. Normal and abnormal detachment of body and gut from the blastoderm in the chick embryo, with remarks on the early development of the allantois. *J. Morphol., 69*, 83–125.

Gruenwald, P. 1941b. Early human twin embryo attached to other twin and not to the chorion. *Anat. Rec., 79*, Suppl., pp. 27–28.

Gruenwald, P. 1942. Early human twins with peculiar relations to each other and the chorion. *Anat. Rec., 83*, 267–279.

Guyot, R. 1985. *Théorie nouvelle sur les âges de la vie.* Barré & Dayez, Paris (2nd ed.).

Häggström, P. 1922. Über degenerative "parthenogenetische" Teilungen von Eizellen in normalen Ovarien des Menschen. *Acta gynecol. scand., 1*, 137–168.

Hamilton, W. J. 1946. The first findings of a pronuclear stage in man. *J. Anat., 80*, 224.

Hamilton, W. J. 1949. Early stages of human development. *Ann. Roy. Coll. Surg. Engl., 4*, 281–294.

Hamilton, W. J., Barnes, J., and Dodds, G. H. 1943. Phases of maturation, fertilization and early development in man. *J. Obstet. Gynaecol., Brit. Emp., 50*, 241–245.

Hamilton, W. J., and Boyd, J. D. 1950. Phases of human development. Ch. 8 in K. Bowes (ed.), *Modern Trends in Obstetrics and Gynaecology.* Butterworth, London, pp. 114–137.

Hamilton, W. J., and Boyd, J. D. 1960. Development of the human placenta in the first three months of gestation. *J. Anat., 94*, 297–328.

Hamilton, W. J., Boyd, J. D., and Misch, K. A. 1967. A very early monozygotic abnormal twin pregnancy. *Proc. Roy. Soc. Med., 60*, 995–998.

Hamilton, W. J., and Gladstone, R. J. 1942. A presomite human embryo (Shaw): the implantation. *J. Anat., 76*, 187–203.

Hamlett, G. W. D. 1935. Primordial germ cells in a 4.5 mm. human embryo. *Anat. Rec., 61*, 273–279.

Heard, O. O. 1957. Methods used by C. H. Heuser in preparing and sectioning early embryos. *Carnegie Instn. Wash. Publ. 611, Contrib. Embryol., 36*, 1–18.

Heine, Dr., and Hofbauer, J. 1911. Beitrag zur frühesten Entwicklung. *Z. Geburtsh. Gynäkol., 68*, 665–688.

Hendrickx, A. G. 1971. *Embryology of the Baboon.* University of Chicago Press, Chicago.

Hendrickx, A. G., Houston, M. L., and Kraemer, D. C. 1968. Observations on twin baboon embryos (*Papio sp.*). *Anat. Rec., 160*, 181–186.

Hendrickx, A. G., and Sawyer, R. H. 1975. Embryology of the rhesus monkey. *In* Bourne, G. H. (ed.). *The Rhesus Monkey.* Academic Press, New York, pp. 141–169.

Harris, J. W. S., and Ramsey, E. M. 1966. The morphology of human uteroplacental vasculature. *Carnegie Instn. Wash. Publ. 625, Contrib. Embryol., 38*, 43–58.

Harrison, R. G., and Jeffcoate, T. N. A. 1953. A presomite human embryo showing an early stage of the primitive streak. *J. Anat., 87*, 124–129.

Harrison, R. G., Jones, C. H., and Jones, E. P. 1966. A pathological presomite human embryo. *J. Pathol. Bacteriol., 92*, 583–584.

Herranz, G., and Vázquez, J. J. Partenogénesis rudimentaria en el óvulo humano. *Rev. Med. Univ. Navarra, 8*, 115–120.

Hertig, A. T. 1935. Angiogenesis in the early human chorion and in the primary placenta of the macaque monkey. *Carnegie Instn. Wash. Publ. 459, Contrib. Embryol., 25*, 37–81.

Hertig, A. T. 1968. *Human Trophoblast.* Thomas, Springfield, Illinois.

Hertig, A. T., Adams, E. C., McKay, D. G., Rock, J., Mulligan, W. J., and Menkin, M. F. 1958. A thirteen-day human ovum studied histochemically. *Amer. J. Obstet. Gynecol., 76*, 1025–1043.

Hertig, A. T., and Rock, J. 1941. Two human ova of the previllous stage, having an ovulation age of about eleven and twelve days respectively. *Carnegie Instn. Wash. Publ. 525, Contrib. Embryol., 29*, 127–156.

Hertig, A. T., and Rock, J. 1944. On the development of the early human ovum, with special reference to the trophoblast of the previllous stage: a description of 7 normal and 5 pathologic human ova. *Amer. J. Obstet. Gynecol., 47*, 149–184.

Hertig, A. T., and Rock, J. 1945a. Two human ova of the pre-villous stage, having a developmental age of about seven and nine days respectively. *Carnegie Instn. Wash. Publ. 557, Contrib. Embryol., 31*, 65–84.

Hertig, A. T., and Rock, J. 1945b. On a normal human ovum not over 7½ days of age. *Anat. Rec., 91*, 281.

Hertig, A. T., and Rock J. 1945c. On a normal ovum of approximately 9 to 10 days of age. *Anat. Rec., 91*, 281.

Hertig, A. T., and Rock, J. 1949. Two human ova of the pre-villous stage, having a developmental age of about eight and nine days respectively. *Carnegie Instn. Wash. Publ. 583, Contrib. Embryol., 33*, 169–186.

Hertig, A. T., and Rock, J. 1973. Searching for early fertilized human ova. *Gynecol. Invest., 4*, 121–139.

Hertig, A. T., Rock, J., and Adams, E. C. 1956. A description of 34 human ova within the first 17 days of development. *Amer. J. Anat., 98*, 435–493.

Hertig, A. T., Rock, J., Adams, E. C., and Mulligan, W. J. 1954. On the preimplantation stages of the human ovum: a description of four normal and four abnormal specimens ranging from the second to the fifth day of development. *Carnegie Instn. Wash. Publ. 603, Contrib. Embryol., 35*, 199–220.

Herzog, M. 1909. A contribution to our knowledge of the earliest known stages of placentation and embryonic development in man. *Amer. J. Anat., 9*, 361–400.

Hesseldahl, H., and Larsen, J. F. 1969. Ultrastructure of human yolk sac: endoderm, mesenchyme, tubules and mesothelium. *Amer. J. Anat., 126*, 315–335.

Hesseldahl, H., and Larsen, J. F. 1971. Hemopoiesis and blood vessels in human yolk sac. An electron microscopic study. *Acta anat., 78*, 274–294.

Heuser, C. H. 1930. A human embryo with 14 pairs of somites. *Carnegie Instn. Wash. Publ. 414, Contrib. Embryol., 22*, 135–153.

Heuser, C. H. 1932a. An intrachorionic mesothelial membrane in young stages of the monkey (Macacus rhesus). *Anat. Rec., 52*, Suppl., 15–16.

Heuser, C. H. 1932b. A presomite human embryo with a definite chorda canal. *Carnegie Instn. Wash. Publ. 433, Contrib. Embryol., 23*, 251–267.

Heuser, C. H. 1954. Monozygotic twin human embryos with an estimated ovulation age of 17 days. *Anat. Rec., 118*, 310.

Heuser, C. H. 1956. A human ovum with an estimated ovulation age of about nine days. *Anat. Rec., 124*, 459.

Heuser, C. H., and Corner, G. W. 1957. Developmental horizons in human embryos. Description of age group X, 4 to 12 somites. *Carnegie Instn. Wash. Publ. 611, Contrib. Embryol., 36*, 29–39.

Heuser, C. H., Rock, J., and Hertig, A. T. 1945. Two human embryos showing early stages of the definitive yolk sac. *Carnegie Instn. Wash. Publ. 557, Contrib. Embryol., 31*, 85–99.

Heuser, C. H., and Streeter, G. L. 1929. Early stages in the development of pig embryos, from the period of initial cleavage to the time of the appearance of limb-buds. *Carnegie Instn. Wash. Publ. 394, Contrib. Embryol., 20*, 1–29.

Heuser, C. H., and Streeter, G. L. 1941. Development of the macaque embryo. Carnegie Instn. Wash. Publ. 525, Contrib. Embryol., 29, 15–55.

Hill, J. P. 1932. The developmental history of the Primates. *Phil. Trans. Roy. Soc. London* B, *221*, 45–178.

Hill, J. P., and Florian, J. 1931a. The development of head-process and prochordal plate in man. *J. Anat., 45*, 242–246.

Hill, J. P., and Florian, J. 1931b. A young human embryo (embryo Dobbin) with head-process and prochordal plate. *Phil. Trans. Roy. Soc. London* B, *219*, 443–486.

Hill, J. P., and Florian, J. 1931c. Further note on the prochordal plate in man. *J. Anat., 46*, 46–47.

Hill, J. P., and Florian, J. 1963. The development of the primitive streak, head-process and annular zone in *Tarsius*, with comparative notes on *Loris. Bibliog. Primatol., 2*, 1–90.

Hill, J. P., and Tribe, M. 1924. The early development of the cat (Felis domestica). *Quart. J. Microsc. Sci., 68*, 513–602.

Hines, M. 1922. Studies in the growth and differentiation of the telencephalon in man. The fissura hippocampi. *J. Comp. Neurol., 34*, 73–171.

Hinrichsen, K. 1985. The early development of morphology and patterns of the face in the human embryo. *Adv. Anat. Embryol. Cell Biol., 98*, 1–79.

Hiramatsu, K. 1936. Ein junges Menschenei (Ei-Andô). *Folia anat. jap., 14*, 15–45.

Hirschland, L. 1898. Beiträge zur ersten Entwicklung der Mammarorgane beim Menschen. *Anat. Hefte*, Abt. I, Heft 34, 35 (Vol. II). Cited by Streeter (1945).

His, W. 1880–1885. *Anatomie menschlicher Embryonen.* Vogel, Leipzig.

Hochstetter, F. 1907. *Atlas.* Munich. Cited by Streeter (1945).

Hochstetter, F. 1919. *Beiträge zur Entwicklungsgeschichte des menschlichen Gehirns. 1. Teil.* Deuticke, Vienna.

Hochstetter, F. 1948. Entwicklungsgeschichte der Ohrmuschel und des äusseren Gehörganges des Menschen. *Denkschr. Akad. Wissensch. Wien Math.-Naturwiss. Klasse, 108*, 1–50.

Holmdahl, D. E. 1934. Neuralleiste und Ganglienleiste beim Menschen. *Z. mikr.-anat. Forsch., 36*, 137–178.

Holmdahl, D. E. 1939. Eine ganz junge (etwa 10 Tage alte) menschliche Embryonalanlage. *Upsala Läkareför. Förhandl., 45*, 363–371.

Holmdahl, D. E. 1943. Beitrag zur Kenntnis der Entwicklung des Blutgefässsystems und Blutes beim Menschen. *Z. mikr.-anat. Forsch., 54*, 219–296.

Hoyes, A. D. 1969. The human foetal yolk sac. An ultrastructural study of four specimens. *Z. Zellforsch., 99*, 469–490.

Hughes, E. C. 1958. *In* Discussion (pp. 1041–1042) of Hertig, A. T., Adams, E. C., McKay, D. G., Rock, J., Mulligan, W. J., and Menkin, M. F. A thirteen-day human ovum studied histochemically. *Amer. J. Obstet. Gynecol., 76*, 1025–1043.

Ilieş, A. 1967. La topographie et la dynamique des zones nécrotiques normales chez l'embryon humain. I. *Rev. roum. Embryol. Cytol., Sér. Embryol., 4*, 51–84.

Ingalls, N. W. 1907. Beschreibung eines menschlichen Embryos von 4.9 mm. *Arch. mikr.-anat. Entw., 70*, 506–576.

Ingalls, N. W. 1908. A contribution to the embryology of the liver and vascular system in man. *Anat. Rec., 2*, 338–344. Cited by Streeter (1945).

Ingalls, N. W. 1918. A human embryo before the appearance of the myotomes. *Carnegie Instn. Wash. Publ. 227, Contrib. Embryol., 7*, 111–134.

Ingalls, N. W. 1920. A human embryo at the beginning of segmentation, with special reference to the vascular system. *Carnegie Instn. Wash. Publ. 274, Contrib. Embryol., 11*, 61–90.

Jacobson, C. B., Sites, J. G., and Arias-Bernal, L. F. 1970. In vitro maturation and fertilization of human follicular oocytes. *Int. J. Fertil., 15*, 103–114.

Jahnke, V., and Stegner, H.-E. 1964. Ein menschlicher Keim von 15 bis 16 Tagen in situ. *Arch. Gynäkol., 200*, 88–98.

Jankelowitz, A. 1895. Ein junger menschlicher Embryo und die Entwicklung des Pancreas bei demselben. *Arch mikr.-anat. Entw., 46*, 702–708. Cited by Streeter (1945).

Janošík, J. 1887. Zwei junge menschliche Embryonen. *Arch. mikr.-anat. Entw., 30*, 559–595.

Jellinger, K., Gross, H., Kaltenbäck, E. and Grisold, W. 1981. Holoprosencephaly and agenesis of the corpus callosum: frequency of associated malformations. *Acta neuropathol., 55*, 1–10.

Jiménez Collado, J., and Ruano Gil, D. 1963. Descripcion de un embrion humano normal de 3 pares de somitos. *An. Desarrollo, 11*, 151–158.

Jirásek, J. E. 1971. *Development of the Genital System and Male Pseudohermaphroditism.* Johns Hopkins Press, Baltimore.

Jirásek, J. E., Uher, J., and Uhrová, M. 1966. Water and nitrogen content of the body of young human embryos. *Amer. J. Obstet. Gynecol., 96*, 869–871.

Johnson, F. P. 1910. The development of the mucous membrane of the oesophagus, stomach and small intestine in the human embryo. *Amer. J. Anat., 10*, 521–559.

Johnson, F. P. 1917. A human embryo of twenty-four pairs of somites. *Carnegie Instn. Wash. Publ. 226, Contrib. Embryol., 6*, 125–168.

Johnston, J. B. 1909. The morphology of the forebrain vesicle in vertebrates. *J. Comp. Neurol., 19*, 457–539.

Johnston, T. B. 1940. An early human embryo, with 0.55 mm. long embryonic shield. *J. Anat., 75*, 1–49.

Johnston, T. B. 1941. The chorion and endometrium of the embryo H.R.1. *J. Anat., 75*, 153–163.

Johnstone, R. W. 1914. Contribution to the study of the early human ovum based upon the investigation of I. A very early ovum embedded in the uterus and II. A very early ovum in the infundibulum of the tube. *J. Obstet. Gynaec. Brit. Emp., 26*, 231–276.

Jones, H. O., and Brewer, J. I. 1941. A human embryo in the primitive-streak stage (Jones-Brewer ovum I). *Carnegie Instn. Wash. Publ. 525, Contrib. Embryol., 29*, 157–165.

Jung, P. 1908. *Beiträge zur frühesten Ei-Einbettung beim menschlichen Weibe.* Karger, Berlin.

Kampmeier, C. F. 1929. On the problem of "parthenogenesis" in the mammalian ovary. *Amer. J. Anat., 43*, 45–76.

Kanagasuntheram, R. 1967. A note on the development of the tubotympanic recess in the human embryo. *J. Anat., 101*, 731–741.

Keibel, F. 1890. Ein sehr junges menschliches Ei. *Arch. Anat. Physiol., Anat. Abth., 250–267.*

Keibel, [F.] 1907. Ueber ein junges, operativ gewonnenes menschliches Ei in situ. *Verh. Anat. Ges., Erg. Heft Anat. Anz., 30*, 111–114.

Keibel, F., and Elze, C. 1908. *Normentafeln zur Entwicklungsgeschichte der Wirbeltiere. 8. Heft Normentafeln zur Entwicklungsgeschichte des Menschen.* Fisher, Jena.

Keibel, F., and Mall, F. P. 1910 and 1912. *Manual of Human Embryology.* Volume 1 and Volume 2, Lippincott, Philadelphia.

Keller, R., and Keller, B. 1954. Implantation eines sehr jungen menschlichen Eise (wahrscheinlich weniger als 13 Tage alt) am äusseren Muttermund. *Zbl. Gynäkol., 76*, 1–4.

Kennedy, J. F., and Donahue, R. P. 1969. Human oocytes: maturation in chemically defined media. *Science, 164*, 1292–1293.

Khvatov, B. P. 1959. New data on fecundation in man [in Russian]. *Arkh. Anat. Gistol. Embriol, 36*, 42–43.

Khvatov, B. P. 1967. Human embryo at the stage of blastodermic vesicle [in Russian]. *Arkh. Anat. Gistol. Embriol., 53*, 51–56.

Khvatov, B. P. 1968. Phenomenon of parthenogenesis in atretic follicle of human ovary [in Russian]. *Arkh. Anat. Gistol. Embriol., 54*, 93–96.

Kindred, J. E. 1933. A human embryo of the presomite period from the uterine tube. *Amer. J. Anat., 53*, 221–241.

Kistner, R. W. 1953. A thirteen-day normal human embryo showing early villous and yolk-sac development. *Amer. J. Obstet. Gynecol., 65*, 24–29.

Knorre, A. G. 1956. Cited by Mazanec (1959).

Knoth, M. 1968. Ultrastructure of chorionic villi from a four somite human embryo. *J. Ultrastruct. Res., 25*, 423–440.

Knoth, M., and Larsen, J. F. 1972. Ultrastructure of a human implantation site. *Acta obstet. gynecol. scand., 51*, 385–393.

Koff, A. 1933. Development of the vagina in the human fetus. *Carnegie Instn. Publ. 443, Contrib. Embryol., 24*, 59–60.

Koga, A. 1971. Morphogenesis of intrahepatic bile ducts of the human fetus. *Z. Anat. Entw., 135*, 156–184.

Kollmann, J. 1889. Die Körperform menschlicher normaler und pathologischer Embryonen. *Arch. Anat. Entw., Anat. Abth.*, Suppl. Band, 105–138. Cited by Streeter (1942).

Kollmann, J. 1907. *Handatlas der Entwicklungsgeschichte des Menschen*, 2 vols., Fischer, Jena.

Krafka, J. 1939. Parthenogenic cleavage in the human ovary. *Anat. Rec., 75*, 19–21.

Krafka, J. 1941. The Torpin ovum, a presomite human embryo. *Carnegie Instn. Wash. Publ. 525, Contrib. Embryol., 29*, 167–193.

Krafka, J. 1942. A free human tubal ovum in a late cleavage stage. *Anat. Rec., 82*, 426.

Kramer, T. C. 1942. The partitioning of the truncus and conus and the formation of the membranous portion of the interventricular septum in the human heart. *Amer. J. Anat., 71*, 343–370.

Krause, W. 1952. Ein menschliches Ei mit 0,32 mm Keimschildlänge in Situ. *Z. mikr.-anat. Forsch., 59*, 29–119.

Kroemer, P. 1903. Wachsmodell eines jungen menschlichen Embryo. *Verh. deutsch. Gesellsch. Gynäkol.*, Würzburg, p. 537.

Krukenberg. 1922. Ein junges menschliches Ei. *Zbl. Gynäkol., 46*, 193–194.

Kunitomo, K. 1918. The development and reduction of the tail, and of the caudal end of the spinal cord. *Carnegie Instn. Wash. Publ. 271, Contrib. Embryol., 8*, 161–198.

Laane, H. M. 1974. The nomenclature of the arterial pole of the embryonic heart. *Acta morphol. neerl.-scand., 12*, 167–209.

Langemeijer, R. A. T. M. 1976. Le coelome et son revêtement comme organoblastème. *Bull. Ass. Anat., 60*, 547–558.

Larsen, J. F. 1970. Electron microscopy of nidation in the rabbit and observations on the human tropohoblastic invasion. In *Ovo-implantation. Human Gonadotropins and Prolactin*. Karger, Basel, pp. 38–51.

Larsen, J. F., and Fuchs, F. 1963. Human embryo with four somites recovered for electron microscopy. Preliminary communication. *Dan. Med. Bull., 10*, 191–195.

Lassau, J.-P., and Hureau, J. 1967. Remarque sur l'organogenèse des voies biliaires de l'homme. *C.R. Ass. Anat., 52*, 750–754.

Lee, S. 1971. High incidence of true hermaphroditism in the early human embryo. *Biol. Neonate, 18*, 418–425.

Lemire, R. J. 1969. Variations in development of the caudal neural tube in human embryos (horizons XIV–XXI). *Teratology, 2*, 361–369.

Lemire, R. J., Loeser, J. D., Leech, R. W., and Alvord, E. C. 1975. *Normal and Abnormal Development of the Human Nervous System*. Harper & Row, Hagerstown, Maryland.

Lemire, R. J., Shepard, T. H., and Alvord, E. C. 1965. Caudal myeloschisis (lumbo-sacral spina bifida cystica in a five millimeter (horizon XIV) human embryo. *Anat. Rec., 152*, 9–16.

Lewis, B. V., and Harrison, R. G. 1966. A presomite human embryo showing a yolk-sac duct. *J. Anat., 100*, 389–396.

Lewis, W. H. 1920. The cartilaginous skull of a human embryo twenty-one millimeters in length. *Carnegie Instn. Wash. Publ. 272, Contrib. Embryol., 9*, 299–324.

Licata, R. H. 1954. The embryonic heart in the ninth week. *Amer. J. Anat., 94*, 73–125.

Linzenmeier, G. 1914. Ein junges menschliches Ei in situ. *Arch. Gynäk., 102*, 1–17.

Lipp, W. 1952. Die frühe Strukturentwicklung des Leberparenchyms beim Menschen, *Z. mikr.-anat. Forsch., 59*, 161–186.

Litzenberg, J. C. 1933. A young human ovum of the early somite period. *Amer. J. Obstet. Gynecol., 26*, 519–529.

Lopata, A., Kohlman, D., and Johnston, I. 1983. The fine structure of normal and abnormal human embryos developed in culture. *In* Beier, H. M., and Lindner, H. R. (ed.). *Fertilization of the Human Egg in vitro*. Springer, Berlin, pp. 189–210.

Lopata, A., Kohlman, D. J., and Kellow, G. N. 1982. The fine structure of human blastocysts developed in culture. *In* Burger, M. M., and Weber, R. (ed.). *Embryonic Development, Part B*. Liss, New York, pp. 69–85.

Lopata, A., McMaster, R., McBain, J. C., and Johnston, W. I. H. 1978. In-vitro fertilization of preovulatory human eggs. *J. Reprod. Fertil., 52*, 339–342.

Lopata, A., Sathananthan, A. H., McBain, J. C., Johnston, W. I. H., and Speirs, A. L. 1980. The ultrastructure of the preovulatory human egg fertilized in vitro. *Fertil. Steril., 33*, 12–20.

Lordy, C. 1931. A human ovum in its early phases of development. *Ann. Fac. Med. São Paulo, 6*, 29–35.

Los, J.-A. 1965. Le cloisonnement du tronc artériel chez l'embryon humain. *Bull. Ass. Anat., 50*, 682–686.

Los, J. A. 1978. Cardiac septation and development of the aorta, pulmonary trunk, and pulmonary veins. *In* Rosenquist, G. C., and Bergsma, D. (ed.). *Morphogenesis and Malformation of the Cardiovascular System.* Liss, New York, pp. 109–138.

Low, A. 1908. Description of a human embryo of 13–14 mesodermic somites. *J. Anat. Physiol., 42*, 237–251.

Luckett, W. P. 1971. The origin of extraembyronic mesoderm in the early human and rhesus monkey embryos. *Anat. Rec., 169*, 369–370.

Luckett, W. P. 1973. Amniogenesis in the early human and rhesus monkey embryos. *Anat. Rec., 175*, 375.

Luckett, W. P. 1975. The development of primordial and definitive amniotic cavities in early rhesus monkey and human embryos. *Amer. J. Anat., 144*, 149–167.

Luckett, W. P. 1978. Origin and differentiation of the yolk sac and extraembryonic mesoderm in presomite human and rhesus monkey embryos. *Amer. J. Anat., 152*, 59–97.

Ludwig, E. 1928. Über einen operativ gewonnenen menschlichen Embryo mit einem Ursegmente (Embryo Da 1). *Morph. Jahrb., 59*, 41–104.

Ludwig, E. 1929. Embryon humain avec dix paires de somites mésoblastiques. *C. R. Ass. Anat., 24*, 580–585.

M'Intyre, D. 1926. The development of the vascular system in the human embryo prior to the establishment of the heart. *Trans. Roy. Soc. Edinburgh, 55*, 77–113.

McBride, R. E., Moore, G. W., and Hutchins, G. M. 1981. Development of the outflow tract and closure of the interventricular septum in the normal human heart. *Amer. J. Anat., 160*, 1609–1631.

McClure, C. F. W., and Butler, E. G. 1925. The development of the vena cava inferior in man. *Amer. J. Anat., 35*, 331–383.

McKay, D. G., Adams, E. C., Hertig, A. T., and Danziger, S. 1955. Histochemical horizons in human embryos. I. Five millimeter embryo—Streeter horizon XIII. *Anat. Rec., 122*, 125–151.

McKay, D. G., Adams, E. C., Hertig, A. T., and Danziger, S. 1956. Histochemical horizons in human embryos. II. 6 and 7 millimeter embryos—Streeter horizon XIV. *Anat. Rec., 126*, 433–463.

Magovern, J. H., Moore, G. W., and Hutchins, G. M. 1986. Development of the atrioventricular valve region in the human embryo. *Anat. Rec., 215*, 167–181.

Mall, F. P. 1891. A human embryo twenty-six days old. *J. Morph., 5*, 459–480.

Mall, F. P. 1897. Development of the human coelom. *J. Morphol., 12*, 395–453.

Mall, F. P. 1900. A contribution to the study of the pathology of early human embryos. *Johns Hopkins Hosp. Rep., 9*, 1–68.

Mall, F. P. 1907. On measuring human embryos. *Anat. Rec., 1*, 129–140.

Mall, F. P. 1912. On the development of the human heart. *Amer. J. Anat., 13*, 249–298.

Mall, F. P. 1913. A plea for an institute of human embryology. *J. Amer. Med. Ass., 60*, 1599–1601.

Mall, F. P. 1914. On stages in the development of human embryos from 2 to 25 mm. long. *Anat. Anz., 46*, 78–84.

Mall, F. P. 1916. The human magma réticulé in normal and in pathological development. *Carnegie Instn. Wash. Publ. 224, Contrib. Embryol., 4*, 5–26.

Mall, F. P. 1918. On the age of human embryos. *Amer. J. Anat., 23*, 397–422.

Mall, F. P., and Meyer, A. W. 1921. Studies on abortuses: a survey of pathologic ova in the Carnegie Embryological Collection. *Carnegie Instn. Wash. Publ. 275, Contrib. Embryol., 12*, 1–364.

Mandarim-de-Lacerda, C. A., Le Floch-Prigent, P., and Hureau, J. 1985. Étude du tissu de conduction atrial chez l'embryon humain de 17 mm V-C. *Arch. Mal. Coeur, 78*, 1504–1509.

Marchetti, A. A. 1945. A pre-villous human ovum accidentally recovered from a curettage specimen. *Carnegie Instn. Wash. Publ. 557, Contrib. Embryol., 31*, 107–115.

Mari Martínez. 1950. Embrión humano (Ca) con nueve pares de segmentos primitivos. Contribución al estudio de las primeras fases de la diferenciación somítica en el embrión humano. *Arch. españ. morfol., 8*, 225–242.

Martin, C. P., and Falkiner, N. McI. 1938. The Falkiner ovum. *Amer. J. Anat., 63*, 251–271.

Martínez Rovira, J. 1953. Estudio de la notocorda ("Chorda dorsalis") en un embrión humano de nueve pares de somitos. *Arch. españ. morfol., 10*, 179–191.

Masy, S. 1955. Le système nerveux péripherique crânien de l'embryon humain de 9 mm. *J. Embryol. Exp. Morphol., 3*, 30–43.

Mazanec, K. 1949. A young human embryo "Pha I" with the headprocess 0.090 mm long. *Bull. internat. Acad. tchèque Sci., 50*, 1–18.

Mazanec, K. 1953. *Blastogenesa člověka.* Státní Zdravotnické Nakladatelství, Prague.

Mazanec, K. 1959. *Blastogenese des Menschen.* Fischer, Jena.

Mazanec, K. 1960. A young human embryo "HEB-18" with a

Hensen's node 0.071 mm long, before the Anlage of a head process. *Scripta med., 33*, 185–194.

Mazanec, K., and Musilová, M. 1959. A young human presomite embryo "HEB-42" with a headprocess 0.250 mm long (preliminary report). *Scripta med., 32*, 261–270.

Meier, S., and Tam, P. P. L. 1982. Metameric pattern development in the embryonic axis of the mouse. 1. Differentiation of the cranial segments. *Differentiation, 21*, 95–108.

Menkin, M. F., and Rock, J. 1948. In vitro fertilization and cleavage of human ovarian eggs. *Amer. J. Obstet. Gynecol., 55*, 440–452.

Meyer, A. W. 1904. On the structure of the human umbilical vesicle. *Amer. J. Anat., 3*, 155–166.

Meyer, A. W. 1953. The elusive human allantois in older literature. In *Science, Medicine and History*. Oxford University Press, Oxford, pp. 510–520.

Meyer, P. 1924. Ein junges menschliches Ei mit 0,4 mm langem Embryonalschild. *Arch. Gynäk., 122*, 38–87.

Moffett, B. C. 1957. The prenatal development of the human temporomandibular joint. *Carnegie Instn. Wash. Publ. 611, Contrib. Embryol., 36*, 19–28.

Mohr, L., and Trounson, A. 1984. In vitro fertilization and embryo growth. *In* Wood, C., and Trounson, A. (ed.). *Clinical in Vitro Fertilization*. Springer, Berlin. pp. 99–115.

Moore, G. W., Hutchins, G. M., and O'Rahilly, R. 1981. The estimated age of staged human embryos and early fetuses. *Amer. J. Obstet. Gynecol., 139*, 500–506.

Mori, T. 1959a. Histochemical studies on the distribution of alkaline phosphatase in the early human embryos. I. Observations on two embryos in early somite stage, Streeter's horizon X. *Arch. histol. jap., 16*, 169–193.

Mori, T. 1959b. Histochemical studies on the distribution of alkaline phosphatase in early human embryos. II. Observations on an embryo with 13–14 somites. *Arch. histol. jap., 18*, 197–209.

Mori, T. 1965. Histochemical studies on the distribution of alkaline phosphatase in early human embryos. III. Embryos in Streeter's horizon XII. *Okajimas Folia anat. jap., 40*, 765–793.

Morton, W. R. M. 1949. Two early human embryos. *J. Anat., 83*, 308–314.

Mossman, H. W. 1937. Comparative morphogenesis of the fetal membranes and accessory uterine structures. *Carnegie Instn. Wash. Publ. 479, Contrib. Embryol., 26*, 129–246.

Müller, F., and O'Rahilly, R. 1980a. The early development of the nervous system in staged insectivore and primate embryos. *J. Comp. Neurol., 193*, 741–751.

Müller, F. and O'Rahilly, R. 1980b. The human chondrocran-

ium at the end of the embryonic period proper, with particular reference to the nervous system. *Amer. J. Anat., 159*, 33–58.

Müller, F., and O'Rahilly, R. 1983. The first appearance of the major divisions of the human brain at stage 9. *Anat. Embryol., 168*, 419–432.

Müller, F., and O'Rahilly, R. 1984. Cerebral dysraphia (future anencephaly) in a human twin embryo at stage 13. *Teratology, 30*, 167–177.

Müller, F., and O'Rahilly, R. 1985. The first appearance of the neural tube and optic primordium in the human embryo at stage 10. *Anat. Embryol., 172*, 157–169.

Müller, F., and O'Rahilly, R. 1986a. Wilhelm His und 100 Jahre Embryologie des Menschen. *Acta anat., 125*, 73–75.

Müller, F., and O'Rahilly, R. 1986b. Somitic-vertebral correlation and vertebral levels in the human embryo. *Amer. J. Anat., 177*, 1–19.

Müller, F., and O'Rahilly, R. 1986c. The development of the human brain and the closure of the rostral neuropore at stage 11. *Anat. Embryol., 175*, 205–222.

Müller, F., O'Rahilly, R., and Tucker, J. A. 1981. The human larynx at the end of the embryonic period proper. I. The laryngeal and infrahyoid muscles and their innervation. *Acta otolaryngol., 91*, 323–336.

Müller, F., O'Rahilly, R., and Tucker, J. A. 1985. The human larynx at the end of the embryonic period proper. 2. The laryngeal cavity and the innervation of its lining. *Ann. Otol. Rhinol. Laryngol., 94*, 607–617.

Müller, S. 1930. Ein jüngstes menschliches Ei. *Z. mikr.-anat. Forsch., 20*, 175–184.

Neill, C. A. 1956. Development of the pulmonary veins, with reference to the embryology of anomalies of pulmonary venous return. *Pediatrics, 18*, 880–887.

Nery, E. B., Kraus, B. S., and Croup, M. 1970. Timing and topography of early human tooth development. *Arch. Oral Biol., 15*, 1315–1326.

Nishimura, H., Takano, K., Tanimura, T., and Yasuda, M. 1968. Normal and abnormal development of human embryos. *Teratology, 1*, 281–290.

Noback, C. R., Paff, G. H., and Poppiti, R. J. 1968. A bilaminar human ovum. *Acta. anat., 69*, 485–496.

Noyes, R. W., Dickmann, Z., Clewe, T. H., and Bonney, W. A. 1965. Pronuclear ovum from a patient using an intrauterine contraceptive device. *Science, 147*, 744–745.

Odgers, P. N. B. 1930. Some observations on the development of the ventral pancreas in man. *J. Anat., 65*, 1–7.

Odgers, P. N. B. 1937. An early human ovum (Thomson) *in situ. J. Anat., 71*, 161–168.

Odgers, P. N. B. 1941. A presomite human embryo with a neurenteric canal (embryo R. S.). *J. Anat., 75*, 381–388.

Okamoto, N., Akimoto, N., Satow, Y., Hidaka, N., and Miyabara, S. 1981. Role of cell death in conal ridges of developing human heart. *Perspect. Cardiovasc. Res., 5*, 127–137.

Olivier, G., and Pineau, H. 1962. Horizons de Streeter et âge embryonnaire. *Bull. Ass. Anat., 47*, 573–576.

O'Rahilly, R. 1963. The early development of the otic vesicle in staged human embryos. *J. Embryol. Exp. Morphol., 11*, 741–755.

O'Rahilly, R. 1965. The optic, vestibulocochlear, and terminal-vomeronasal neural crest in staged human embryos. *In* Rohen, J. W. (ed.) *Second Symposium on Eye Structure.* Schattauer, Stuttgart.

O'Rahilly, R. 1966. The early development of the eye in staged human embryos. *Carnegie Instn. Wash. Publ. 625, Contrib. Embryol., 38*, 1–42.

O'Rahilly, R. 1968. The development of the epiphysis cerebri and the subcommissural complex in staged human embryos. *Anat. Rec., 160*, 488–489.

O'Rahilly, R. 1970. The manifestation of the axes of the human embryo. *Z. Anat. Entw., 132*, 50–57.

O'Rahilly, R. 1971. The timing and sequence of events in human cardiogenesis. *Acta anat., 79*, 70–75.

O'Rahilly, R. 1973. *Developmental Stages in Human Embryos, Including a Survey of the Carnegie Collection. Part A: Embryos of the First Three Weeks (Stages 1 to 9).* Carnegie Instn. Wash. Publ. 631. Washington, D.C.

O'Rahilly, R. 1979. Early human development and the chief sources of information on staged human embryos. *Europ. J. Obstet. Gynec. Reprod. Biol., 9*, 273–280.

O'Rahilly, R. 1983a. The timing and sequence of events in the development of the human endocrine system during the embryonic period proper. *Anat. Embryol., 166*, 439–451.

O'Rahilly, R. 1983b. The timing and sequence of events in the development of the human eye and ear during the embryonic period proper. *Anat. Embryol., 168*, 419–432.

O'Rahilly, R., and Boyden, E. A. 1973. The timing and sequence of events in the development of the human respiratory system during the embryonic period proper. *Z. Anat. Entw., 141*, 237–250.

O'Rahilly, R., and Gardner, E. 1971. The timing and sequence of events in the development of the human nervous system during the embryonic period proper. *Z. Anat. Entw., 134*, 1–12.

O'Rahilly, R., and Gardner, E. 1972. The initial appearance of ossification in staged human embryos. *Amer. J. Anat., 134*, 291–307.

O'Rahilly, R., and Gardner, E. 1975. The timing and sequence of events in the development of the limbs in the human embryo. *Anat. Embryol., 148*, 1–23.

O'Rahilly, R., and Gardner, E. 1979. The initial development of the human brain. *Acta anat., 104*, 123–133.

O'Rahilly, R., and Müller, F. 1981. The first appearance of the human nervous system at stage 8. *Anat. Embryol., 163*, 1–13.

O'Rahilly, R., and Müller, F. 1984a. Embryonic length and cerebral landmarks in staged human embryos. *Anat. Rec., 209*, 265–271.

O'Rahilly, R., and Müller, F. 1984b. The early development of the hypoglossal nerve and occipital somites in staged human embryos. *Amer. J. Anat., 169*, 237–257.

O'Rahilly, R., and Müller, F. 1984c. Respiratory and alimentary relations in staged human embryos. New embryological data and congenital anomalies. *Ann. Otol. Rhinol. Laryngol., 93*, 421–429.

O'Rahilly, R., and F. Müller, 1985. The origin of the ectodermal ring in staged human embryos of the first 5 weeks. *Acta anat., 122*, 145–157.

O'Rahilly, R., and Müller, F. 1986a. Human growth during the embryonic period proper. *In* Falkner, F., and Tanner, J. M. (ed.). *Human Growth.* Vol. 1, 2nd ed. Plenum, New York. Ch. 15, pp. 245–253.

O'Rahilly, R., and Müller, F. 1986b. The meninges in human development. *J. Neuropathol. Exp. Neurol., 45*, 588–608.

O'Rahilly, R., and Müller, F. 1987. Stages in early human development. *In* Feichtinger, W., and Kemeter, P. (ed.). *Future Aspects in Human in vitro Fertilization.* Springer, Berlin, in press.

O'Rahilly, R., Müller, F., and Bossy, J. 1982. Atlas des stades du développement du système nerveux chez l'embryon humain intact. *Arch. Anat. Histol. Embryol., 65*, 57–76.

O'Rahilly, R., Müller, F., Hutchins, G. M., and Moore, G. W. 1984. Computer ranking of the sequence of appearance of 100 features of the brain and related structures in staged human embryos during the first 5 weeks of development. *Amer. J. Anat., 171*, 243–257.

O'Rahilly, R., Müller, F., and Meyer, D. B. 1980. The human vertebral column at the end of the embryonic period proper. I. The column as a whole. *J. Anat., 131*, 567–575.

O'Rahilly, R., Müller, F., and Meyer, D. B. 1983. The human vertebral column at the end of the embryonic period proper. 2. The occipitocervical region. *J. Anat., 136*, 181–195.

O'Rahilly, R., and Tucker, J. A. 1973. The early development of the larynx in staged human embryos. *Ann. Otol. Rhinol. Laryngol., 82*, Suppl. 7, 1–27.

Ortmann, R. 1938. Über die Placenta einer in situ fixierten menschlichen Keimblase aus der 4. Woche. *Z. Anat. Entw., 108*, 427–458.

Orts Llorca, F. 1934. Beschreibung eines menschlichen Embryo mit 4 Urwirbelpaaren. *Z. Anat. Entw., 103*, 765–792.

Orts Llorca, F., Jiménez Collado, J., and Ruano Gil, D. 1960. La fase plexiforme del desarrollo cardiaco en el hombre. Embriones de 21 ± 1 dia. *An. Desarrollo, 8*, 79–98.

Orts-Llorca, F., and Lopez Rodriguez, A. 1957. La curva dorsal en los embriones humanos del periodo somitico. *Cirug. Ginecol. Urol., 11*, 1–6.

Orts-Llorca, F., Lopez Rodriguez, A., and Cano Monasterio, A. 1958. Embrion humano de 14 pares de somitos. *Cirug. Ginecol. Urol., 12*, 226–232.

Osaka, K., Matsumoto, S., and Tanimura, T. 1978. Myeloschisis in early human embryos. *Child's Brain, 4*, 347–359.

Park, W. W. 1957. The occurrence of sex chromatin in early human and macaque embryos. *J. Anat., 91*, 369–373.

Patten, B. M. 1961. The normal development of the facial region. *In* Pruzansky, S. (ed.). *Congenital Anomalies of the Face and Associated Structures.* Thomas, Springfield, Illinois, pp. 11–45.

Patten, B. M., and Philpott, R. 1921. The shrinkage of embryos in the processes preparatory to sectioning. *Anat. Rec., 93*, 393–413.

Payne, F. 1925. General description of a 7-somite human embryo. *Carnegie Instn. Wash. Publ. 361, Contrib. Embryol., 16*, 115–124.

Pearson, A. A. 1980. The development of the eyelids. Part I. External features. *J. Anat., 130*, 33–42.

Pearson, A. A., Nishimura, H., Tanimura, T., and Sauter, R. W. 1968. Observations on the development of the external form of the Japanese embryo. *Anat. Rec., 160*, 489–490.

Penkert. 1910. Über ein sehr junges Ei in der Tube. *Zbl. Gynäk., 34*, 345–347.

Pereda, J., and Coppo, M. 1984. Ultrastructure of the cumulus cell mass surrounding a human egg in the pronuclear stage. *Anat. Embryol., 170*, 107–112.

Pereda, J., and Coppo, M. 1985. Ultrastructure of a two-cell human embryo fertilized *in vivo. Ann. N.Y. Acad. Sci., 442*, 416–419.

Peter, K. 1913. *Atlas der Entwicklung der Nase und des Gaumens beim Menschen.* Fischer, Jena.

Peters, H. 1899. *Über die Einbettung des menschlichen Eies und das früheste bisher bekannte menschliche Placentationsstadium.* Deuticke, Leipzig.

Petrov, G. N. 1958. Fertilization and the first cleavage stages in the human ovum outside the organism [in Russian]. *Arkh. Anat. Gistol. Embriol., 35*, 88–91.

Pexieder, T. 1975. Cell death in the morphogenesis and teratogenesis of the heart. *Adv. Anat. Embryol. Cell Biol., 51*, 1–100.

Pexieder, T. 1978. Development of the outflow tract of the embryonic heart. *In* Rosenquist, G. C., and Bergsma, D. (ed.). *Morphogenesis and Malformation of the Cardio-*

vascular System. Liss, New York, pp. 29–68.

Pexieder, T. 1982. La solution de deux énigmes de l'organogénèse du coeur. *Bull. Fond. suisse Cardiol., 13*, 39–50.

Piersol, W. H. 1938. A human embryo of two somites, in situ. *Anat. Rec., 67 suppl.*, 39–40.

Pillet, J. 1966. Reconstruction des organes pelviens d'embryons humains de 12,5 et de 25 mm. *Bull. Ass. Anat., 51*, 819–827.

Pillet, J. 1968. Reconstruction du pelvis d'un embryon humain de 7,5 mm (stade XVI de Streeter). *C.R. Ass. Anat., 52*, 1013–1023.

Pinner, B., and Swinyard, C. A. 1969. Histochemical studies of limb development. *In* Swinyard, C. A. (ed.). *Limb Development and Deformity.* Thomas, Springfield, Illinois, pp. 56–70.

Piper, H. 1900. Ein menschlicher Embryo von 6.8 mm. Nakkenlinie. *Arch. Anat. Physiol., Anat. Abth.* Cited by Streeter (1945).

Politzer, G. 1928a. Über einen menschlichen Embryo mit 18 Ursegmentpaaren. *Z. Anat. Entw., 87*, 674–727.

Politzer, G. 1928b. Über Zahl, Lage und Beschaffenheit der "Urkeimzellen" eines menschlichen Embryo mit 26–27 Ursegmentpaaren. *Z. Anat. Entw., 87*, 766–780.

Politzer, G. 1930. Ueber einen menschlichen Embryo mit sieben Urwirbelpaaren. *Z. Anat. Entw., 93*, 386–428.

Politzer, G. 1933. Die Keimbahn des Menschen. *Z. Anat. Entw., 100*, 331–361.

Politzer, G. 1936. Die Grenzfurche des Oberkieferfortsatzes und die Tränennasenrinne. *Z. Anat. Entw., 105*, 329–332.

Politzer, G., and Hann, F. 1935. Über die Entwicklung der branchiogenen Organe beim Menschen. *Z. Anat. Entw., 104*, 670–708.

Politzer, G., and Sternberg, H. 1930. Ueber die Entwicklung der ventralen Körperwand und des Nabelstranges beim Menschen. *Z. Anat. Entw., 92*, 279–376.

Pommerenke, W. T. 1958. A twelfth night ovum. *Fertil. Steril., 9*, 400–406.

Potter, E. L. 1965. Development of the human glomerulus. *Arch. Pathol., 80*, 241–255.

Potter, E. L. 1972. *Normal and Abnormal Development of the Kidney.* Year Book, Chicago.

Puerta Fonollá, A. J., and Orts Llorca, F. 1978. Origin and development of the septum primum. *Acta anat., 100*, 250–257.

Puerta Fonollá, A. J., and Ribes Blanquer, R. 1973. Primer esbozo del foramen primum en el embrion humano (embrion Pu, horizonte XIV). *Rev. esp. Cardiol., 26*, 255–260.

Puerta Fonollá, A. J., and Ribes Blanquer, R. 1977. Participación de tejido extracardiaco en la embriogénesis del corazón humano. *An. Desarrollo, 21*, 19–22.

Rabl, C. 1902. *Tafeln zur Entwicklungsgeschichte der äussern Körperform der Wirbeltiere.* Leipzig. Cited by Streeter (1945).

Ramsey, E. M. 1937. The Lockyer embryo: an early human embryo *in situ. Carnegie Instn. Wash. Publ. 479, Contrib. Embryol., 26*, 99–120.

Ramsey, E. M. 1938. The Yale embryo. *Carnegie Instn. Wash. Publ. 496, Contrib. Embryol., 27*, 67–84.

Ramsey, E. M. 1975. *The Placenta of Laboratory Animals and Man.* Holt, Rinehart & Winston.

Ramsey, E. M., and Donner, M. W. 1980. *Placental Vasculature and Circulation.* Thieme, Stuttgart.

Rewell, R. E., and Harrison, R. G. 1976. A presomite human embryo of Horizon VII. *J. Anat., 121*, 65–70.

Reynolds, S. R. M. 1954. Developmental changes and future requirements. *In* The Mammalian Fetus: Physiological Aspects of Development. *Cold Spring Harbor Symp. Quant. Biol., 19*, 1–2.

Richter, K. M. 1952. A new human embryo having an estimated age of fifteen days. *Anat. Rec., 112*, 462.

Robertson, G. G., O'Neill, S. L., and Chappell, R. H. 1948. On a normal human embryo of 17 days development. *Anat. Rec., 100*, 9–28.

Rock, J., and Hertig, A. T. 1941. Two human ova of the previllous stage, having an ovulation age of about eleven and twelve days respectively. *Carnegie Instn. Wash. Publ. 525, Contrib. Embryol., 29*, 127–156.

Rock, J., and Hertig, A. T. 1942. Some aspects of early human development. *Amer. J. Obstet. Gynecol., 44*, 973–983.

Rock, J., and Hertig, A. T. 1944. Information regarding the time of human ovulation derived from a study of 3 unfertilized and 11 fertilized ova. *Amer. J. Obstet. Gynecol., 47*, 343–356.

Rock, J., and Hertig, A T. 1945. Two human ova of the previllous stage, having a developmental age of about seven and nine days respectively. *Carnegie Instn. Wash. Publ. 557, Contrib. Embryol., 31*, 65–84.

Rock, J., and Hertig, A. T. 1948. The human conceptus during the first two weeks of gestation. *Amer. J. Obstet. Gynecol., 55*, 6–17.

Rock, J., and Hertig, A. T. 1949. Two human ova of the previllous stage, having a developmental age of about 8 and 9 days respectively. *Carnegie Instn. Wash. Publ. 583, Contrib. Embryol., 33*, 169–186.

Rodríguez-García, S. 1965. Estudio comparativo de dos embriones humanos de 2,5 y 5 mm de longitud, reconstruidos por el método de Born al "plástico espumoso." *Am. Anat. (Zaragoza), 14*, 341–379.

Rosenbauer, K. A. 1955. Untersuchung eines menschlichen Embryos mit 24 Somiten, unter besonderer Berücksichti-

gung des Blutgefässsystems. *Z. Anat. Entw., 118*, 236–276.

Rossenbeck, H. 1923. Ein junges menschliches Ei. Ovum humanum Peh. 1-Hochstetter. *Z. Anat. Entw., 68*, 325–385.

Rossi, F., Pescetto, G., and Reale, E. 1957. Enzymatic activities in human ontogenesis: first synoptic tables of histochemical research. *J. Histochem. Cytochem., 5*, 221–235.

Rossi, F., and Reale, E. 1957. The somite stage of human development studied with the histochemical reaction for the demonstration of alkaline glycerophosphatase. *Acta anat., 30*, 656–681.

Ruano Gil, D. 1963. Malformacion diencefalica en un embrion humano de 6 mm. a consecuencia de un transtorno en el mecanismo de cierre del neuroporo anterior. *An. Desarrollo, 11*, 57–62.

Sarrazin, R., Mallard, G., and Charignon, G. 1971. Intérêt topographique des relevés de niveaux autorisant une interprétation sagittale de coupes transversales. *C.R. Ass. Anat., 54* (No. 146), 610–614.

Sarrazin, R., Mallard, G., and Faure, G. 1971. Les préparatifs de fermeture de la cavité péricardique chez l'embryon du XVe horizon. *Bull. Ass. Anat., 54*, 615–624.

Sathananthan, A. H., and Trounson, A. O. 1982. Ultrastructure of cortical granule release and zona interaction in monospermic and polyspermic human ova fertilized in vitro. *Gamete Res., 6*, 225–234.

Sathananthan, A. H., and Trounson, A. O. 1985. The human pronuclear ovum: fine structure of monospermic and polyspermic fertilization in vitro. *Gamete Res., 12*, 385–398.

Sathananthan, A. H., Trounson, A. O., and Wood, C. 1986. *Atlas of Fine Structure of Human Sperm Penetration, Eggs and Embryos Cultured in vitro.* Praeger, New York.

Sathananthan, A. H., Wood, C., and Leeton, J. F. 1982. Ultrastructural evaluation of 8–16 cell human embryos cultured in vitro. *Micron, 13*, 193–203.

Saunders, R. L. de C. H. 1943. Combined anterior and posterior spina bifida in a living neonatal human female. *Anat. Rec., 87*, 255–278.

Schenck, R. 1954. Beschreibung eines menschlichen Keimlings mit 5 Ursegmentpaaren. *Acta anat., 22*, 236–271.

Schlafke, S., and Enders, A. C. 1967. Cytological changes during cleavage and blastocyst formation in the rat. *J. Anat., 102*, 13–32.

Schlagenhaufer, [F.], and Verocay, [F.] 1916. Ein junges menschliches Ei. *Arch. Gynäk., 105*, 151–168.

Schmitt, H. 1898. Über die Entwicklung der Milchdrüse und die Hyperthelie menschlicher Embryonen. *Morphol. Arb., Jena, 8*, 236–303.

Schuster, G. 1965. Untersuchungen an einem Embryo von Papio doguera Pucheran (7-Somiten-Stadium) (Mam. Primates, Cercopithecidae). *Anat. Anz., 117*, 447–475.

Scipiades, E. 1938. Young human ovum detected in uterine scraping. *Carnegie Instn. Wash. Publ. 496, Contrib. Embryol., 27*, 95–105.

Sensenig, E. C. 1949. The early development of the human vertebral column. *Carnegie Instn. Wash. Publ. 583, Contrib. Embryol., 33*, 21–41.

Severn, C. B. 1968. The morphological development of the hepatic diverticulum in staged human embryos. *Anat. Rec., 160*, 427.

Severn, C. B. 1971. A morphological study of the development of the human liver. I. Development of the hepatic diverticulum. *Amer. J. Anat., 131*, 133–158.

Severn, C. B. 1972. A morphological study of the development of the human liver. II. Establishment of liver parenchyma, extrahepatic ducts and associated venous channels. *Amer. J. Anat., 133*, 85–107.

Shaner, R. F. 1945. A human embryo of two to three pairs of somites. *Canad. J. Res., 23*, 235–243.

Shaw, W. 1932. Observations on two specimens of early human ova. *Brit. Med. J., 1*, 411–415.

Shettles, L. B. 1956. A morula stage of human ovum developed in vitro. *Clin. Excerpts, 18*, 92–93.

Shettles, L. B. 1957. Parthenogenetic cleavage of the human ovum. *Bull. Sloane Hosp. Women, 3*, 59–61.

Shettles, L. B. 1958. The living human ovum. *Amer. J. Obstet. Gynecol., 76*, 398–406.

Shettles, L. B. 1960. *Ovum Humanum*. Hafner, New York.

Shikinami, J. 1926. Detailed form of the Wolffian body in human embryos of the first eight weeks. *Carnegie Instn. Wash. Publ. 363, Contrib. Embryol., 18*, 46–61.

Silverman, H. 1969. Über die Entwicklung der Epithelplatten in den Corpuscula renalia der menschlichen Urniere. *Acta anat., 74*, 36–43.

Smith, D. W. 1970. *Recognizable Patterns of Human Malformation. Genetic, Embryologic, and Clinical Aspects.* Saunders, Philadelphia.

Soupart, P., and Morgenstern, L. L. 1973. Human sperm capacitation and in vitro fertilization. *Fertil. Steril., 24*, 462–478.

Soupart, P., and Strong, P. A. 1974. Ultrastructural observations on human oocytes fertilized in vitro. *Fertil. Steril., 25*, 11–44.

Springer, M. 1972. Der Canalis neurentericus beim Menschen. *Z. Kinderchir., 11*, 183–189 and 192–194.

Starck, D. 1956. Die Frühphase der menschlichen Embryonalentwicklung und ihre Bedeutung für die Beurteilung der Säugerontogenese. *Ergeb. Anat. Entwicklungsgesch., 35*, 133–175.

Steptoe, P. C., Edwards, R. G., and Purdy, J. M. 1971. Human blastocysts grown in culture. *Nature, 229*, 132–133.

Sternberg, H. 1927. Beschreibung eines menschlichen Embryo mit vier Ursegmentpaaren, nebst Bemerkungen über die Anlage und früheste Entwicklung einiger Organe beim Menschen. *Z. Anat. Entw., 82*, 142–240.

Sternberg, H. 1929. Modell eines menschlichen Embryo mit 4 Ursegmentpaaren, 2,3 mm gr. L. *Anat. Anz., 67*, 397–399.

Stewart, H. I. 1952. Duration of pregnancy and postmaturity. *J. Amer. Med. Ass., 148*, 1079–1083.

Stieve, H. 1926a. Ein 13½-Tage altes, in der Gebärmutter erhaltenes und durch Eingriff gewonnenes menschliches Ei. *Z. mikr.-anat. Forsch., 7*, 295–402.

Stieve, H. 1926b. Ein menschliches Ei vom Ende der 2. Woche. *Verb. Anat. Ges., Jena.*

Stieve, H. 1931. Die Dottersackbildung beim Ei des Menschen. *Anat. Anz., 72*, 44–56.

Stieve, H. 1936. Ein ganz junges, in der Gebärmutter erhaltenes menschliches Ei (Keimling Werner). *Z. mikr.-anat. Forsch., 40*, 281–322.

Strahl, H. 1916. Über einen jungen menschlichen Embryo nebst Bemerkungen zu C. Rabl's Gastrulationstheorie. *Anat. Hefte, 54*, 113–147.

Strahl, H., and Beneke, R. 1910. *Ein junger menschlicher Embryo.* Bergmann, Wiesbaden.

Strauss, F. 1945. Gedanken zur Entwicklung des Amnions und des Dottersackes beim Menschen. *Rev. Suisse Zool., 52*, 213–229.

Streeter, G. L. 1906. On the development of the membranous labyrinth and the acoustic and facial nerves in the human embryo. *Amer. J. Anat., 6*, 139–165.

Streeter, G. L. 1908a. The nuclei of origin of the cranial nerves in the 10 mm human embryo. *Anat. Rec., 2*, 111–115.

Streeter, G. L. 1908b. The peripheral nervous system in the human embryo at the end of the first month (10 mm). *Amer. J. Anat., 8*, 285–301.

Streeter, G. L. 1920a. A human embryo (Mateer) of the presomite period. *Carnegie Instn. Wash. Publ. 272, Contrib. Embryol., 9*, 389–424.

Streeter, G. L. 1920b. Weight, sitting height, head size, foot length and menstrual age of the human embryo. *Carnegie Instn. Wash. Publ. 274, Contrib. Embryol., 11*, 143–170.

Streeter, G. L. 1922. Development of the auricle in the human embryo. *Carnegie Instn. Wash. Publ. 277, Contrib. Embryol., 14*, 111–138.

Streeter, G. L. 1926. The "Miller" ovum—the youngest normal human embryo thus far known. *Carnegie Instn. Wash. Publ. 363, Contrib. Embryol., 18*, 31–48.

Streeter, G. L. 1927a. Development of the mesoblast and notochord in pig embryos. *Carnegie Instn. Wash. Publ. 380, Contrib. Embryol., 19*, 73–92.

Streeter, G. L. 1927b. Archetypes and symbolism. *Science, 65,* 405–412.

Streeter, G. L. 1937. Origin of the yolk sac in primates. *Anat. Rec., 70* suppl., 53–54.

Streeter, G. L. 1939a. A new profile reconstruction of the Miller ovum. *Anat. Rec., 73* suppl., 75.

Streeter, G. L. 1939b. New reconstruction of the Miller ovum. *Carnegie Instn. Wash. Year Book 38,* 149.

Streeter, G. L. 1942. Developmental horizons in human embryos. Description of age group XI, 13 to 20 somites, and age group XII, 21 to 29 somites. *Carnegie Instn. Wash. Publ. 541, Contrib. Embryol., 30,* 211–245.

Streeter, G. L. 1945. Developmental horizons in human embryos. Description of age group XIII, embryos about 4 or 5 millimeters long, and age group XIV, period of indentation of the lens vesicle. *Carnegie Instn. Wash. Publ. 557, Contrib. Embryol., 31,* 27–63.

Streeter, G. L. 1948. Developmental horizons in human embryos. Description of age groups XV, XVI, XVII, and XVIII, being the third issue of a survey of the Carnegie Collection. *Carnegie Instn. Wash. Publ. 575, Contrib. Embryol., 32,* 133–203.

Streeter, G. L. 1949. Developmental horizons in human embryos (fourth issue). A review of the histogenesis of cartilage and bone. *Carnegie Instn. Wash. Publ. 583, Contrib. Embryol., 33,* 149–169.

Streeter, G. L. 1951. Developmental horizons in human embryos. Description of age groups XIX, XX, XXI, XXII, and XXIII, being the fifth issue of a survey of the Carnegie Collection (prepared for publication by C. H. Heuser and G. W. Corner). *Carnegie Instn. Wash. Publ. 592, Contrib. Embryol., 34,* 165–196.

Streiter, A. 1951. Ein menschlicher Keimling mit 7 Urwirbelpaaren (Keimling Ludwig). *Z. mikr.-anat. Forsch., 57,* 181–248.

Studnička, F. K. 1929. Über den Zusammenhang des Cytoplasmas bei jungen menschlichen Embryonen. *Z. mikr.-anat. Forsch., 18,* 553–656.

Studnička, F. K., and Florian, J. 1928. Les cytodesmes et le mésostroma chez quelques jeunes embryons humains. *C. R. Ass. Anat., 23,* 437–443.

Stump, C. W. 1929. A human blastocyst *in situ. Trans. Roy. Soc. Edinburgh, 56,* 191–202.

Sundström, P., Nilsson, O., and Liedholm, P. 1981. Cleavage rate and morphology of early human embryos obtained after artificial fertilization and culture. *Acta obstet. gynecol. scand., 60,* 109–120.

Szabo, S. P., and O'Day, D. H. 1983. The fusion of sexual nuclei. *Biol. Rev., 58,* 323–342.

Tandler, J. 1907. Ueber einen menschlichen Embryo vom 38. Tage. *Anat. Anz., 31,* 49–56.

Teacher, J. H. 1925. On the implantation of the human ovum and the early development of the trophoblast. *Z. Anat. Entw., 76,* 360–385.

Teal, S. I., Moore, G. W., and Hutchins, G. M. 1986. Development of aortic and mitral valve continuity in the human embryonic heart. *Amer. J. Anat., 176,* 447–460.

Tesařík, J. 1986. From the cellular to the molecular dimension: the actual challenge for human fertilization research. *Gamete Res., 13,* 47–89.

Tesařík, J., Kopečný, V., Plachot, M., Mandelbaum, J., DaLage, C., and Fléchon, J.-E. 1986. Nucleologenesis in the human embryo developing *in vitro:* ultrastructural and autoradiographic analysis. *Devel. Biol., 115,* 193–203.

Thomas, F., and van Campenhout, E. 1953. Étude d'un oeuf humain d'approximativement 17 jours. Découverte d'autopsie médico-légale. *Ann. méd. légale,* Paris, *33,* 193–199.

Thomas, F., and van Campenhout, E. 1963. Untersuchung eines, bei einer gerichtlichen Sektion nachgewiesenen, etwa 11 Tage alten menschlichen Eies. *Deutsche Z. gerichtl. Med., 54,* 119–123.

Thompson, P. 1907 and 1908. Description of a human embryo of 23 paired somites. *J. Anat., 41,* 159–171, and *42,* 170–175.

Thompson, P. 1915. Description of a human embryo, 7 mm. greatest length. *Studies in Anatomy.* University of Birmingham, pp. 1–50.

Thompson, P., and Brash, J. C. 1923. A human embryo with head-process and commencing archenteric canal. *J. Anat., 58,* 1–20.

Thyng, F. W. 1914. The anatomy of a 17.8 mm human embryo. *Amer. J. Anat., 17,* 31–112.

Torrey, T. W. 1954. The early development of the human nephros. *Carnegie Instn. Wash. Publ. 603, Contrib. Embryol., 35,* 175–197.

Treloar, A. E., Behn, G. B., and Cowan, D. W. 1967. Analysis of gestational interval. *Amer. J. Obstet. Gynecol., 99,* 34–45.

Treutler, K. 1931. Ueber das wahre Alter junger menschlicher Embryonen. *Anat. Anz., 71,* 245–258. Cited by Heuser and Corner (1957).

Triepel, H. 1916. Ein menschlicher Embryo mit Canalis neurentericus. Chordulation. *Anat. Hefte, 54,* 149–185.

Tucker, J. A., and O'Rahilly, R. 1972. Observations on the embryology of the human larynx. *Ann. Otol. Rhinol. Laryngol., 81,* 520–523.

Turner, C. L. 1920. A wax model of a presomite human embryo. *Anat. Rec., 19,* 372–412.

Van Beneden, E. 1899. Sur la présence, chez l'homme, d'un canal archentérique. *Anat. Anz., 15,* 349–356.

van den Broek, A. J. P. 1911. Zur Kasuistik junger menschlicher Embryonen. *Anat. Hefte, I. Abt., 44,* 275–304.

van Heukelom, S. 1898. Ueber die menschliche Placentation. *Arch. Anat. Physiol., Anat. Abth.,* 1–35.

van Oordt, G. J. 1921. Early developmental stages of Manis javanica Desm. *Verh. Konink. Akad. Wetensch. Amsterdam, 21,* pp. 102.

Veit, O., and Esch, P. 1922. Untersuchung eines in situ fixierten, operativ gewonnenen menschlichen Eies der vierten Woche. *Z. Anat. Entw., 63,* 343–414.

Vernall, D. G. 1962. The human embryonic heart in the seventh week. *Amer. J. Anat., 111,* 17–24.

v. Hayek, H. 1931. Ein menschlicher Embryo mit 16 Urwirbeln, 25 Tage alt. *Anat. Anz., 71,* 194–202.

v. Hayek, H. 1934. Ein menschlicher Embryo vom 40. Tage. *Anat. Anz., 78,* 315–320.

Vogl, E. 1925. Rudimente des branchialen Cöloms bei einem menschlichen Embryo. *Z. Anat. Entw., 77,* 226–233.

Volcher, R. 1959. Le système nerveux périphérique crânien d'un embryon humain de 12 mm. *Arch. Biol. (Liège), 70,* 179–215.

Volcher, R. 1963. Le système nerveux périphérique d'un embryon humain de 8 mm. *Arch. Biol. (Liège), 74,* 95–127.

Vollman, R. F. 1977. *The Menstrual Cycle.* Saunders, Philadelphia.

von Möllendorff, W. 1921a. Über das jüngste bisher bekannte menschliche Abortivei (Ei Sch.). Ein Beitrag zur Lehre von der Einbettung des menschlichen Eies. *Z. Anat. Entwicklungsgesch., 62,* 352–405.

von Möllendorff, W. 1921b. Über einen jungen, operativ gewonnenen menschlichen Keim (Ei OP.). *Z. Anat. Entw., 62,* 406–432.

von Möllendorff, W. 1925. Das menschliche Ei WO(lfring). Implantation, Verschluss der Implantationsöffnung und Keimesentwicklung beim Menschen vor Bildung des Primitivstreifens. *Z. Anat. Entw., 76,* 16–42.

von Spee, F. Graf 1887. Ueber einen menschlichen Embryo von 2.69 mm. längstem geraden Durchmesser. *Mitth. Vereines Schleswig-Holsteiner Aerzte,* part II, No. 8.

von Spee, F. Graf 1896. Neue Beobachtungen über sehr frühe Entwicklungsstufen des menschlichen Eies. *Arch. Anat. Physiol., Anat. Abth.,* 1–30.

von Spee, F. Graf. 1889. Beobachtungen an einer menschlichen Keimscheibe mit offener Medullarrinne und Canalis neurentericus. *Arch. Anat. Physiol., Anat. Abth.,* 159–176.

Waldeyer, A. 1929a. Ein junges menschliches Ei in situ [Schö(nholz)]. *Z. Anat. Entw., 90,* 412–457.

Waldeyer, A. 1929b. Mesodermbildung bei einem jungen menschlichen Embryo. *Anat. Anz., 35,* 145–151.

Wallin, I. E. 1913. A human embryo of thirteen somites. *Amer. J. Anat., 15,* 319–331.

Waterman, R. E., and Meller, S. M. 1974. Alterations in the epithelial surface of human palatal shelves prior to and during fusion: a scanning electron microscopic study. *Anat. Rec., 180,* 111–135.

Waterston, D. 1914. A human embryo of 27 pairs of somites. *J. Anat. Physiol., 49,* 90–118.

Watt, J. C. 1915. Description of two young human embryos with 17–19 paired somites. *Carnegie Instn. Wash. Publ. 222, Contrib. Embryol., 2,* 5–44.

Way, S., and Dawson, N. 1959. A human ovum in a vaginal smear. *J. Obstet. Gynaec. Brit. Emp., 66,* 491.

Weller, G. L. 1933. Development of the thyroid, parathyroid and thymus glands in man. *Carnegie Instn. Wash. Publ. 443, Contrib. Embryol., 24,* 93–139.

Wells, L. J. 1954. Development of the human diaphragm and pleural sacs. *Carnegie Instn. Wash. Publ. 603, Contrib. Embryol., 35,* 107–134.

Wells, L. J., and Boyden, E. A. 1954. The development of the bronchopulmonary segments in human embryos of horizons XVII to XIX. *Amer. J. Anat., 95,* 163–201.

Wells, L. J., and Kaiser, I. H. 1959. Two choice human embryos at Streeter's horizons XI and XIV. *Obstet. Gynecol., 14,* 411–416.

Wen, I. C. 1928. The anatomy of human embryos with seventeen to twenty-three pairs of somites. *J. Comp. Neurol., 45,* 301–376.

Wenink, A. C. G. 1971. Some details on the final stages of heart septation in the human embryo. Thesis, Luctor et Emergo, Leiden (76 pp).

West, C. M. 1930. Description of a human embryo of eight somites. *Carnegie Instn. Wash. Publ. 407, Contrib. Embryol., 21,* 25–35.

West, C. M. 1937. A human embryo of twenty-five somites. *J. Anat., 71,* 169–201.

West, C. M. 1952. Two presomite human embryos. *J. Obstet. Gynaecol. Brit. Emp., 59,* 336–351.

Wharton, L. R. 1949. Double ureters and associated renal anomalies in early human embryos. *Carnegie Instn. Wash. Publ. 583, Contrib. Embryol., 33,* 103–112.

Wilder, H. H. 1904. Duplicate twins and double monsters. *Amer. J. Anat., 3,* 387–472.

Wilens, S. (ed.). 1969. *R. G. Harrison: Organization and Development of the Embryo.* Yale Univ. Press, New Haven, Connecticut.

Willis, R. A. 1962. *The Borderland of Embryology and Pathology,* 2nd edition, Butterworths, London.

Wilson, D. B., and Hendrickx, A. G. 1984. Fine structural aspects of the cranial neuroepithelium in early embryos of the rhesus monkey. *J. Craniofacial Genet. Develop. Biol.,* 4, 85–94.

Wilson, J. T. 1914. Observations upon young human embryos. *J. Anat.,* 48, 315–351.

Wilson, K. M. 1926a. Origin and development of the rete ovarii and the rete testis in the human embryo. *Carnegie Instn. Wash. Publ. 362, Contrib. Embryol.,* 17, 69–88.

Wilson, K. M. 1926b. Correlation of external genitalia and sex-glands in the human embryo. *Carnegie Instn. Wash. Publ. 363, Contrib. Embryol.,* 18, 23–30.

Wilson, K. M. 1945. A normal human ovum of sixteen days development (the Rochester ovum). *Carnegie Instn. Wash. Publ. 557, Contrib. Embryol.,* 31, 101–106.

Wilson, K. M. 1954. A previllous ovum of eleven days development. *Amer. J. Obstet. Gynecol.,* 68, 63–68.

Windle, W. F. 1970. Development of neural elements in human embryos of four to seven weeks gestation. *Exp. Neurol., Suppl. 5,* 44–83.

Windle, W. F., and Fitzgerald, J. E. 1942. Development of the human mesencephalic trigeminal root and related neurons. *J. Comp. Neurol.,* 77, 597–608.

Witschi, E. 1948. Migration of the germ cells of human embryos from the yolk sac to the primitive gonadal folds.

Carnegie Instn. Wash. Publ. 575, Contrib. Embryol., 32, 67–80.

Witschi, E. 1956. *Development of Vertebrates.* Saunders, Philadelphia.

Woźniak, W., and O'Rahilly, R. 1980. The times of appearance and the developmental sequence of the cranial parasympathetic ganglia in staged human embryos. *Anat. Rec., 196,* 255A–256A.

Yamauchi, A. 1965. Electron microscopic observations on the development of S—A and A—V nodal tissues in the human embryonic heart. *Z. Anat. Entw., 124,* 562–587.

Yokoh, Y. 1970. Differentiation of the dorsal mesentery in man. *Acta anat., 76,* 56–67.

Yokoh, Y. 1971. Early formation of nerve fibers in the human otocyst. *Acta anat., 80,* 99–106.

Young, M. P., Whicher, J. T., and Potts, D. M. 1968. The ultrastructure of implantation in the golden hamster *(Cricetus auratus). J. Embryol. Exp. Morphol., 19,* 341–345.

Zamboni, L. 1971. *Fine Morphology of Mammalian Fertilization.* Harper & Row, New York.

Zamboni, L., Mishell, D. R., Bell, J. H., and Baca, M. 1966. Fine structure of the human ovum in the pronuclear stage. *J. Cell Biol., 30,* 579–600.

Zechel, G. 1924. Über Muskelknospen beim Menschen, ein Beitrag zur Lehre von der Differenzierung des Myotoms. *Z. Anat. Entw., 74,* 593–607.